STUDIES IN THE ARCADIAN LIBRARY

NO. 3

ايحو الحلبة تكون على ضربين ان منها الورق والاخضر الذي لم يبزر بعد ومنها ما ينبت في المنازل والدور
والنقية والرمل على حاله قوة مزارته ولذلك صار رفعه اذا طبخ ليغسل به حرارة وشرب نفع المعي المرارة
من الفصول العفلية والالبان المنتنة وطلب رائحة الثقل وقد تتخذ منه دهن يحمر الشعر ويقويه

الاسم		تفسيرها باختلاف اللغات	
حنا	بارد يابس في الاولى	هو اليرقون ورقان من اللغة وبالعجمية الحنا هو نور الحنا وراتب وبالعجمية الحنا نوار الحنا وكل نوار وبالعجمية ابو حنيفة اجود الحنا حماه واصله المهز بعال حنات تخمى بالحنا وقال اليرنا واليرنا هما الغشان في الحنا المولف رايت يطرح من كل	...
حسك	حار يابس في ...	هو السكوبح وهو باليونانية وهو الامير وبعاله ديل اعور ويعرف بالعجمية غاله جافه وبعجمية ديل الجمل وهو بالعجمية ايضا قطيا الثر من عمل الام ينفع من القولنج اضراره بالراس اضاجه ترمهو للحل السمريه من درهم الى درهم	...
حلبة	حار في الثانية يابس في الاولى	ذكر ان عرب الشام يسمونها الفريقه قال ابو حنيفة اخبرني بعض الشيوخ ان عرب الشام يسمونها الفريقه ولذلك يسمى النقوع الذي يتخذ منها ومن التمر ومن اخلاط اخر فيسقى المريض الفريقه	...
حزاز الصخر	بارد يابس	هو الذي يكون على صخور ندية يقع عليها الندا والطل وهو شبيه بالطحلب اخضر وهو كثير في الصخور الندية	الطحلب
حماحم	حار يابس	هو الحبق العريض الورق الشامي الذي يستعمل في الاشربة واللعاقات ويسمى بالشام الحبق النبطي وهو بالرومية البلسليقن ابو حنيفة حماحم بقلة ... مغروفه والواحدة حماحمة	...
حب الفلفل	حار يابس في الرابعة	هو الفلفل والفافل وهو باليونانية ارمنيس وقال صاحب النبات الفلفل حب مثل اللوبيا تكون في غلف اغبر اللون وقيل انه حب القنبم ولم يصح وهو الاسباسو ... واصله هو الزند ليعرب المقادح	...

يسحه اخرى ومن السعتر رطل ينقع ذلك في الزيت سبعة ايام ويحول كل يوم ثلاث مرات ويعصر ويرمى
حقنة الرحم المراة له قد عسر عليها الولادة اذا احتبس الولد امراط خروج الرطوبات من الرحم

botri: cipro

fenug

xasm

ocim

piper

IBN BAKLARISH'S BOOK OF SIMPLES

MEDICAL REMEDIES BETWEEN THREE FAITHS IN TWELFTH-CENTURY SPAIN

edited by
Charles Burnett

THE ARCADIAN LIBRARY
in association with
OXFORD UNIVERSITY PRESS

OPPOSITE TITLE PAGE
The Arcadian Library
manuscript, p. 120

The Arcadian Library in association with Oxford University Press

The Arcadian Library, London, is an affiliate of
The Arcadian Group S.A., Case Postale 200, 1211 Geneva 12, Switzerland

The Arcadian Library is a private, family library specializing in the historic influences of the Levant upon Europe. Its aim is to promote this cultural transfer through exhibition and through publication

Oxford University Press, Great Clarendon Street, Oxford OX2 6DP

Oxford University Press is a department of the University of Oxford.
It furthers the University's objective of excellence in research, scholarship, and education by publishing worldwide in Oxford New York Auckland Cape Town Dar es Salaam Hong Kong Karachi Kuala Lumpur Madrid Melbourne Mexico City Nairobi New Delhi Shanghai Taipei Toronto
With offices in Argentina Austria Brazil Chile Czech Republic France Greece Guatemala Hungary Italy Japan Poland Portugal Singapore South Korea Switzerland Thailand Turkey Ukraine Vietnam

Oxford is a registered trade mark of Oxford University Press
in the UK and in certain other countries

Published in the United States by Oxford University Press Inc., New York

First published 2008

British Library Cataloguing in Publication Data (data available)

Library of Congress Cataloguing in Publication Data (data available)

ISBN 978-0-19-954306-9

Project management by Robert Jones, Series editor Alastair Hamilton, Academic editor Charles Burnett
Copy-editor Bernard Dod, Designed and typeset by Phil Cleaver and Emily Berry of etal-design.com ltd
Photography at the Arcadian Library: John Stone and Karem Ibrahim
Printed in Great Britain by Cambridge University Press, on Stow Book Wove, free from chlorine (TCF) and OBA, and resistant to ageing in accordance with ISO 97006
Typeset in Monotype Arcadian Bembo

TABLE OF CONTENTS

THE CONTRIBUTORS

Charles Burnett
Professor of the History of Arabic/Islamic Influences in Europe, Warburg Institute, University of London

Ana Labarta
Professor of Arabic, University of Valencia

Joëlle Ricordel
Private scholar, Paris

Juan Carlos Villaverde Amieva
Professor of Arabic, University of Oviedo

Jan Just Witkam
Professor of Palaeography and Codicology of the Islamic World, Leiden University

Geoffrey Khan
Professor of Semitic Philology, University of Cambridge

David J. Wasserstein
Professor of History and of Jewish Studies, Vanderbilt University

Emilie Savage-Smith
Professor of the History of Islamic Science, University of Oxford

Anna Contadini
Senior Lecturer in the Arts and Archaeology of Islam, School of Oriental and African Studies, London

CHARLES BURNETT

PREFACE

In October 2003 the Arcadian Library acquired an Arabic manuscript consisting entirely of a previously unnoticed copy of the *Kitāb al-Mustaʿīnī* of Ibn Baklarish, an important book of *materia medica* written in the Iberian peninsula at the turn of the eleventh to the twelfth century. It is reported that the manuscript was bought in Paris in the 1960s by a Middle Eastern historian of medicine and thence came by family descent to the United Kingdom. Its earlier history is unknown. It excited attention not only because it was a complete and clearly written copy of the work, but also because in the colophon the anonymous scribe states that he completed his copy on 18 January 1130 A.D., that is within a generation of the composition of the original text. It was decided that a group of scholars should be brought together to share their expertise on the content of this manuscript and to assess its significance in relation to other manuscripts of the *Kitāb al-Mustaʿīnī* and within the context of eleventh- and twelfth-century medicine in Islamic Spain. The symposium took place on 10 September 2005, and the participants willingly revised their articles for inclusion in this volume. We are grateful to the Patron of the Arcadian Library for making the symposium and the publication possible, to Robert Jones for overseeing the whole process and taking care of the manuscript, to Helen Loveday for its paper conservation and to Kathy Abbott for its binding, to John Stone and Karem Ibrahim for taking the photographs, to Alice Bailey and Daniela Reimers for their administrative help, to Phil Cleaver, the designer, who has mastered the intricacies of typesetting in several Oriental languages, and to Bernard Dod for his diligent reading of the text. Alastair Hamilton, as well as steering the book through its various stages of preparation, has translated the articles of Ricordel and Villaverde and provided valuable guidance throughout.

Before proceeding to the individual papers, most of which concentrate on the content of the manuscript, it would be helpful to consider the appearance of the manuscript as a whole.[1] It is a codex of 140 folios, paginated in a modern hand, bound in gatherings of eight paper folios, with no sign of an original cover. On p. 1 is a title, *kitāb al-adwiya al-mufrada li-l-Isrāʾīlī* ('the book of simple medicines by the Israeli') written in the hand of the main scribe of the text in ornate black letters with vowels marked in red ink surrounded by later notes on a variety of subjects, including metrology, which have been partially obliterated. These notes continue on pp. 2–3, while the text proper of the *Kitāb al-Mustaʿīnī* begins at the top of p. 4. The long Introduction extends from p. 4 until the top of p. 30. It is written with titles in a thicker stroke and *materia medica* in rubric. The rest, and major part, of p. 30 and the whole of p. 31 are blank. Then the synoptic tables fill almost all the rest of the manuscript, pp. 32–273. The headings of the columns are written in alternate brown and red ink, and red ink is also used for the *abjad* numerals and the names of authorities. The colophon, which includes the date—'the middle ten days of the month of *yannayr* which is Ṣafar of the year 524 [= 18 January 1130 A.D.]'—occurs on p. 273. A grid for a table had been prepared on the following page (p. 274) but

1. The following paragraphs include information supplied in the entry of the Sotheby's London Sales Catalogue, *Arts of the Islamic World*, 15 October 2003, lot 11, for which Marvin Colker supplied valuable information.

was not needed for *materia medica*. In the central cell on the top row is written *kamāl bi-ʿawni'llāh* ('finished with the help of God') and in the central cell on the lowest row there is a recipe for making ink with lead and gold (including a word in Latin script, possibly 'istanu' = 'stannum', 'tin') written in the same hand as the rest of the text. An incomplete classification of medical simples according to their effects, which is not part of the *Kitāb al-Mustaʿīnī*, but, again, is written in the same hand, fills pp. 275–8 (headings are in rubric). Later notes in several hands have added further recipes and some magical signs on pp. 279 and 280. On the last page (p. 280) these are mostly obliterated, but a passage in Latin and Arabic has been written at the top of the page in the hand of the main scribe, and may have had some apotropaic significance (I shall return to this below).

The paper is a smooth, cream, lightly burnished Spanish laid paper with five laid lines to the centimetre and with full-length chain lines occasionally visible at intervals of 25 mm. It is similar to the Spanish paper of MS Oxford, Bodleian Library, Marsh 292, which contains part of the *Sunan* of Ibn Abi Da'ud al-Sijistani and is dated 22 Ramadan 585 (3 November 1189 A.D.). Another manuscript written on 'bright and yellowish' paper with chain lines clearly visible is the well-known Leiden Arabic–Latin glossary.[2] The pages of the Arcadian manuscript are 29.8 x 22 cm, while the writing space for the Introduction is 23.5 x 16.1 cm, and for the tables is 20.9 x 15.4 cm. The manuscript is stained by damp and mould and it has suffered some small losses, tears and worm damage.

The interest of this manuscript is enhanced by the number of words in Latin script that are found throughout the text, and that attest to the composition and reception of the manuscript in contexts in which Latin was used alongside Arabic (see Villaverde, pp. 72–4 below). The Latin words within the text have been written on the same line and in the same ink as the Arabic, and are presumably by the same scribe as the Arabic text itself; they appear in Visigothic script (p. 92 'sanguinis canis' [Fig. 1], p. 118 'triticum', p. 150 'bettonica'; also a marginal gloss on p. 94), Carolingian script (p. 258 'furmentu' [Fig. 2], p. 284 'istanu'), and in a mixture of the two (p. 258 'falernum'). In Carolingian script have also been added synonyms for the *materia medica* (in the margins on pp. 21, 32, 34, 38, 40, 44, 58, 94, 96, 102, 182, 208, 210, 214, 216, 220, 224, 264). The Visigothic script closely resembles that of the Leiden glossary,[3] while the script in the margins is not unlike that of an early manuscript of a translation from Arabic made by Hugo of Santalla, who used the library of the Saragossa royal family, the Banu Hud, in the 1140s.[4] A bold hand has written numerous synonyms in Latin script from the beginning of the tables up to p. 146, using a thick pen and bold strokes. This script is distinctive because it includes ticks indicating the stressed syllable within a word [Fig. 3]. It is quite crude, and

2. Pieter Sjoerd van Koningsveld, *The Latin–Arabic Glossary of the Leiden University Library*, Leiden 1977, p. 24. Van Koningsveld states that this is the type of paper referred to as 'al-waraq al-Ṣāṭibī' (paper from Játiva), 'whose finest specimens, like Cod. Or. 2073 of the Leiden University Library, are almost identical to vellum in their bright yellowish colour and their smoothness' (ibid., p. 25).

3. Van Koningsveld, in his plausible interpretation of the barely legible inscription at the end of the Leiden glossary, reads the place of the copying of the manuscript as 'the city of Toledo', and conjectures from the information in this inscription and other features of the manuscript that it was copied in c. 1175: see pp. 40, 42.

4. Paris, Bibliothèque Nationale de France, MS lat. 13951, a manuscript of Apollonius, *De secretis naturae*.

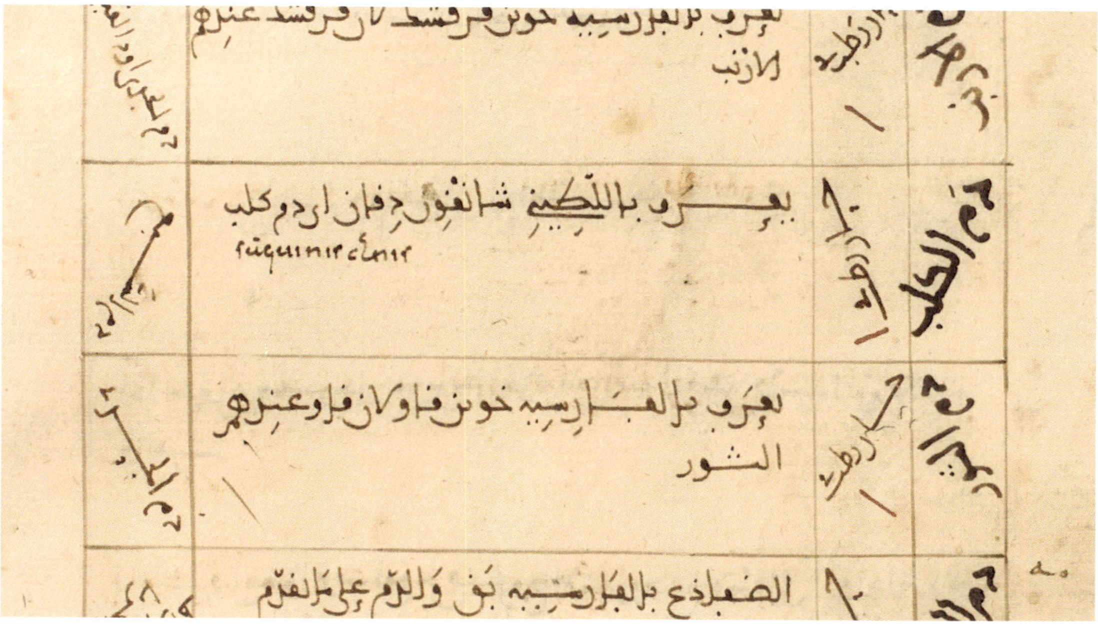

Fig. 1.
'Sanguinis canis' written in Visigothic script. The Arcadian Library manuscript, p. 92

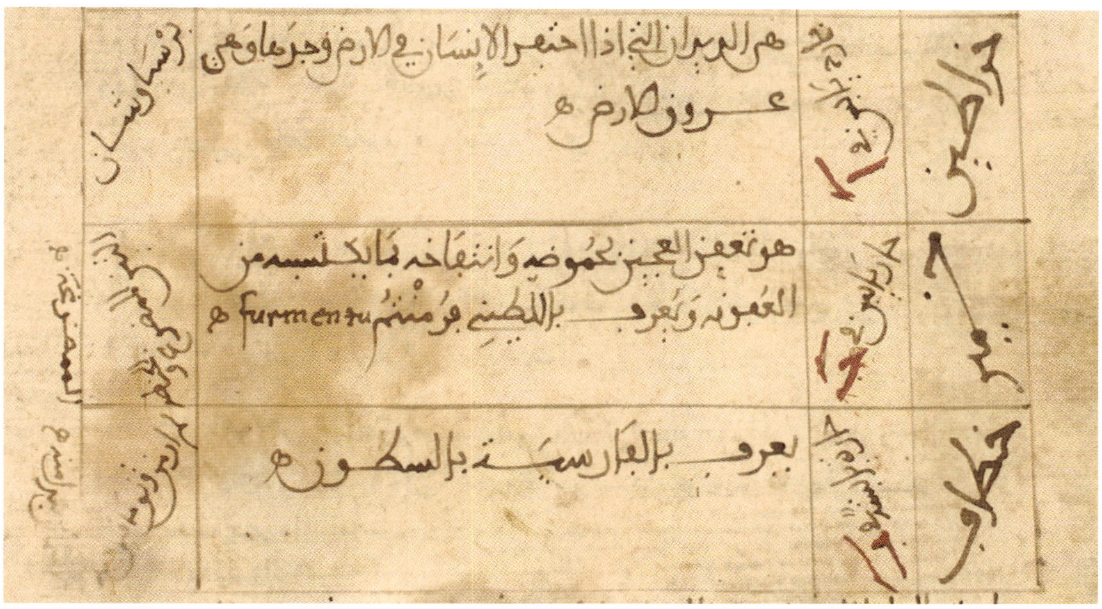

Fig. 2.
'Furmentu' written in Carolingian script. The Arcadian Library manuscript, p. 258

Fig. 3.
The Latin and Arabic glosses.
The Arcadian Library
manuscript, p. 36

favours capital letter forms. It may be the same hand as that of the Arabic script used in the glosses on pp. 36, 80, 124, if not the hand of the Arabic entries naming the *materia medica* written with a thicker pen in the first columns of the tables. Other Arabic glosses evidently were added by different, later, hands. The gloss in Greek letters ἀετίτης (derived from the transcription in Latin script which was definitely written before it: 'aetítis') on p. 134 must be later, but the Arabic gloss in Hebrew characters on p. 236 ([Fig. 4]; see also p. 108 below) may be early.

The early Carolingian hand also wrote the mysterious passage on the final page of the manuscript (p. 280; [Fig. 5]. The Arabic equivalent that follows it is likely to have been written after the Latin, although it is fuller than the Latin.[5] But that it was written in the same context (perhaps by the same person) is indicated by the facts that both the Latin and Arabic are written in the same black ink, and that the scribe of the Latin text has added 'pe' above most of the occurrences of the free-standing *bāʾ* in the Arabic. So this bilingual text neatly corroborates the evidence scattered throughout this manuscript of the *Kitāb al-Mustaʿīnī* of an origin in a mixed Arabic and Latin-Romance culture. Unfortunately not all the words of the Arabic or Latin text can be read because this last page has been subject to the most wear and a corner of the page is missing. Nevertheless, the Latin word can sometimes be reconstructed from the Arabic, and *vice versa*. The whole text may be a commentary on the row of 'p's which follow rows of capital 'r's and 'm's respectively, immediately above. The central portion of this text reads:

pe ante pe pe post pe magister legi pe si legis pe laudo te et si non legis pe error erit

which corresponds to the following passage of the Arabic immediately below it:

با قبل ب با بعد ب يا معلم اقرا ب انك ان قريت البا فاني مادح لك ... البا فاني مستجهلك لاجل الغلط

and which may be translated:

The p *before the* p, *the* p *after the* p. *Master, read the* p! *If you read the* p, *I praise you. If you do not read the* p, *it will be wrong* [Arabic: *I will regard you as ignorant because of the mistake*].

The articles follow in order. Ana Labarta, to whom we are indebted for the first edition and translation of a substantial part of the *Kitāb al-Mustaʿīnī*, namely the Introduction,[6] summarizes the history of scholarship concerning Ibn Baklarish, and compares the data provided by the Arcadian manuscript with what is already known about Ibn Baklarish and his book. She also briefly runs through the sources used by Ibn Baklarish. Mention is made of two proposed editions of the *Kitāb al-Mustaʿīnī* which never saw the light of day. The first was undertaken by Henri Renaud, who was a pioneer in the study of Arabic medicine in the 1930s, and was the first scholar

5. One indication of this is that a Latin 'p' (the main subject of the text) would be expected to be transliterated as 'b' in Arabic, whereas an Arabic 'b' would be transliterated as a Latin 'b'.
6. Ana Labarta, 'El prólogo de *al-Kitāb al-Mustaʿīnī de Ibn Buklāriš*', in Juan Vernet (ed.), *Estudios sobre historia de la ciencia árabe*, Barcelona 1981, pp. 181–316.

وزعم قوم من الاطباء ان الصنف الاول اللازورد في مكان اغاليس اذا
للسبب الرجعة سكن وجعها **د** . من اكليل الملك ما لونه الى لون الزعفران طيب الرائحة
ويحلل **ج** طعم الاشنة فابض باعتدال وهو نقا الاول قوة لليبس باردة ... قوية

الاسماء	الطبائع	تفسير ما في اختلاف اللغات	ابدالها	
اناغاليس	حار يابس في **٢**	هي حشيشة الحلق ونبا العجمية الفرذنالة والشنتيلة وهما صنفان ذكر وانثى فالذكر هو الشنتالة والانثى هو الفرذنالة في اللازورد هو الانثى والاحمر هو الذكر	[illegible]	anagalus
اكليل الملك	حار يابس في **١**	قيل هو شجرة الحب ونبا العجمية القرقلية وقيل هو القرط **الزهراوي** ليس القرقلية لان بينهما فرق فلان اكليل الملك هو القرط واخالبه املس واكليل القرقلية خرش ... وبقال له مليلوطس وهو نبات منتشر	[illegible]	Melilotu وهو حلبة برّية
الاشنة	حار يابس في **١**	هي شيبة العجوز وهي التي تصير على شجر البلوط والجوز والشربين واجود ما كان موجودا على الشربين الجبلي وكان طيب الرائحة ابيضا وخاصتها النفع من البلغم والسوداء اقراره بالمعا اصلاحها بالانيسون ... ه	[illegible]	Vrion:
قبر	حار يابس في **٢**	هو الكبر وهو القبار ويسمى بالرومية القبوس ويعرفه العامة الكبار بالكاف والالف . ويعرف ايضا باللام	[illegible]	Caparis:
ابريسم	حار يابس في **١**	هو الحرير **ان ما سوده** اذا انسج دود الحرير على نفسه ولم يقشر ... وخرج منه كان منه الابريسم والقز وان ترك في الشمس حتى يموت كان منه الحرير وهو الخام ه	[illegible]	Serico; metaxi:
انيسون	حار يابس في **٢**	هو الانيسون وهو الحبة الحلوة وهو الرازيانج الرومي ❀ ومن زعم انه اقراره بالمعا اصلاحه بالرازيانج بزره	[illegible]	Aniso

مركب من طعوم ثلاثة مرارة وحرافة وعفوصة والمرارة والحرافة فيه اكثر والعفوصة ❀
اقل ... ولمصمصة نفع من وجع الاسنان ❀ **بعض الاطباء** الحرير حار ما كان منه خرير ...
كبير الحبة قوي الرائحة والنفع ما في معرا البراب ... ❀

Fig. 4.
A gloss in Hebrew characters. The Arcadian Library manuscript, p. 236

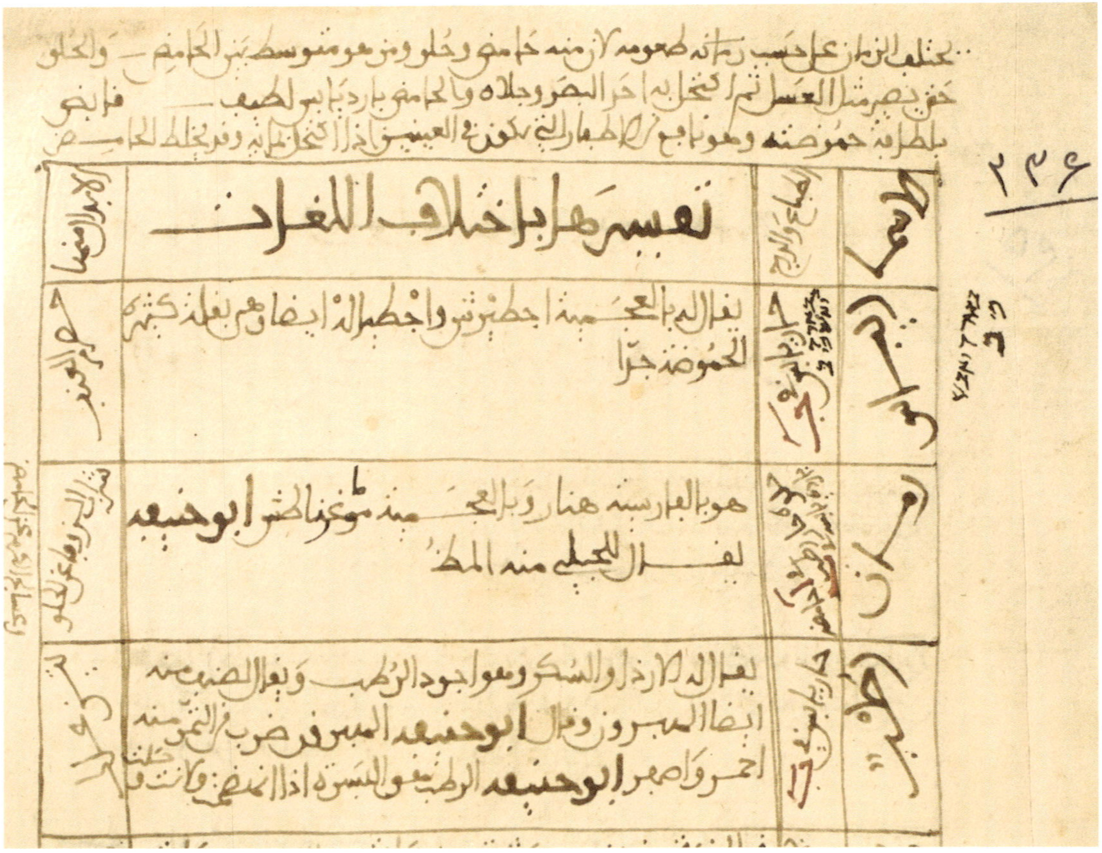

Fig. 5.
An enigmatic Latin and Arabic text. The Arcadian Library manuscript, p. 280

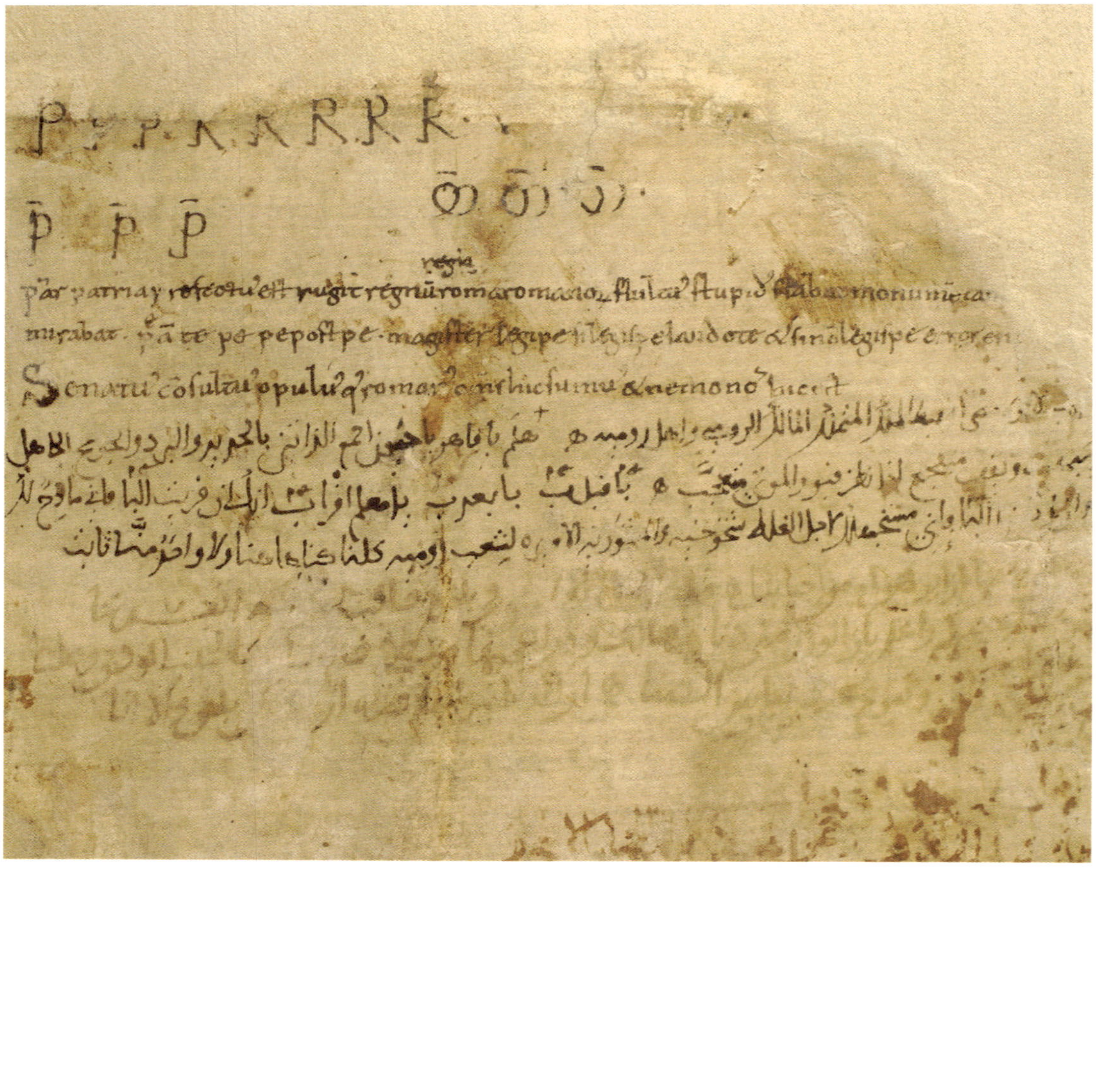

to realize the importance of Ibn Baklarish's work. Another edition and translation was announced as being prepared by Amador Díaz García in 1981, and this was the reason why Ana Labarta herself did not continue to edit the complete work, having completed her edition and translation of the Introduction as her licentiate dissertation (1972). Now we are fortunate in that a critical edition is being prepared by Joëlle Ricordel.

In the second article in this book Ricordel discusses her forthcoming edition and shows how the Arcadian manuscript can contribute to establishing the text. She shows that the diffusion of Ibn Baklarish's work was entirely in the western part of the Islamic world, and that the Arcadian manuscript is closest to the Madrid manuscript.

While Ricordel is concerned with the edition of the Arabic text, Juan Carlos Villaverde Amieva explores the considerable Romance elements in the transmission of the work, both in the main text and in the glosses. He points out that the Romance lexicon varies from manuscript to manuscript, in density, in variety and in linguistic affinity. This fluidity from manuscript to manuscript makes it difficult to identify the 'original' form of the text; and perhaps suggests that it is inappropriate to look for such a form. The Romance (*ʿajamiyya*) words cited in Arabic script in the text which may be regarded as closest in time and place to the author are unlikely to represent the Romance dialect spoken in Ibn Baklarish's milieu (as has been assumed in the past), but are rather there by the chance selection of the different sources brought into service in the book, while the glosses in Latin script attest to the use of the text in various parts of the Iberian peninsula and beyond the Pyrenees. He hypothesizes that the peculiar language mix of the Arcadian manuscript, and in particular the simultaneous presence of Latin and Arabic in the manuscript, point to its being written in Toledo, the centre of the translations from Arabic into Latin in the period.

Jan Just Witkam describes the Leiden manuscript of the *Kitāb al-Mustaʿīnī* and reveals the existence of at least two further copies of the text, against which *al-Kitāb al-Mustaʿīnī* was collated. He compares the format and some of the readings of the Leiden manuscript with the Arcadian one. His findings attest to the popularity of the work in North Africa in the seventeenth century, and its appeal to Jacobus Golius, the renowned Dutch Orientalist and mathematician (1596–1667), who wanted to have his own copy of the work.

Geoffrey Khan's article considers the 31 citations of 'Syriac' (*suryāniyya*) synonyms for the *materia medica* in the Arcadian manuscript and shows that they belong to different dialects, thus corroborating the findings that Ibn Baklarish used a variety of written sources (in which these Syriac synonyms were included), rather than his own direct experience.

David Wasserstein returns to the possible connection of 'Biklarish' with 'Biclaro/Valclaro', raised but dismissed by Labarta, and examines the significance of the epithet 'Isra'ili' applied to Ibn Baklarish. He sees little evidence of Ibn Baklarish being involved in Hebrew culture in Spain, but considers that his work should be seen as forming part of the Islamic cultural tradition.

Emilie Savage-Smith, drawing on her wide experience of cataloguing Arabic medical manuscripts and assessing the doctrine contained in them, explores the place of the *Kitāb al-Mustaʿīnī* in the didactic tradition of presenting medical material in synoptic tables, and the concern for establishing synonyms for a medicinal substance.

After showing how several texts adopt the same format, but differ quite considerably in content, she raises the question of whether the similarities shared uniquely by Maimonides and Ibn Baklarish might suggest some connection between Jewish doctors within al-Andalus.

Finally, Anna Contadini catalogues and classifies the references in the *Kitāb al-Mustaʿīnī* to medicaments taken from animals, and compares recipes using these ingredients to what is found in encyclopedias concerning animals. She shows that, although the general format of the recipes is the same, there is little correspondence in the details, and the professed sources of the material are different.

Since, in most cases, the references in the articles are to the head words in the tables, rather than to page numbers of the manuscript, it may be helpful to give a list of the alphabetical order and the page numbers of the changes from each letter to the next (there is no alphabetical order within each letter):

Alif pp. 32–53, *bā'* pp. 52–71, *jīm* pp. 70–81, *dāl* pp. 80–95, *hā'* pp. 94–9, *wāw* pp. 98–103, *zāy* pp. 102–17, *ḥā'* pp. 116–43, *ṭā'* pp. 142–7, *yā'* pp. 146–9, *kāf* pp. 148–65, *lām* pp. 164–75, *mīm* pp. 174–91, *nūn* pp. 190–7, *sīn* pp. 196–209, *ʿayn* pp. 208–15, *fā'* pp. 214–21, *qāf* pp. 220–35, *rā'* pp. 234–41, *ṣād* pp. 240–45, *tā'* pp. 244–9, *thā'* pp. 248–51, *khā'* pp. 250–61, *dhāl* pp. 260–1, *ghayn* pp. 262–3, *shīn* pp. 262–73.

Photographic acknowledgments. Figs. 18, 19, 24, 29–34, 42, 44: copyright University of Leiden; Fig. 28: reproduced by courtesy of the University Librarian and Director, The John Rylands University Library, the University of Manchester; Figs. 36, 37, 38, 41: copyright University of Oxford; Fig. 43: by kind permission of the Library of the Topkapı Sarayi, Istanbul; Figs. 47, 49: copyright British Library; Figs. 48, 50: copyright Biblioteca Real, San Lorenzo del Escorial.

ANA LABARTA

IBN BAKLARISH'S *KITĀB AL-MUSTAʿĪNĪ*: THE HISTORICAL CONTEXT TO THE DISCOVERY OF A NEW MANUSCRIPT

A new manuscript

The Arcadian Library's recently acquired manuscript of the *Kitāb al-adwiya al-mufrada li-l-Isrā'īlī* ('The Book on Simple Medicines by al-Isra'ili'), dealing with simple medicines, i.e., with the individual natural substances used to heal (as opposed to books on compound medicines), is in two different parts: a substantial introduction and more than 100 folios of synoptic tables (*jadāwil*).[1] If we start reading the Introduction, we soon find a more exact title and the explanation for it: the author decided to name his book '*al-Mustaʿīnī*' because he dedicated it to 'al-Mustaʿīn bi-llāh Abū Jaʿfar Aḥmad, the son of al-Mu'tamin bi-llāh ibn Hūd'. He also says that he saw al-Mustaʿin when he had reached the peak of his glory, and he wishes God to make his rule last. As we know, Abu Jaʿfar Ahmad al-Mustaʿin bi-llah, the son of al-Mu'tamin bi-llah, of the Banu Hud dynasty, was a *ṭā'ifa* king who ruled in Saragossa from 1085 to 1110. The book must therefore have been written between these two dates, during the lifetime and reign of the king. The author adds that he had already written a *Risālat al-tabyīn wa-l-tartīb*, i.e. a book on dietetics. But what else do we know about the book and its author?

Arabic biographical sources

In the Arabic sources we find only three references:

(a) In about the middle of the fourteenth century, a Moroccan author, possibly from Fez, ʿAli ibn Yusuf al-Hakim, writing about the mint (*sikka*), gives some information about silver according to 'al-ḥakīm fī adwiyati-hi al-mufrada al-mujadwala' ('the scholar in his simple drugs arranged in tables').[2] This description suggests he may be referring to our book, and a comparison with the article on *fiḍḍa* ('silver') in the Arcadian manuscript pp. 220–1 confirms this.

(b) The seventeenth-century bibliographer, Hajji Khalifa, refers to '*al-Mustaʿīnī* on medicine'.[3] This would only have been useful had the book been lost. He does not give any further information about the work or the name of its author.

These two references show that the book was known and used in North Africa and in the Middle East some centuries after its composition.

1. For a brief description, see above, pp. 7–8.
2. ʿAli B. Yusuf Al-Hakim, *al-Ḍawḥa al-mushtabika fī ḍawābiṭ dār al-sikka*, ed. Husayn Mu'nis, *Revista del Instituto de Estudios Islámicos en Madrid*, 6, 1958, pp. 63–204 (printed separately, Madrid 1960): '*ammā al-fiḍḍa ʿalā mā qāla-hu al-ḥakīm fī adwiyati-hi al-mufrada al-mujadwala …*' (p. 102).
3. Hajji Khalifa, *Kashf al-ẓunūn*, Teheran 1387/1967: '*al-Mustaʿīnī, fī-l-ṭibb*' (vol. 2, col. 1764).

(c) In the *'Uyun al-anbā'*, a biographical dictionary of physicians by the thirteenth-century Syro-Egyptian Ibn Abi Usaybiʿa, we find the following statement: 'Ibn B·klār·sh was a Jew and one of the wisest men of al-Andalus with regard to the practice of medicine, endowed with great experience and a profound knowledge of simple medicines. He served as physician to the [dynasty of the] Banū Hūd. He wrote a synoptic treatise on simples at Almería for al-Mustaʿīn bi-llāh Abū Jaʿfar Aḥmad, the son of al-Mu'tamin bi-llāh ibn Hūd.'[4] It seems clear that this refers to the author of our book, and Ibn Abi Usaybiʿa gives us some relevant new information: his *shuhra* was Ibn B·klar·sh, a Jew (and this justifies the *laqab* 'al-Isra'īlī' we see in our manuscript) who lived in Muslim Spain (al-Andalus). He was one of the wisest men with regard to the *practice* of medicine, with great experience and a profound knowledge of simple medicines, and served as physician to the dynasty of the Banu Hud. He wrote his synoptic treatise on simples (the *Kitāb al-Mustaʿīnī*) at Almería. We do not know where Ibn Abi Usaybiʿa derived this information, but we do not have any other Arabic source.

In what follows I shall try to describe briefly the contribution of modern scholarship to our subject.

History of scholarship concerning the Kitāb al-Mustaʿīnī

Now that we know the name of the author, we can turn to the modern bio-bibliographical manuals, starting with Brockelmann. In his *Geschichte*, we see that Jusuf b. Ishaq b. Beklaresh al-Isra'ili is 'ein jüdischer Artz, [der] schrieb u.d. J.500 /1106'.[5] He refers to the *Kitāb al-Mustaʿīnī*, and directs us to the text of Ibn Abi Usaybiʿa and to the catalogues of the libraries of Leiden and Naples. From this reference we can deduce there are two more manuscripts: one in Leiden and one in Naples. Brockelmann reads the *shuhra* as Beklaresh, and adds that his *ism* was Jusuf and his *nasab* Ibn Ishaq. In the *Supplementband* we read: 'Yūnus b. Isḥaq b. Beklāresh al-Isrā'īlī um 500/1106'. He then mentions a new manuscript: '*K. al-Mustaʿīnī* noch Rabat 481',[6] and an article by Renaud published in *Hespéris*.[7] Note that the *ism* of our author has become 'Yunus'.

The Leiden catalogue by De Jong and De Goeje reads: *'al-Mustaʿini. Liber Mos-*

4. Ibn Abi Usaybiʿa, *'Uyūn al-Anbā' fī ṭabaqāt al-aṭibbā'. Sources d'informations sur les classes des médecins*, ed. and trans. Henri Jahier and Abdelkader Noureddine, Algiers 1377/1958: 'Ibn Baklarich était un juif des plus savants médecins d'Andalousie, qui avait une grande expérience et une très grande connaissance des médicaments simples. Il servit comme médecin la dynastie des Banū Hūd. Il a écrit un traité synoptique sur les médicaments simples à Alméria, pour al-Mustaʿīn Billāh' (no. LVII, p. 54).

5. Carl Brockelmann, *Geschichte der arabischen Litteratur*, 2 vols., Weimar 1898–1902: 'Jūsuf b. Isḥāq b. Beklāresh al-Isrā'īlī, ein jüdischer Artz, schrieb u. d. J. 500 /1106 [...] *Kitāb al-Mustaʿīnī* über die einfachen Heilmittel in Tabellenform, gewidmet dem Fürsten von Saragossa al *Mustaʿīnī* billāh. A. b. Hud (478 bis 503 / 1085-1109) [Leid. 1339, cat. Ital. 237 nr. 96; vgl. Uṣ [IAU] II 52]' (vol. I, p. 486).'

6. Carl Brockelmann, *Geschichte der arabischen Litteratur. Supplementbände*, 3 vols., Leiden 1937–42: 'Yūnus b. Isḥāq b. Beklāresh al-Isrā'īlī um 500/1106 *kitāb al-Mustaʿīnī* noch Rabāṭ 481, s. H. P. J. Renaud [1930]' (vol. I, p. 889).

7. Henri P. J. Renaud, 'Trois études d'histoire de la médecine arabe en Occident: I. Le *Mustaʿīnī* d'Ibn Beklāreš', *Hespéris*, 10, 1930, pp. 135–50.

taïniticus, auctore Junos [i.e. Yunus] ibn Isḥák ibn-Beklárisch al-Isráïlí (circa a.500), de medicamentis simplicibus'.[8] There follows a good description of the work and two very long extracts in Arabic from the Introduction. The manuscript is undated; it was sent from Morocco by Golius and has an old part and a modern one that completes it.[9] Here the *ism* and *nasab* 'Junos ibn Isḥák' appear for the first time in the modern literature: they are at the beginning of the Leiden manuscript, but written in a modern, seventeenth-century, Moroccan hand.

Buonazia describes the manuscript in the Biblioteca Nazionale of Naples as a complete although badly bound copy.[10] The colophon (fol. 79a) gives the name of the copyist and the place and date of the copy: Leria (?) 14 Dhū-l-Qaʿdah 888 A.H. It is based on an earlier copy written in Córdoba on 5 February 1303, corresponding to 15 Rabīʿ II 663 A.H. Buonazia also says that we can find an extensive description in the Leiden catalogue. And indeed, he takes part of the preceding information, which is not in the Naples manuscript, from the Leiden catalogue. In fact, here we only read (fol. 1a): 'kitāb al-mustaʿīnī wa li-B·[amended to li-Ibn] qlār·sh al-mutaṭabbib'. There is no *ism*, *nasab*, or *laqab*, and the *shuhra* is written with a 'q' (with a *sukūn* over it). Moreover, the place and date of the copy must be corrected to: completed in Almeria, on Monday 14 Dhū-l-Ḥijja of 888 A.H. [= 11 January 1482 A.D.] from a manuscript completed in Córdova on 17 Rabīʿ II 663, i.e. 5 February 1303 of the Ṣufr era [=1265 A.D.].

The excellent article by Renaud gives a totally new point of view: a complete bibliography, references to the extant manuscripts, a discussion of the author, a commentary on the manuscript of Rabat and a study of the Berber words found in the *Kitāb al-Mustaʿīnī*. The Rabat manuscript is described as a fine but very late copy, dated 29 Muḥarram 1309 or 4 September 1891. Renaud begins his article by saying that this book was used as a source by Dozy for his *Dictionnaire*[11] and by Simonet for his *Glosario*.[12] Referring to the manuscripts, Renaud adds that, until Lévi-Provençal's *Catalogue*[13] of the Rabat manuscripts revealed the presence of a new one, there were only three known copies in European libraries: Leiden, Madrid and Naples. This is the first reference to a manuscript in Madrid.

Dozy names the book, but not the author. He used the manuscripts from both Leiden and Naples, and explains in his *Supplément aux dictionnaires arabes* (1881) that the

8. Piet De Jong, and Michael Jan De Goeje, *Catalogus Codicum Orientalium Bibliothecae Academiae Lugduno Batavae*, vol. 3, Leiden 1865.

9. For a discussion of the Leiden manuscript, see the chapter by Witkam in this volume.

10. Lupo Buonazia, 'Biblioteca Nazionale di Napoli: codici arabi' in: *Cataloghi dei codici orientali di alcune biblioteche d'Italia*, 7 fascicles, Florence 1878–1904: '[Pos., III, F. 65] In carta bambagina, di 143 fogli, alto 28c, largo 21c; caratteri magrebini [...] *al-Mustaʿīnī*, scritto da Jūnis b. Ishāq Beklariz al-Israīlī, per Mustaʿīn billāh b. Mu'tamin billāh b. Hūd, che regnó in Saragozza dall'anno 478 all'anno 503 dell'Egira. L'opera é completa, ma stata mal rilegata, come si vede facilmente dall'ordine alfabetico turbato, e dal fine che si trova al f. 79 r., dove é anche la chiusa, nella quale si legge che questa copia la fece per sé Hasan bin Jūsuf bin Hasan bin Ahmad bin Sālih bin S'uʿaʿ ad-Din al-Ansārī, e la finí in Leria (?) il 14 di Dhū'l Qaʿdah, dell'anno 888 dell'Egira, copiandola da un manoscritto che aveva nella chiusa la data di Cordova al 5 Febbraio dell'anno 1303 di G.C., corrispondente al 15 di Rabīʿ II dell'anno 663 dell'Egira' (Fasc. II, p. 237, nr. 96).

11. Reinhardt Dozy, *Supplément aux dictionnaires arabes*, 2 vols., Leiden 1881; 2nd edn., Paris 1927.

12. Francisco Javier Simonet, *Glosario de voces ibéricas y latinas usadas entre los mozárabes*, Madrid 1888; reprinted Madrid 1982.

13. Evariste Lévi-Provençal, *Catalogue de la Bibliothéque Génerale du Protectorat français au Maroc*, Paris 1913.

Naples manuscript was lent to him thanks to Michele Amari. In the quotations from the Leiden manuscript he distinguishes between the old and the modern parts. He did not use the manuscript from Madrid, even though he was in close contact with Simonet.

The Madrid manuscript of the *Kitāb al-Mustaʿīnī* was one of the sources used by Simonet (1888) in compiling his *Glosario*. He calls this manuscript 'toledano', because it had previously been in the library of Toledo Cathedral (Pluteo XCVII, no. 17). The manuscript bears an old number: Gg [i.e., Gayangos] 149. Simonet believes that the manuscript 'perteneció a los Hebreos de Toledo y no es posterior al siglo XIII'. I do not know what made him think the manuscript belonged to the Toledan Jews. Admittedly the presence of glosses and annotations in Spanish, Hebrew and Arabic in the margins and on the first folios show that the book passed through many different hands. Yet the scribe did not register the date of the copy. Simonet's idea that it was no later than the thirteenth century has become, in Renaud's article, 'no later than the twelfth century'.

The Madrid Catalogue by Guillén Robles reads: 'Yunos Ben Ishak Ben Buclarex Alisraelí. *Kitāb al-Mustaʿīnī*'.[14] The description of the manuscript draws attention to an annotation at the beginning, in a late sixteenth-century hand: *Las melezinas simples de buclares*. The manuscript lacks an author's name and it was through a comparison of its text with the Leiden manuscript that the identification was made after the title had been recognized in the Introduction.

So, whereas the existence of three manuscripts (those in Madrid, Leiden and Naples) was known in Spain, in the rest of the world the Madrid manuscript was ignored. Brockelmann does not mention it in his *Supplement*, although Renaud's article—his source on the Rabat manuscript—lists the four codices known in his time (Madrid, Leiden, Naples and Rabat). Even Levey and Souryal[15] omit the Madrid manuscript, as does Ullmann.[16]

In 1940 Max Meyerhof used the *Kitāb al-Mustaʿīnī* to annotate his edition of Maimonides's glossary.[17] In the introduction (p. xxviii) he thanked Renaud, who was preparing the edition and annotated translation of the *Kitāb al-Mustaʿīnī*, for his help. In 1968 Martin Levey and Safwat Souryal published an English translation of the Introduction to the *Kitāb al-Mustaʿīnī*, based on the Rabat and Leiden manuscripts.[18] Levey completed his work by publishing two articles in 1969 and

14. Francisco Guillén Robles, *Catálogo de los manuscritos árabes existentes en la Biblioteca Nacional de Madrid*, Madrid 1889: 'Yunos Ben Ishak Ben Buclarex Alisraelí. *Kitāb al-Mustaʿīnī. Libro (titulado) Almostainí*. Fol: papel. [...] 139 fol.: foliación castell.: al principio 3 fol. de papel más moderno que el del texto, y en uno de ellos esta nota en letra del s. XVIII: *De simplicibus medicamentis*: después 2 fol. de igual papel al del texto, con varias notas sobre Medicina, y entre ellas, en letra del s. XVI ó principios del XVII, esta otra nota: *Las melezinas simples de buclares*: falto al comedio (p. 63, nr. cxxvii). No consta en el códice el nombre de su autor; pero por la nota castellana, que se ha indicado en sus primeros folios, y por la comparación con el que se ha mencionado de la Bibl. Leyd., perfectamente descrito por los autores de su catálogo, puede afirmarse que es del autor á quien se asigna: si alguna duda quedara, la hubiera resuelto el título de la obra, que aparece en la introducción' (p. 64).

15. Martin Levey and Safwat S. Souryal, 'The Introduction to the *Kitāb al-Mustaʿīnī* of Ibn Biklārish (fl. 1106)', *Janus*, 55, 1968, pp. 134–66.

16. Manfred Ullmann, *Die Medizin im Islam*, Leiden–Cologne 1970: 'Yūsuf (Yūnus?) ibn Isḥāq ibn Biklāriš schrieb in Almeria um die Wende vom 11. zum 12. Jhdt. [...] *K. al-Mustaʿīnī* [Mss.: Naples, Rabat; Lit.: Renaud 1930, Dozy]' (p. 275).

17. Max Meyerhof, *Sharḥ asmāʾ al-ʿuqqār (L'explication des noms des drogues): un glossaire de matière médicale composé par Maïmonide*, Cairo 1940.

18. Levey and Souryal, 'The Introduction to the *Kitāb al-Mustaʿīnī* of Ibn Biklārish'.

1971: one about the pharmacology of Ibn Baklarish in the Introduction[19] and another describing the pharmacological tables.[20] According to Levey and Souryal the *Kitāb al-Mustaʿīnī* 'is composed almost entirely of synoptic tables which are now being studied and translated' (p. 134).

Unaware of Levey's work, I myself started working on the Introduction of *al-Mustaʿīnī*, and in 1972 I presented the Arabic edition based on the Madrid and Naples manuscripts, with a Spanish translation and a study, notes and indexes.[21] My work was published some years later, in 1980, as 'El prólogo de *al-Kitāb al-Mustaʿīnī de Ibn Buklārish* [Texto árabe y traducción anotada]' in a collective volume.[22] The next year I published the entry on 'Ibn Buklāriš' in an article entitled 'Corpus medicorum arabico-hispanorum' in which a group of Spanish scholars tried to put together all the material known to us on physicians in al-Andalus: the basic biographical data, the extant manuscripts and the bibliography.[23] To my surprise, somebody added to the text I submitted the reference to a manuscript located at Hyderabad in the Salar Jang Library (I do not know if this is correct or not) and stated at the end: 'an edition and translation are being prepared by Amador Díaz'. My study on the sources of the *Kitāb al-Mustaʿīnī* appeared in 1983,[24] having been presented at a conference some years before.

In 2002 a good and complete summary of all available information on Ibn Buklārish, his work, manuscripts and bibliography was published by Ildefonso Garijo in the *Enciclopedia de al-Andalus*.[25]

More recently the *Kitāb al-Mustaʿīnī* has been studied by Joëlle Ricordel, who has examined the theory of compound drugs, the 'stones' named in it and the system of *jadwal* arrangement.[26] In 2004 she defended her thesis on the tables of the *Kitāb al-Mustaʿīnī* in an edition, French translation and analysis of the letters *alif* to *zāy*.[27]

It is perhaps just as well that the edition of the full text has not yet been published. For the appearance of new library catalogues has brought to light the existence of

19. Martin Levey, 'The Pharmacology of Ibn Biklārish in the Introduction to his *Kitāb al-Mustaʿīnī*', *Studia Islamica*, 6, 1969, pp. 98–104.

20. 'The Pharmacological Table of Ibn Biklārish (fl. 1106)', *Journal of the History of Medicine*, 26, 1971, pp. 413–21.

21. Ana Labarta, 'El prólogo de "al-*Mustaʿīnī*" de Ibn Buklāriš según los manuscritos de Madrid y Nápoles. Transcripción, traducción y estudio', Universidad de Barcelona 1972 (unpublished Thesis de licenciatura).

22. Ana Labarta, 'El prólogo de *al-Kitāb al-Mustaʿīnī de Ibn Buklāriš* (texto árabe y traducción anotada)' in: Juan Vernet (ed.), *Estudios sobre historia de la ciencia árabe*, Barcelona 1980, pp. 181–316.

23. Ana Labarta, 'Ibn Buklāriš' in: Carmen Peña *et al.*, 'Corpus medicorum arabico-hispanorum', *Awrāq*, 4, 1981, pp. 79–111.

24. Ana Labarta, 'La farmacología de Ibn Buklāriš: sus fuentes' in: *Actas del IV Coloquio Hispano-Tunecino (Palma de Mallorca, 1979)*, Madrid 1983, pp. 165–74.

25. Ildefonso Garijo, 'Ibn Buklāriš' in: *Enciclopedia de al-Andalus. Diccionario de autores y obras andalusíes*, Granada 2002, I, pp. 667–8.

26. Joëlle Ricordel, 'Le médicament composé: théories andalouses sur l'évaluation de son degré (XIIe siècle)', *Revue d'Histoire de la Pharmacie*, 49, nr. 330, 2001, pp. 135–48; 'Les "pierres" dans les tables médicales d'Ibn Biklārish (fin 11ᵉ / début 12ᵉ s.)' in: 'Identité culturelle des sciences et des philosophies arabes: auteurs, œuvres et transmissions', Colloque International, Namur–Brussels, 15–18 January 2003 (unpublished); 'Le catalogue médical d'Ibn Biklārish: une formulation nouvelle pour les connaissances pharmaceutiques andalousiennes' (in press).

27. Joëlle Ricordel, 'Les Tables des medicaments simples d'Isḥāḳ ibn Biklārish. Édition, traduction française et analyse (des lettres alif à zāy)', 3 vols., November 2004, Université Paris VII-Denis Diderot (unpublished thesis).

several previously unknown manuscripts. The latest arrival, the Arcadian Library manuscript, is an early copy and by far the best of the manuscripts I know. As I shall explain later, I believe it should be used as the basis of the critical edition.

The author's name and life

SHUHRA

We have no explanation for the last element of the author's name, which is meaningless in Arabic, and this makes the vocalization uncertain. Even though we do not have any evidence that the name was Romance, there is a general tendency to make of it a Latin or Romance adjective. Modern authors have either read it according to what they suppose is its etymology, or have simply followed what others have proposed.

In brief, we have the following variants: B·klār·sh in Ibn Abi Usaybiʿa in Arabic without short vowels; B·qlār·sh in the Naples manuscript in Arabic without short vowels. The older Latin transcriptions try to avoid the problem of the short vowels by inserting one or two neutral 'e's. Beclaris without the 'ibn' is found in Hottinger;[28] Beklariz without the 'ibn' in Buonazia[29] and Steinschneider;[30] Beclárix and Buclárix in Simonet;[31] Beklarisch in Wüstenfeld,[32] De Jong and De Goeje,[33] and Simonet; Beklāresh in Brockelmann (1898 and 1937)[34] and Renaud (1930);[35] Boclaris and Buclaris in Steinschneider; Buclares without the 'ibn' in the Madrid manuscript (sixteenth century); Buclarex in Guillén Robles (1889);[36] and Buclarís in Ribera (1896)[37] (the accent must be a misprint).

Buklārish, which looks like the 'academic' version of the names listed above, is

28. Joh. Henricus Hottinger, *Promtuarium sive bibliotheca orientalis exhibens Catalogum, sive, Centurias aliquot, tam Authorum, quam librorum Hebraicorum, Syriacorum, Arabicorum, Aegyptiacorum, Aethiopicorum etc.*, Heidelberg 1658: '*Kitāb al-mustaʿīnī fī-l-mufradāt al-ṭibbiyya li-Ibn Isḥāq Bklārsh al-Isrāylī*. Isacides, fil. Beclaris, Israëlita, de Simplicium Medicamentorum facultatibus' (p. 215, no. 16).

29. See above, n. 10.

30. Moritz Steinschneider, *Hebraeische Bibliographie*, Berlin 1880: '[...] darunter S. 237 No. 96 das vielsprachliche Werk des Juden Junis b. Ishaq „Beklariz", wovon bisher nur das Leydener Exemplar bekannt war (s. Virchow's Archiv Bd. 39, S. 317); es wird als „Boclaris" oder „Buclaris" angeführt im latein. Gafiki, worüber mehr in meinem II. Artikel Gafiki, der nahezu fertig ist. Sollte der Namen nicht mit einem Orte Biclar ... in Portugal zusammenhängen? In Dozy's Supplem. aux Dictionn. ar. scheint das Werk noch nicht benutzt', vol. 20, p. 90.

31. Simonet, *Glosario*, p. CXLV: 'El copioso diccionario de materia médica que un Hebreo llamado Jonás, hijo de Isaac (en Árabe Yunos ben Ishác), y apellidado *Ibn Buclárix* (ó Beclárix), escribió en lengua arábiga hácia el año 500-1106, y tituló *Almostainí* por haberlo dedicado al rey moro de Zaragoza Ahmed Almostaín ibn Hud.'

32. Ferdinand Wüstenfeld, *Geschichte der arabischen Ärzte und Naturforscher*, Göttingen 1846: 'Isaac Ibn Beklārisch, ein jüdischer Arzt in Spanien ums J. 520 (1126). O. [= Ibn Abi Usaybiʿa] XIII, 58. Liber auxilii indigentium de medicamentis simplicibus. K. [= Hottinger] 215' (p. 88, no. 155).

33. See above, pp. 16–17 and n. 8.

34. See above, nn. 5, 6.

35. Renaud, 'Trois études', p. 135: 'Yūsuf (ou mieux Yūnus) b. Isḥāḳ Ibn Beklāresh [J'adopte ici la transcription de l'arabe parlé, comme le fait Brockelmann [...] ce qui a l'avantage de ne rien préjuger relativement à la vocalisation de ce nom propre, dont l'origine est controversée.]'

36. Francisco Guillén Robles, *Catálogo de los manuscritos árabes existentes en la Biblioteca Nacional de Madrid*, Madrid 1889.

37. Julián Ribera, *Bibliófilos y bibliotecas en la España musulmana*, Saragossa 1896; reprinted in idem, *Dis-*

the spelling traditionally employed by Spanish scholars. Renaud and Colin used it too, and it may contain an echo of a fictive *kunya*: *Abū* or *Bū*.[38] The vocalization of Biklārish was invented by Steinschneider (1880) who tried to relate the name to a Visigothic place-name: the no longer extant 'Biclaro'.[39] His hypothetical adjective 'biclarese' is unacceptable for several reasons: the Arabic long vowel should be in the same place as the Spanish accent, which is not the case, nor does such an adjective exist in Spanish. Moreover, it goes against the normal formation. Nevertheless, Meyerhof (1940),[40] Mieli (1966),[41] Levey and Souryal (1968),[42] Ullmann (1970),[43] Dietrich (1993)[44] and Ricordel[45] all follow this vocalization. In their French translation of Ibn Abi Usaybiʿa Jahier and Noureddine use the vocalization Baklārich,[46] which has reappeared in the London auctioneer's description of the Arcadian Library manuscript.[47] I suspect that the name retains an echo of the Arabic word *baql* ('herbs').

As we have seen, there is a large range of possibilities: the 'b' followed by 'a, e, i, o or u'. Surprisingly enough, 'k' is never vocalized; 'l' is always followed by a long 'ā'; after 'r' we find only 'i' or 'e', and 'sh' is never followed by a vowel.

Nobody has ever thought the 'b' could represent a /p/ (Hebrew or Romance). The 'k'/'q' variant may reflect a sound that does not exist in Arabic, maybe a /g/, and the 'ā' could be read /e/ as in *aljamiado* texts. The 'r' could equally well be followed by 'a, o, u', and 'k' could be vocalized too. At least one of the consonants could be geminated. And to complicate matters a little more, some late Moroccan sources pointed out by Renaud refer to him as B·k·lāw·sh· with a 'w' in the place of the 'r'. There is ample room for conjecture and fantasy, and the Arcadian Library manuscript, the best witness to the text, unfortunately does not name the author.

ISM

There is no *ism* in the Arabic or European sources. The only place where it appears is in the opening of the Leiden manuscript, written by the seventeenth-century Moroccan copyist—a very late piece of information.

'Yunus' is given by De Jong and De Goeje following the Leiden manuscript.[48]

---

ertaciones y opúsculos, Madrid 1928, I, pp. 181–228: '[...] Almostaín, al que Abenbuclarís dedicó su famoso libro de materia médica *Al-Mostainí*, con cuya posesión se envanecen algunas bibliotecas europeas (Véase Glosario de Simonet, página CXLVI.)' (p. 213).

38. P.J. Renaud and Georges S. Colin, *Tuḥfat al-Aḥbāb. Glossaire de la matière médicale marocaine*, Paris 1934: 'Dozy s'est peut être plus largement servi encore des manuscrits de Leyde et de Naples du *Mustaʿīnī* d'Ibn Buklārish' (p. XII); 'Bkl. *al-Mustaʿīnī fī ṭ-ṭibb*, par Yūsuf b. Isḥāq Ibn Buklārish, ms. no. 55 [= Rabat]' (p. XXIII).

39. See above, n. 30.

40. Meyerhof, *Sharḥ asmaʾ al ʿuqqār*: Yūnus (Yōnah) ibn Isḥāq ibn Biklārish.

41. Aldo Mieli, *La science arabe et son rôle dans l'évolution scientifique mondiale*, Leiden 1966.

42. Levey and Souryal, 'The Introduction to the *Kitāb al-Mustaʿīnī* of Ibn Biklārish'.

43. Ullmann, *Die Medizin im Islam*.

44. Albert Dietrich (ed.), *Dioscurides triumphans: ein anonymer arabischer Kommentar (Ende 12. Jahr. nach Chr.) zur Materia Medica*, Göttingen 1988, vol. 6, p. 246.

45. Ricordel, 'Les Tables des medicaments simples d'Isḥāḳ ibn Biklāri̲s̲h̲'.

46. Ibn Abi Usaybiʿa, *ʿUyūn al-Anbāʾ fī ṭabaqāt al-aṭibbāʾ*.

47. Sotheby's London Sale Catalogue, *Arts of the Islamic World*, 15 October 2003, lot 11.

48. See above, p. 17 and n. 8.

After them this is the usually accepted name. They are the first to call him so since Hottinger omitted the *ism*.[49] Where the name 'Ishaq' is concerned we see that Wüstenfeld calls him Isaac Ibn Beklārisch,[50] misreading Hottinger. But what Hottinger had was 'Isacides', a Greco-Latin form signifying 'Ibn Ishaq'. As for 'Yusuf', this name appears for the first time in Brockelmann,[51] probably as a misprint, since Brockelmann himself calls him 'Yunus' (with no alternative *ism*) in the *Supplement*, published later.[52] Since Brockelmann is a basic work of reference, some authors have hesitated between these two possibilities, and, like Renaud, have finally adopted both *isms*. And, as Renaud was—and still is—the basic source of information,[53] this mistake was consolidated and spread in Mieli and Ullmann for example.[54]

NASAB

Ibn Ishaq is used everywhere after Hottinger, following the Leiden manuscript.

LAQAB

al-Isra'ili appears almost everywhere after Hottinger, following the Leiden manuscript. The Arcadian manuscript corroborates this.

DATE AND PLACE OF BIRTH AND DEATH

The dates are unknown. We can estimate that our author lived approximately between the second half of the eleventh and the first half of the twelfth century. Many scholars place his *floruit*, his death, or even the year of composition of his book in 500 A.H./1106 A.D. This date can only be an approximate one, proposed by De Jong and De Goeje, while Wüstenfeld places it around 520 (1126).[55]

Ibn Baklarish clearly arrived in Saragossa after 1085. Before Saragossa he seems to have been in Almeria, where he wrote his book. That is all we know. References that make him 'de Zaragoza' (of Saragossa) or 'zaragozano' must be understood as referring to the place where he worked, not to his birthplace.

DATE AND PLACE OF COMPOSITION OF THE BOOK

The *Kitāb al-Mustaʿīnī* was written during the life and reign of al-Mustaʿin II Ibn Hud of Saragossa (ruled 1085–1110). Ibn Baklarish wrote it 'as a way to reach him'. He apparently succeeded, since we read that 'he served as physician to the [dynasty of the] Banū Hūd'. This must be situated between 1085 and 1110. It is impossible to be more precise and any specific year is merely speculative.

According to Ibn Abi Usaybiʿa, the *Kitāb al-Mustaʿīnī* was written in Almería.[56] Renaud found it strange that Ibn Baklarish should have composed his book there and suggested that Ibn Abi Usaybiʿa might have mistaken 'copied' for 'composed',

49. See above, n. 28.
50. See above, n. 32.
51. See above, n. 5.
52. See above, n. 6.
53. See above, n. 35.
54. Mieli, *La science arabe*; Ullmann, *Die Medizin im Islam*.
55. See above, nn. 8, 32.
56. See above, p. 16 and n. 4.

since the Naples manuscript was copied in Almería.[57] He overlooked the fact that Ibn Abi Usaybiʿa died in A.H. 668 and the Naples manuscript was copied in A.H. 888, more than two centuries after his death. Renaud was misled by Steinschneider's theory that related B·klar·sh to the place-name Biclaro (identified with the Vallclara monastery in Tarragona), and for this reason he surmised that Ibn Baklarish or his family came from north-eastern Spain.[58] Naturally enough, Almería, in the south-east, seemed to him to be unlikely. What has to be rejected, however, is not the composition at Almeria but the Steinschneider theory in its entirety.

Some reflections

The *Kitāb al-Mustaʿīnī* is a practical medical book of the utmost interest for the history of science. Ibn Baklarish was both original and comparatively modern in the way in which he collected the material, summarized it, put it in alphabetical order, and arranged it in tables that facilitate quick consultation. Every substance has its degree, its names, its substitute, and its use. There are no gaps. At the same time it is a serious and sober work, with no religion, magic, contradictions, or superfluous wordiness.

In the Introduction, Ibn Baklarish prepares the reader for the tabular section which comprises over 100 folios with the facing pages dealing with the same subjects. On the right-hand page we have: the name of the drug, its nature and degree, its synonyms, and its substitutes: and on the left-hand one its usefulness, properties, and methods of use. The book lists some 700 simple drugs.

We should note that the manuscripts of London, Madrid and Leiden contain six drugs on every page, in exactly the same place. This may show that these three manuscripts reproduce the arrangement in the original book—an arrangement to be adopted in a future critical edition. In the Rabat copy, after the inclusion of later material, there are only three or four items per page, while the Naples manuscript has a larger format, and holds more simples per page.

Ibn Baklarish was a practical physician, with a good knowledge of the simple medicaments. This means that he had studied the works current in his time. But he was neither a botanist nor a linguist. He never talks about his own experiences, observations or travels. His work is made up of quotations, and he insists on pointing out to us that he had to consult a great many books, especially in order to collect the substitutes of the medicaments and their names in different languages. Good editions of the authors and works quoted by Ibn Baklarish will consequently help the editor's task considerably.

57. Renaud, 'Trois études', p. 138, n. 1.

58. Renaud, 'Trois études', p. 137: '[Ibn Beklārеš], ou du moins sa famille, semble avoir été originaire des provinces du nord-est de l'Espagne [...] si, comme l'a suggéré Steinschneider, on rattache étymologiquement ce nom, qui n'a rien d'hébraïque, au toponyme Biclaro, monastère fondé au VIe siècle de J.-C. par saint Jean, évêque de Gérone, dans les montagnes de Tarragone, là où est aujourd'hui la ville de Vallclara ...' See also David Wasserstein's essay in this volume, pp. 105–12 below. My main point, however, is that whatever the possible origin of Ibn Baklarish's name may be, it is not valid to infer from this a local linguistic influence in his work; such an influence cannot be detected.

To start with, we need to establish as nearly as possible the original text, for which an essential preliminary task is to identify and eliminate additional material and marginal glosses that subsequent copyists have introduced into the Tables. Thus, for example, in later manuscripts, such as that of Rabat, there are quotations from Avicenna and Ibn al-Baytar which are not in the London or Madrid manuscripts, and of course do not belong to the original work. It was because of these interpolations that Renaud expressed his doubts about the real date of the work.

The number of authors quoted would suggest that Ibn Baklarish used a large library. At the same time, however, we may assume that many of the quotations are indirect, and that the number of works really used was far smaller. In order to establish the real sources of the *Kitāb al-Mustaʿīnī*, I listed all those named in the Madrid manuscript, identifying the authors and the works, and comparing them—as far as was then possible—with the original.[59] There is no need to repeat the contents of that paper here. It is interesting to point out that when the research was performed in 1979 the bulk of the necessary material was neither available nor published. Since then the situation has changed. Now the whole corpus of Ibn Juljul's works is available. We can use the facsimile of al-Zahrawi; and the *Book of Simples* of Ibn Wafid has been published and translated into Spanish—to mention only the major texts.

The hardest part of the *Kitāb al-Mustaʿīnī* to edit is the column devoted to the synonyms. About some of the words Ibn Baklarish says they are in Syriac, Persian, classical and Byzantine Greek, Arabic, classical and late Latin, or Berber. He was not a polyglot, but was simply copying from other sources, as he himself declares. The information he provides about foreign languages is always second-hand; the spellings are often corrupt and the attribution of a word to this or that language is sometimes wrong. On the other hand, we are not given systematically the equivalents of each drug in all languages. We simply have what he found in addition to some commentaries or discussions. The material does not reflect the language spoken anywhere at his time. Depending on the sources he used, he mixed variants from different periods, and some items of his information were more reliable than others. The copyists, not understanding the exotic words, have contributed to the corruption.

For the different Arabic names of the drugs, Ibn Baklarish quotes mainly the *Kitāb al-Nabāt* of Abu Hanifa (d. 895). It is from this work that he takes data from earlier linguists such as Abu Ziyad al-Kilabi (d. 820) and Abu Nasr al-Bahili (d. 845), the two main sources of Abu Hanifa, and al-Farraʾ (d. 821), Abu ʿUbayda (d. 824), Yaʿqub al-Sikkit (d. 858?), and Abu ʿAmr ibn al-ʿAlaʾ (11th century), as well as notices from Bedouin informants. This allows him to offer some local terms and references concerning Oman, Syria, Iraq, Yemen, and the Hijaz. One term is in Nabataean, and one in Coptic.

Ibn Baklarish mentions three Arabic variants as employed in Ifriqiya, one of them taken from Ibn al-Jazzar (d. 1004) and two Egyptian Arabic forms from Ishaq b. Sulayman al-Isra'ili (d. 932). In two cases he gives a variant used in al-Andalus (s.v. *kumathrà*, *muḥallab*) and in one he refers to Cordova (s.v. *shahsibaram*).

59. Labarta, 'La farmacología de Ibn Buklāriš'.

There are thirty-one terms in 'Syriac' (*suryāniyya*). One of them is taken from al-Zahrawi (*c.* 936–1013) while others are also found in Ibn al-Jazzar. It is noticeable that many of them refer to simples of animal or mineral origin. The Syriac words in the *Kitāb al-Mustaʿīnī* have been studied and commented on in this volume by Geoffrey Khan.

The total number of words in 'Persian' is around 120. The majority are copied again from Abu Hanifa completed by Ibn al-Jazzar, Ibn Juljul (944–94?) and al-Zahrawi. Around thirty words are in 'Berber' (*barbariyya*). Ibn Baklarish says he borrowed them from al-Zahrawi and Ibn Juljul, but he may have used Ibn al-Jazzar too. Renaud studied the Berber lexicon in detail, trying to see if it reflected any particular dialect, but the results were negative.

Although there are many drug names in Greek, only fifteen words are expressly marked as 'Greek' (*yunāniyya*). They probably come from Dioscorides and his commentator Ibn Juljul, directly or via al-Zahrawi who is also mentioned.

Thirty-five terms are also qualified as 'rūmiyya' (i.e. Byzantine Greek). Some are Greek (*kremidia, kreas, gayduri, stafilia*), others Latin (*leporem, crocus*) or Latinized Greek (*mirtus*). Ibn Baklarish here only quotes al-Zahrawi once, although he may have used him in other cases too. Some of the terms are found in al-Razi's *Ḥāwī* (865–?) and in Ibn al-Jazzar, who also refers to the 'rūmiyya' language.

Some 130 words appear as 'ʿajamiyya', i.e., non-Arabic. This means that they can be in any language other than Arabic. Some of them, again, are obviously Greek (*avgá, tirí, kreas, gayduri, neró, krasí*); others are classical Latin (*leporem, asparagus, aramen, ruta, cucumeris*); yet others are in late Latin or Romance. Some words appear twice, once attributed to the 'rūmiyya' and elsewhere to the 'ʿajamiyya', according to the different sources he was using. Some of the material comes from old Oriental works, like that of Abu Hanifa and the *Ḥāwī* of al-Razi, either directly or via Andalusian works. Some of the Romance terms found in Ibn Baklarish are also found in Ibn Wafid and Ibn al-Jazzar, but these are not mentioned as authorities. It is possible that all three authors were using the same sources. Ibn Baklarish explicitly quotes only three authors: Ibn Juljul, al-Zahrawi's *Kitāb al-Taṣrīf* and Ibn Janah.

As Carmen Barceló has shown,[60] this Ibn Janah—who was used as a source by al-Zahrawi and possibly by Ibn Juljul—cannot be the famous Ibn Janah who was born in Córdoba and died in Saragossa (990–1050), but must be earlier. When al-Zahrawi quotes him he calls him 'al-Yahūdī'. But he attributes to him passages that are identical to those Ibn Baklarish attributes to 'Ibn Janah'. Ibn Janah's material probably passed to the *Kitāb al-Mustaʿīnī*—where he is named only four times—by way of al-Zahrawi. It seems clear, in particular, that all the references to the Arabic and Romance language used in and around Saragossa come from Ibn Janah. The *Kitāb al-Mustaʿīnī* contains seven words in 'Latin' (*laṭīnī*) without source ascription (two are in Ibn Juljul and al-Zahrawi, from Ibn Janah).

After a test comparison between some items in the Arcadian and Madrid manuscripts, it is clear to me that between them they show significant variants, and I would like to draw attention to the enormous importance of the Arcadian manuscript in establishing the text of the work. In most of the cases the Arcadian manuscript has

60. Carmen Barceló, 'Romance Lexicon in Pharmacological Treatises Written in Muslim Spain: its Origin and Transmission', *Journal for the History of Arabic Science*, 12, 2001, pp. 111–30.

a better *ductus* than the Madrid one. In some cases it provides a logical reading while we find a meaningless sequence in the Madrid manuscript. Moreover, the Arcadian manuscript sometimes gives the Latin words in Latin characters. The quality of the text found in the Arcadian manuscript should thus enable us to establish a definitive text of the *Kitāb al-Mustaʿīnī* close to the original, and free from later interpolations and misreadings.

JOËLLE RICORDEL

THE MANUSCRIPT TRANSMISSION OF THE *KITĀB AL-MUSTAʿĪNĪ* AND THE CONTRIBUTIONS OF THE ARCADIAN LIBRARY MANUSCRIPT

Although it has been studied relatively little in recent years,[1] the *Kitāb al-Mustaʿīnī* by Ibn Baklarish is of particular interest for the history of science in al-Andalus at the end of the eleventh century. This interest is due as much to its presentation as to its contents. The work is dedicated to Abu Jaʿfar Ahmad al-Mustaʿin bi-llah, the fourth representative of the Banu Hud dynasty which reigned in the Upper March with Saragossa as its capital.[2] Ibn Baklarish, the prince's personal physician,[3] composed his manual with an originality which makes it exceptional in the medical-pharmaceutical tradition of al-Andalus. Indeed, these are the first tables of simple medicines to have been written in this country, concentrating, on facing pages for each medicinal substance, all the information transmitted by the treatises on synonyms, substitutes and *materia medica*. To the practical advantage of rapid consultation—the reader can look up the names of the simple drugs alphabetically—is added the great diversity of the material presented, particularly where the substances of mineral and animal origin are concerned. The Tables, moreover, are preceded by an Introduction in four chapters[4] containing the theories of simple and compound medicines.

Until now all studies of the *Kitāb al-Mustaʿīnī* have been based mainly on four manuscript copies:[5]

~ Madrid, Biblioteca Nacional, MS ar. 5009 (= M)
~ Naples, Biblioteca Nazionale, Vittorio Emanuele II, MS III-F-65 (= N)
~ Rabat, Al-Khizana al-ʿAmma (General Library), MS D 2976 (= R1)
~ Leiden, Bibliotheek der Rijksuniversiteit (University Library), Cod. Or. 15 (= L).

The critical edition which I am preparing led me to add to the inventory five further

1. Its main interest seems to have been due to its lexicographical store which was used extensively by Reinhardt Dozy and Francisco Javier Simonet for the compilation of their *Supplément aux dictionnaires arabes*, Leiden 1881, and *Glosario de voces ibéricas y latinas usadas entre los mozárabes*, Madrid 1888, respectively. Only recently, two partial editions have been made of the Introduction, whereas the tables have only been studied as examples: Ana Labarta, 'El prólogo de *al-Kitāb al-Mustaʿīnī de Ibn Buklāriš* (texto árabe y traducción anotada)' in: Juan Vernet (ed.), *Estudios sobre historia de la ciencia árabe*, Barcelona 1980, pp. 181–316; Al-Faruq ʿUmar al-ʿAsli, '*Kitāb al-Mustaʿīnī fi l-ṭibb* li-Ibn Buklārish', *Al-Ṣaydalī* (Tunis), 40, 1991, pp. 52–4, 41, 1991, pp. 56–9, 42, 1991, pp. 46–51, 44, 1992, pp. 49–51.
2. Al-Mustaʿin II ruled from 1085 to 1110, when he was killed in the battles between his own troops and those of the Christian King Alfonso 'the Battler'.
3. Ibn Abi Usaybiʿa, '*Uyūn al-Anbā' fī ṭabaqāt al-aṭibbā*', ed. August Müller, Cairo 1882–4, reprinted Beyrouth, 1955–6, no. 3, II, p. 52.
4. These chapters are entitled 'On the discovery of the strength of medicines', 'On the knowledge of the natures of compound medicines', 'On laxative medicines according to Galen' and 'On why the Ancients searched for substitutes for drugs'.
5. The siglum given to each manuscript in brackets will be used to indicate it in the rest of the text.

manuscripts and to collate them with the above copies. These are:

~ Rabat, Al-Khizana al-ʿAmma, MS D 2960 (= R2)
~ Rabat, Al-Khizana al-Ḥasaniyya (Royal Library), MS 763 (= R3)
~ Rabat, Al-Khizana al-ʿAmma, MS D 55 (= R4)
~ Tunis, Dar al-Kutub al-Wataniyya (National Library), MS 3575 (= T)
~ Nouakchott, Mauritanian Institute of Scientific Research, MS 589/ Stewart 515 (= Mt)
~ Vatican City, Biblioteca Apostolica Vaticana, MS Vaticano, ebr. 530/1 (= V) (incomplete)

To this list must be added Dublin, Chester Beatty Library, MS Ar. 4506, which I did not use when I was working on the text,[6] and Fez, Qarawiyyin Mosque Library, MS 1652 (Q), which is so damaged as to be extremely difficult to use. The manuscript acquired by the Arcadian Library in London (A) thus brings to twelve the number of recorded copies of Ibn Baklarish's manual, to which we should perhaps add the one in the Salar Jang collection of the Library of Hyderabad in India,[7] the existence of which has not been confirmed.

The manuscript transmission of the Kitāb al-Mustaʿīnī

I shall first discuss the manuscript tradition of Ibn Baklarish as we knew it before the acquisition of a new copy by the Arcadian Library (on which see below, pp. 32ff.). As we can see, the manuscripts of the *Kitāb al-Mustaʿīnī* are at the moment preserved in European libraries and in those of the Maghreb. Do these present locations, which seem to exclude the diffusion of the manual in the area of the Middle East, indicate the geographical origin of the copies?

MANUSCRIPTS IN EUROPEAN LIBRARIES

Before the discovery of the Arcadian Library copy, there were four manuscripts in European libraries: MSS M, N, L and V.

MS L (Leiden, Bibliotheek der Rijksuniversiteit, Cod. Or. 15) is undated, but consists of two parts, respectively written in the fourteenth and the seventeenth century. We know its story.[8] The Dutch scholar Golius acquired it from an inhabitant of Marrakesh, Ahmad b. Qasim al-Andalusi, in the first half of the seventeenth century. The badly mutilated copy was heavily restored at a late stage in order to fill in the lacunae. It has notes which draw attention to variants found in other copies, thus showing that the reconstitution of the text was made from a variety of sources.

MS V (Vaticano, ebr. 530/1) is a composite manuscript which only contains a

6. I owe the reference of this manuscript to the kindness of Professor David Wasserstein.
7. This manuscript is mentioned in Carmen Peña A. Diaz and C. Alvarez de Morales, 'Corpus medicorum arabico-hispanorum', *Awrāq*, 4, 1981, pp. 79–111, see p. 87.
8. This is discussed more fully in the article by Jan Just Witkam in this volume (pp. 75–94).

few leaves of the Introduction to the *Kitāb al-Mustaʿīnī,* in Arabic but in Hebrew characters. It is written in a Sephardic script and could be dated around the fourteenth century. As for its origin, whether Andalusi[9] or Maghribi, this remains unclear.

The other two manuscripts tell us more about the history of the text. They are both of Andalusi origin. We know little about the biography of the author of the *Kitāb al-Mustaʿīnī* other than that he practised his art in Saragossa in the household of al-Mustaʿin II ibn Hud and that he says, in the Introduction, he is dedicating his manual to him. Some remarks made by Ibn Baklarish in the synoptic tables suggest that he stayed, or at least travelled, in the south of al-Andalus.[10] It is thus in the Iberian lands that the author spent his active life, that he wrote his manual, and that its transmission began.

What was, until recently, the earliest known manuscript copy is MS M (Madrid, Biblioteca nacional, MS 5009). There is no colophon but the mark of one of its owners allows us to assume that it was made in the first quarter of the thirteenth century at the latest. Indeed, it belonged to one of the masters of Nahmanides, Yahuda Ibn Yaqar, who set up his Talmudic school in Barcelona in about 1215.[11] It was consequently in this part of Christian Spain that MS M was distributed among the Jewish community—a fact confirmed by marginal notes in Hebrew. It also passed through Christian hands, as is proved by the synonyms in Romance in the margins, the title of the first page in a script said to be of the late sixteenth or early seventeenth century, and the references to the library of the cathedral of Toledo. Three lines of signs and letters on fol. 83b, undoubtedly constituting a talisman, imply that, in the fifteenth or sixteenth century, the manuscript was used by Moriscos accustomed to healing with such magic formulas.[12]

Although the age of the document is not necessarily a valid criterion of quality, the collation of MS M with the other copies known to me at the time showed that it was in fact the most reliable of the manuscripts. It has few omissions and mistakes, and, when the core text is distinguished from the additions, it was probably the closest to the original text, in so far as the plan of the contents and the formal organization are concerned. For these reasons I chose MS M as the base manuscript for my edition.[13]

In N (Naples, MS III-F-65), the *Kitāb al-Mustaʿīnī* forms the first part of the manuscript. The second part contains *Tacuini sanitatis* (*The Almanac of Health according to the Six Causes*)[14] written by Ibn Butlan. The scribe Hasan b. Yusuf b. Hasan b. Ahmad b. Salih b. Shuʿaʿ al-Din al-Ansari says he completed his copy in

9. I.e., of al-Andalus, the part of the Iberian peninsula under Islamic administration.

10. The remarks concern the use of ferns in Córdoba (M, fol. 103b).

11. This mark of ownership appears twice on fol. 1a.

12. For these magic formulas see: Ana Labarta, *Libro de dichos maravillosos (miscelàneo morisco de magia y adivinacíon)*, Madrid 1993.

13. In 2004, I defended a thesis, 'Les Tables des medicaments simples d'Isḥāḳ ibn Biklāri<u>sh</u>. Édition, traduction française et analyse (des lettres alif à zāy)', 3 vols., November 2004, Université Paris VII-Denis Diderot. The manuscript of Madrid Library was then the most reliable of all the manuscripts and I took it as the base of my edition with the assistance of N, T1, R1, R2. After the study of the manuscript of the Arcadian Library that proved the qualities of this new copy, I reworked my critical edition to take it into account. The publication of the whole text of *al-Mustaʿīnī* is envisaged.

14. Hosam Elkhadem, *Le 'Taqwīm al-ṣiḥḥa' (Tacuini sanitatis) d'Ibn Buṭlān: un traité medical du XIe siècle. Histoire du texte, édition critique, traduction, commentaire*, Louvain 1990.

the Andalusi city of Almería on 14 Dhu al-hijja 888 of the Hejira, i.e., 11 January 1482 of the Christian era. This copy undoubtedly circulated among Christians in north-eastern Spain, as we see from the numerous additions of synonyms in Catalan, Aragonese and Castilian in use in the fifteenth century.[15] The collation of MS N shows that it contains many omissions, some of which are significant. None of them are in the other copies studied, which suggests that MS N is independent of these copies. The lack of order among the leaves, which have been displaced, makes it difficult to compare the right-hand pages, which bear the name of the medical substances, with the left-hand ones, which do not have the names and deal with the medicinal properties.

Thanks to the colophon of MS N described above we know that another copy of the *Kitāb al-Musta'īnī* was made in Córdoba, on 17 Rabīʿ al-thānī 663 of the Hejira or 5 February 1303 of the Ṣufr,[16] i.e. 1265 A.D. At that time the former capital of the Umayyad caliphate was already under Christian rule, since it had been conquered by Ferdinand III of Castile in 1236. This manuscript is lost.

Before the discovery of the Arcadian Library manuscript, we had, therefore, only three certain testimonies to the transmission of the *Kitāb al-Musta'īnī* in al-Andalus, since the origin of MS V in Rome has not been confirmed, and MS L of Leiden, in its modern part, and probably also in its earlier part, must belong to the family of manuscripts to which I shall now turn.

MANUSCRIPTS IN NORTH AFRICAN LIBRARIES

The second geographical area of the transmission of Ibn Baklarish's manual is the Maghreb. The lack of biographical information raises questions about the last years of the author's life. Did he, like a number of his compatriots, choose exile under pressure from the Almoravids, who ruled Saragossa after the death of al-Mustaʿin II, or under pressure from the Christians, who conquered it in 1118? This remains an unverifiable hypothesis. But we should observe that most of the manuscripts of the *Kitāb al-Musta'īnī* are to be found in North African libraries. We have noted six, to which we should add the aforesaid MS L and MS Mt preserved in Nouakchott in Mauritania.

One of the copies, MS 3575 (T), is at the National Library in Tunis. It lacks the last two leaves and consequently any colophon. A mark of ownership has been inscribed on the first leaf—that of a bookseller in Tunis, al-ʿAsli, who bought the copy from a private individual in 1963. The bookseller's family subsequently deposited it at the National Library in Tunis.

We have no information about MS 1652 (Q) in the Qarawiyyin Library in Fez, in Morocco, but we should keep in mind that that city was always a haven for Andalusis.

The other manuscripts in Moroccan libraries are very similar to each other, which suggests that they are all based on the same source. The two in the Royal Library in Rabat have dated colophons. They are relatively recent. The copy of MS 55 D (R4) was completed on 29 Muharram 1309 A.H., i.e. 4 September 1891, and MS 763 (R3)

15. Juan Carlos Villaverde Amieva, 'Sobre el estudio del mozárabe en fuentes árabes: a propósito de Ibn Buklāriš' in: *Homenaje a Álvaro Galmés de Fuentes*, III, Oviedo–Madrid, 1987, pp. 703–21.

16. As Dozy writes, the '*ta'rīkh al-ṣufr*' is 'chez les auteurs arabes, l'ère des espagnols qui commence trente huit ans avant la nôtre': Dozy, *Supplément aux dictionnaires arabes*, I, p. 836.

is from the eighteenth century. Its colophon, in so-called *ghubārī* numerals,[17] dates it in 1203, which corresponds to 1788–9.

The relationship between the four manuscripts T, R1, R3 and R4, which already emerges from a comparison of the Introduction, is confirmed by the study of the Tables. In the rubrics of the synonyms and the properties of the simples, the modifications and additions to the text are numerous and identical. The most significant interpolations are quotations of authors later than Ibn Baklarish—anachronisms referring to Ibn al-Baytar[18] and Ibn al-Hashsha'.[19] These manuscripts also have synonyms in Spanish.[20] But despite the elements which lend themselves to comparison, it is not possible to deduce a direct descent or to trace them back to a common source.

MS R2 has differences which classify it outside the manuscripts quoted earlier but which suggest a similarity with the Mauritanian manuscript (Mt)—at least in so far as it is possible to judge from the Introduction alone, since the Tables are missing. It contains the same omissions and errors. The most important omission consists of several pages, and the text thus lacks the end of Chapter 2 'On the knowledge of the natures of compound medicines', as well as the beginning of Chapter 3 'On laxative medicines according to Galen'. At the same time, each of the two copies has individual lacunae which make it impossible that one is the source of the other. This indicates, rather, that they both come from the same secondary source and that the text was reproduced in West Africa, probably via Morocco.

To sum up: the few elements we have gathered define the area of diffusion of Ibn Baklarish's manual and show that it was in regular use from the twelfth to the nineteenth century. The study of the manuscript tradition has not allowed us to establish a definite *stemma*, since the history of the testimonies is uncertain. The collation of the various manuscripts, on the other hand, has isolated MSS N and M, which are independent of one another and have no relationship with the manuscripts preserved in the Maghreb. The synthesis of comparative data makes it possible, provisionally at least, to draw up the following genealogical tree which a more detailed palaeographical and codicological analysis might modify [Fig. 6].

17. These *ghubārī* numerals were used in the Maghreb and in al-Andalus under Muslim rule. The term comes from the little wooden board covered with dust on which they were written; see Georges Ifrah, *Histoire universelle des chiffres*, Paris 1994.

18. Ibn al-Baytar, d. 1248; see Lucien Leclerc, *Ebn al-Beïthār: Traité des simples. Notices et extraits des manuscrits de la Bibliothèque Nationale; traduction française*, Paris 1877–83; new edition: *Ibn al-Bayṭār: Traité des simples, traduction de L. Leclerc*, Paris 1987.

19. Ibn al-Hashsha' compiled his work on the orders of the first Hafsid ruler of Tunisia, Abu Zakariyya, who ruled from 625/1228 to 647/1249; see Georges S. Colin and Henri P. J. Renaud, *Ibn al-H'achcha (13e siècle), Glossaire sur le Mans'uri de Razès (10e siècle): texte arabe établi sur plusieurs manuscrits et publié avec une introduction*, Rabat 1941.

20. See the article by Juan Carlos Villaverde Amieva in this volume (pp. 43–74). I would like to thank Professor Villaverde Amieva for showing me the Spanish version of this article in advance of publication and for helping me in matters concerning Romance terminology in the course of my thesis.

The Arcadian Library manuscript (A)

This study of the copy of the *Kitāb al-Mustaʿīnī* that has been recently acquired by the Arcadian Library has two purposes: to establish its relationship with the other known manuscripts, and to enrich the history of the transmission of the manual.

MS A has the following short colophon which does not indicate the name of the copyist [Fig. 7]:

تم جميع الديوان يوم السبت في العشر الأوسط من شهر ينّير الذي هو صفر عام أربع وعشرين وخمس مائة[21]

According to the information that we can read in the manuscript itself, this copy was completed in '*yannayr* which is Ṣafar 524', i.e. January 1130. It was consequently made within the half-century which followed the composition of the autograph and would be the oldest in existence. This makes it a testimony of essential importance for the knowledge of the history of the text.

My first impression on discovering this manuscript was a sense of *déjà vu*. It appeared to be closely related to MS 5009 of Madrid, the basis of my edition. This impression was tested by analysing the relationship of MS A with all the other manuscripts, first in respect to the presentation of the text and page layout, and then with regard to its contents, taking the Introduction in its entirety and a few pages of the Tables as specimens.

The presentation of the text brings us to the format of the manuscripts, the script and certain editorial characteristics of the Tables (sing. *jadwal* جدول).

THE FORMAT

The written space measures 26 x 15.5 cm in M and 23.5 x 16.1 cm in A on each leaf of the Introduction, and 20.5 to 21 cm x 15.5 cm and 20.9 x 15.4 cm respectively in the Tables. Among all manuscripts examined, the number of lines per page of the Introduction varies from 18 to 29 or 30, but the two manuscripts A and M have 24 and 25 lines respectively. If we look at the Tables, we see that the number of items treated on each of the facing pages also varies. M and A share with most manuscripts six rows of substances, to which is added a row of indications, but the number is reduced to three in R1 and four in R4, while it varies according to the importance of the items in N. These criteria accentuate the resemblance between M and A, but are not sufficient for us to establish a close relationship.

THE SCRIPT

Although all the manuscripts are in a Maghribi hand, the letter forms which are closest to one another are in M and A. The letters are written in the same way, notably where the ح , س , ك and ي appear at the end of the word, as in ينبغي or في. And yet certain letter forms are very different, as we see in the case of هي or the systematic use of لاكن in M and of لكن in A.

21. 'The whole text was completed on Saturday of the middle ten [days] of the month of *yannayr* which is Ṣafar of the year 524 [= 18 January 1130 A.D.]'.

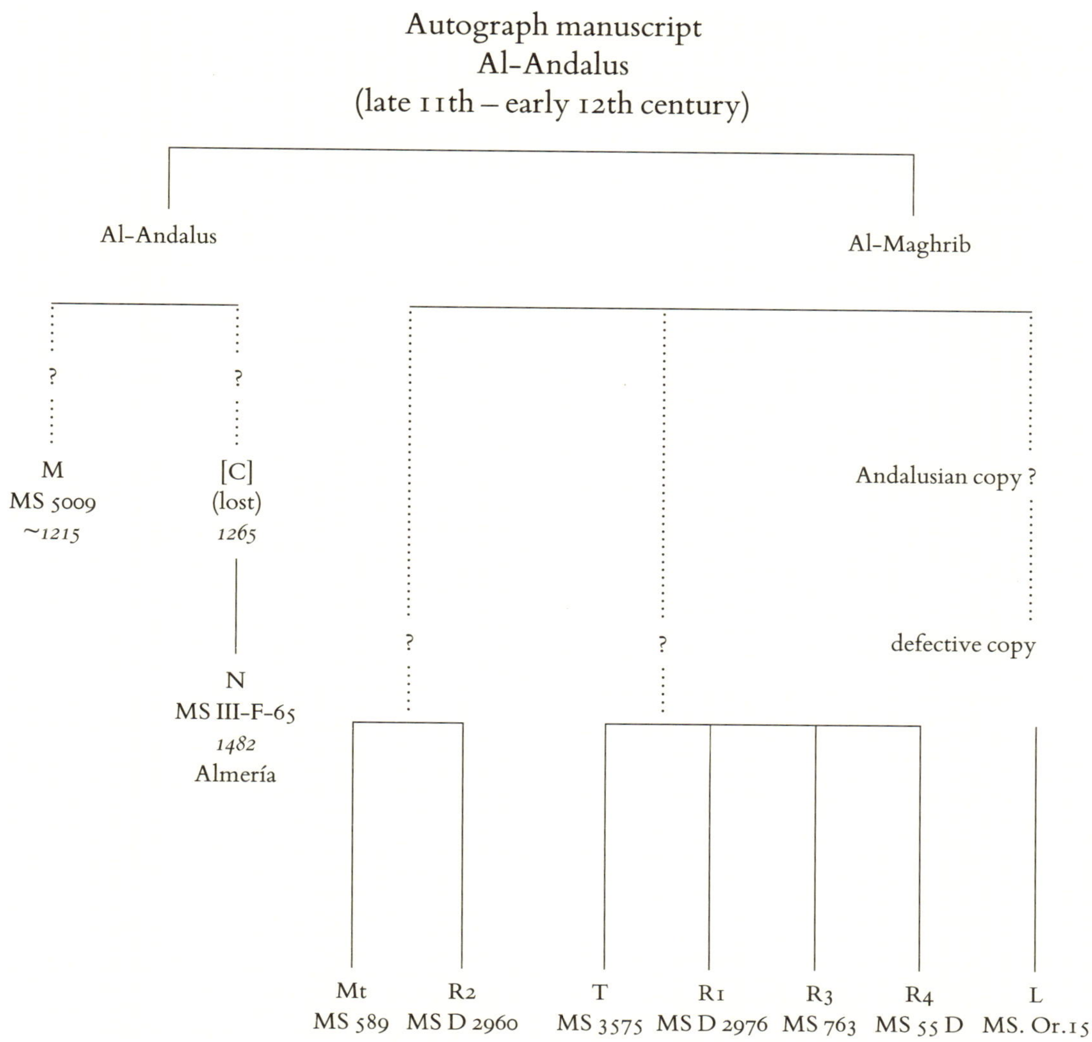

Fig. 6.
Provisional *stemma codicum* of the manuscripts of the *Kitāb al-Mustaʿīnī*. For a further *stemma* based on Romance connections, see below, p. 50

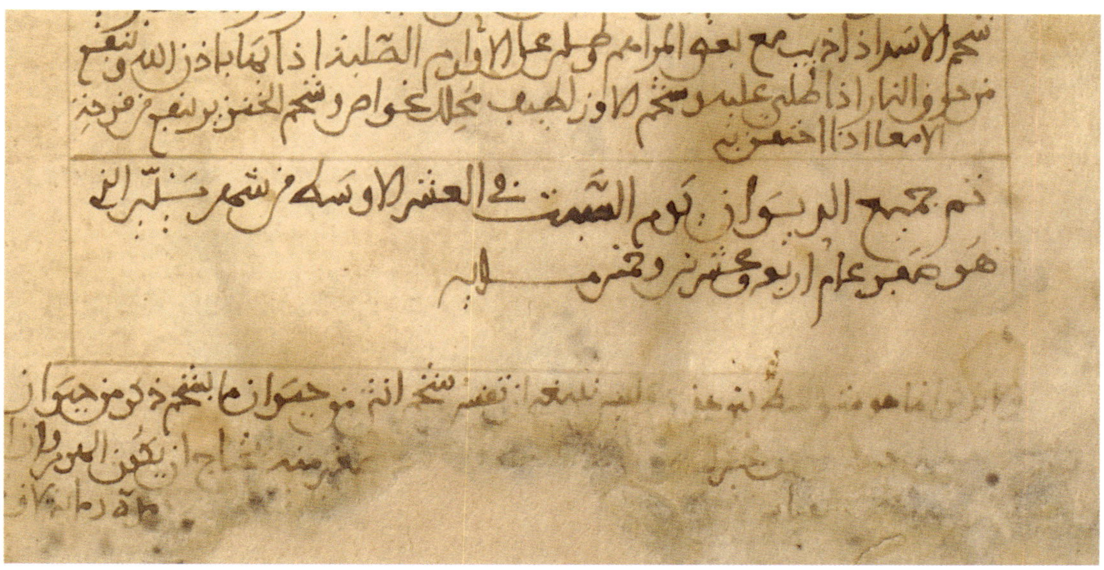

Fig. 7.
The colophon in the Arcadian Library manuscript, pp. 272–3

In these two manuscripts, the rubrics are written in brick red to emphasize the salient elements (the names of substances, the degrees and so on) or the articulations of the text (قال المؤلف : the author said). Palaeographical and codicological studies should narrow down these first impressions.

THE PASSAGE FROM ONE LETTER OF THE ALPHABET TO THE NEXT

There is a more cogent element which allows us to make a closer comparison, since it isolates three copies of the group. As we know, the Tables are classified according to an alphabetical order which is an *abjad maghribī*.[22] The passage from one letter to another is announced regularly within the frame of the table and takes up one of the rows devoted to the simples, but there are five exceptions:

~ the passage from ب to ج is placed in the last line of the lower margins;
~ the passage from ج to د is on the side of the left-hand page;
~ the passage from ه to و is above the row of indications;
~ the passage from ز to ح is below the lower margins [Fig. 9];
~ the passage from ل to م is above the row of indications.

These five exceptions only appear in three copies, M, A and L. The other copyists used a row of the table according to the usual practice in all five cases.

THE VERTICAL ARRANGEMENT OF THE TEXT

There is also another editorial element which particularly isolates M and A from the other copies. The text that does not fit into the narrow space of a cell in the table is arranged vertically, parallel to the frame of the table [Fig. 8]. These are not additions written in the margin but the continuation of the text itself. The procedure is repeated over and over again, and each time the copyist of M uses it, it is also used by the copyist of A, although the latter resorts to it more frequently.

These remarks on criteria emerging from codicology bring out the close relationship between the manuscripts of Madrid and the Arcadian Library. This will no doubt be confirmed by the study of the content of the two copies.

THE INTERPOLATIONS

The study of the Tables leads us to distinguish between three groups of interpolations in the various manuscripts: the ones only to be found in MS N, those common to the manuscripts of Maghrebi origin T, R1, R2, R3, R4 and L, and finally the ones only to be found in M and A.

The interpolations in M and A are sometimes introduced directly in the course of the text (as on M fol. 49a / A p. 95, where the copyist completes a partial quotation of Ibn Masawayh[23] by Ibn Baklarish), or at the end of a cell to add a synonym or a substitute. These additions are usually accompanied by the expression 'from another source' (من غير الأم) and concern the secondary effects of the drugs and their curative properties, as we see in the following example (M fol. 18b / A p. 32):

22. See the article by Jan Just Witkam in this volume (p. 75, n. 1).
23. يشم منه رائحة العود تعلوه صفرة قلية.

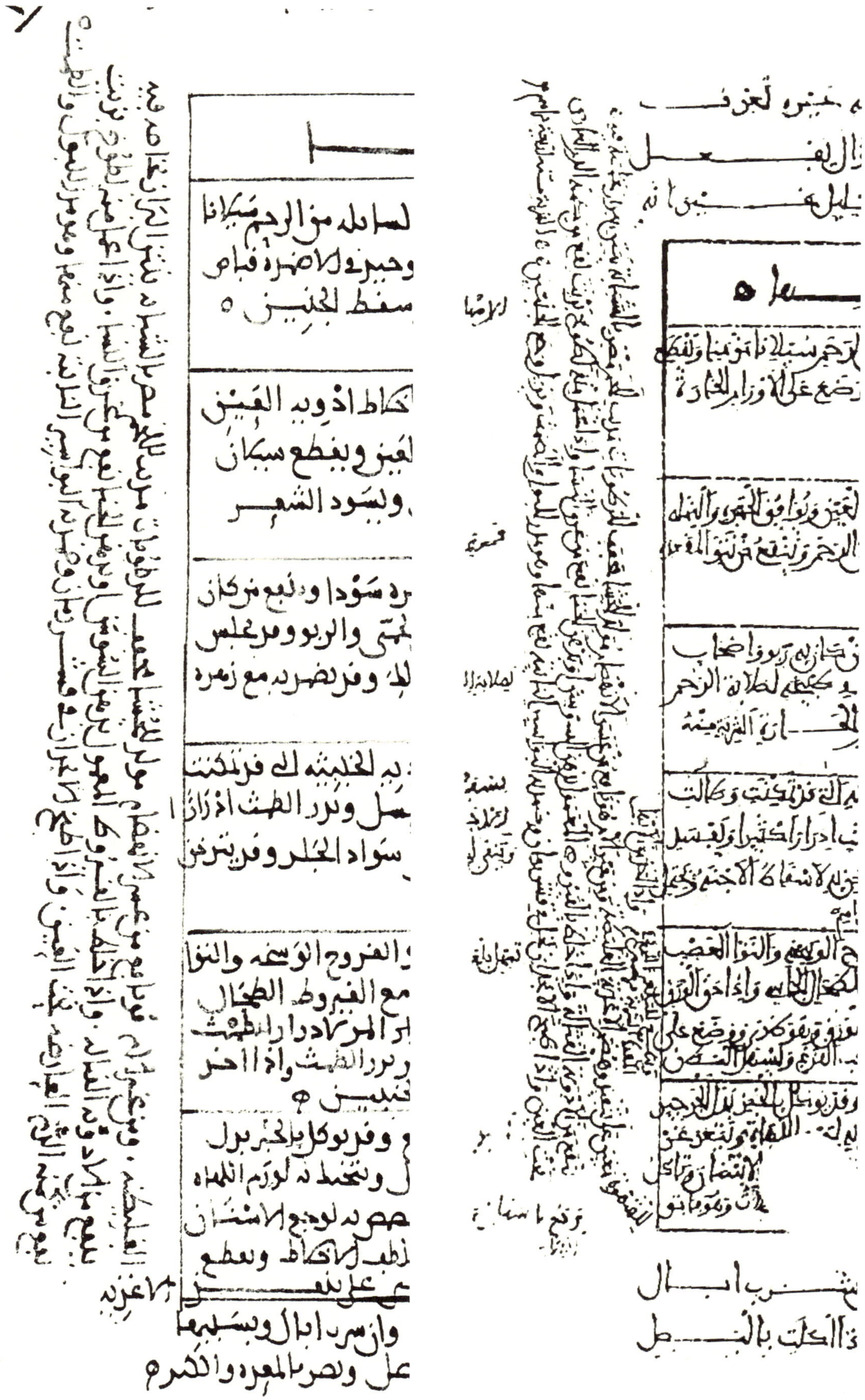

Fig. 8.
Comparison between texts placed vertically in the Arcadian Library manuscript, p. 33, and Madrid, Biblioteca Nacional, MS. ar. 5009, fol. 18a

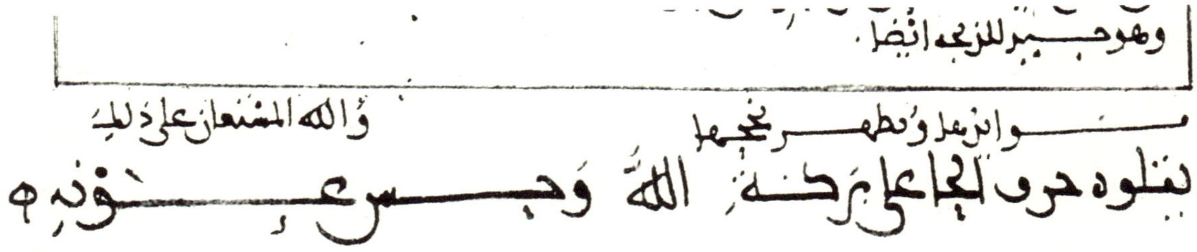

وهو جيد للزنجة أيضا

سوا ابزها وتطهر نجها والله المستعان على ذلك

يتلوه حرف الجاعل بركة الله وحسن عونه

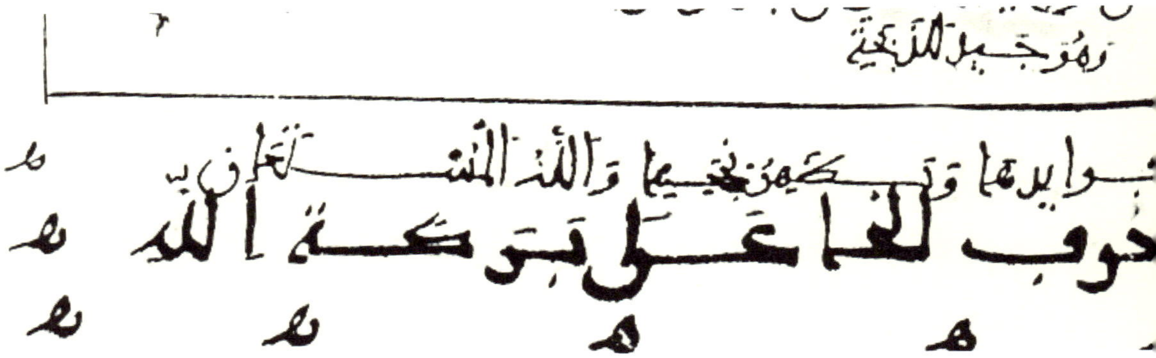

وهو جيد للزنجة

سوا ابزها وتطهير نجها والله المستعان

حروف الجاعل بركة الله

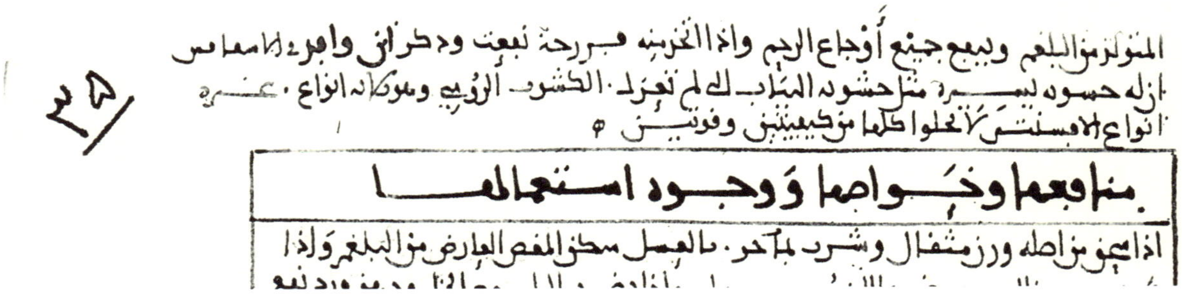

المتولد من البلغم ويبيع جميع أوجاع الرحم وإذا احتملته فرزجة نفعت وذكر ان وافره لا منفعة فيه حسونة ليسيرة مثل حشونة الثياب لكن لم تعرف الكشوث الرومي وهو ثلاثة انواع عشرة انواع الافستين لا تخلوا كلها من كيفيتين وقوتين

منافعها وخواصها ووجوه استعمالها

اذا سحق من اصله ورن مثقال وشرب بماء حار فالعمل سحق المغص العارض من البلغم وإذا

35

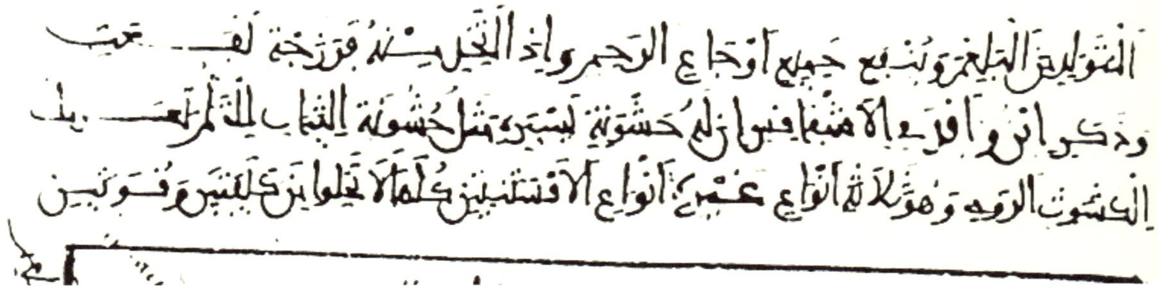

المتولد من البلغم وينبع جميع أوجاع الرحم وإذا احتملته فرزجة نفعت وذكر ان وافرع الا منفعة فيه زالت حشونة يسيرة مثل حشونة الثياب لكن لم تعرف الكشوث الرومي وهو ثلاثة انواع عشرة انواع الافستين كلها لا تخلوا من كيفيتين وقوتين

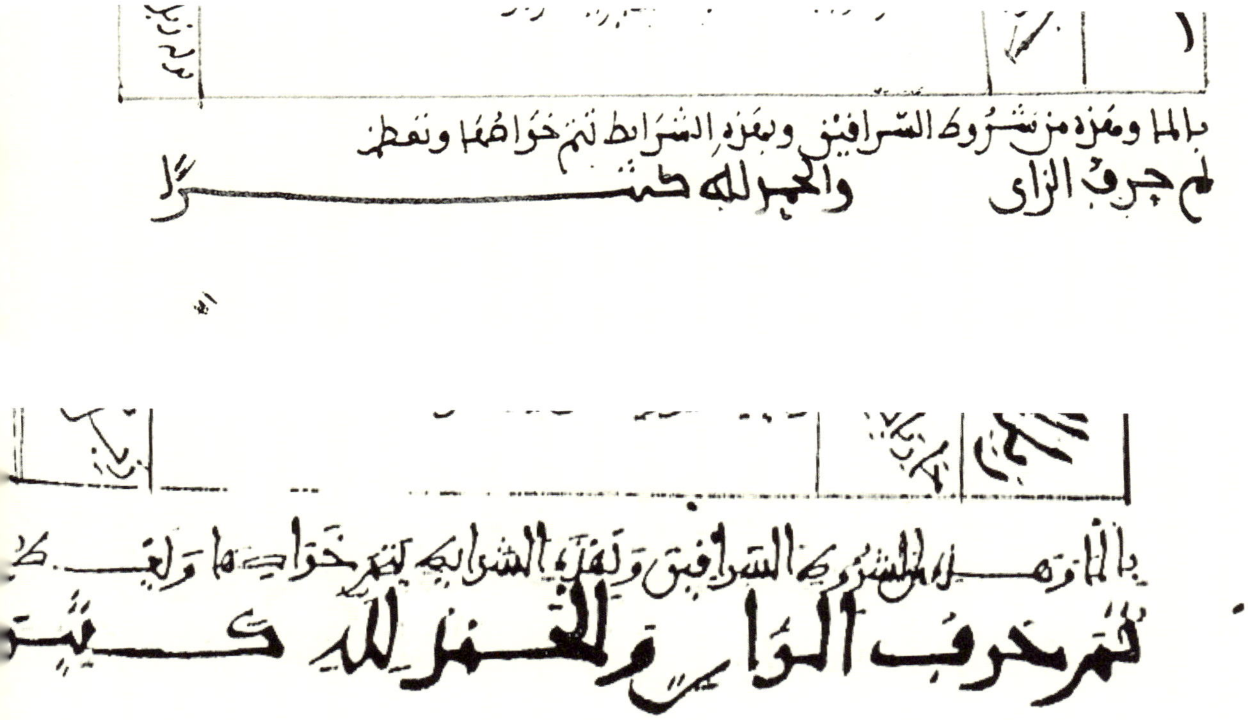

Fig. 9.
Comparison between the passage from *zāy* to *hā'* in the Arcadian Library manuscript, pp. 116–17, and the same passage in Madrid, Biblioteca Nacional, MS ar. 5009, fols. 59b–60a

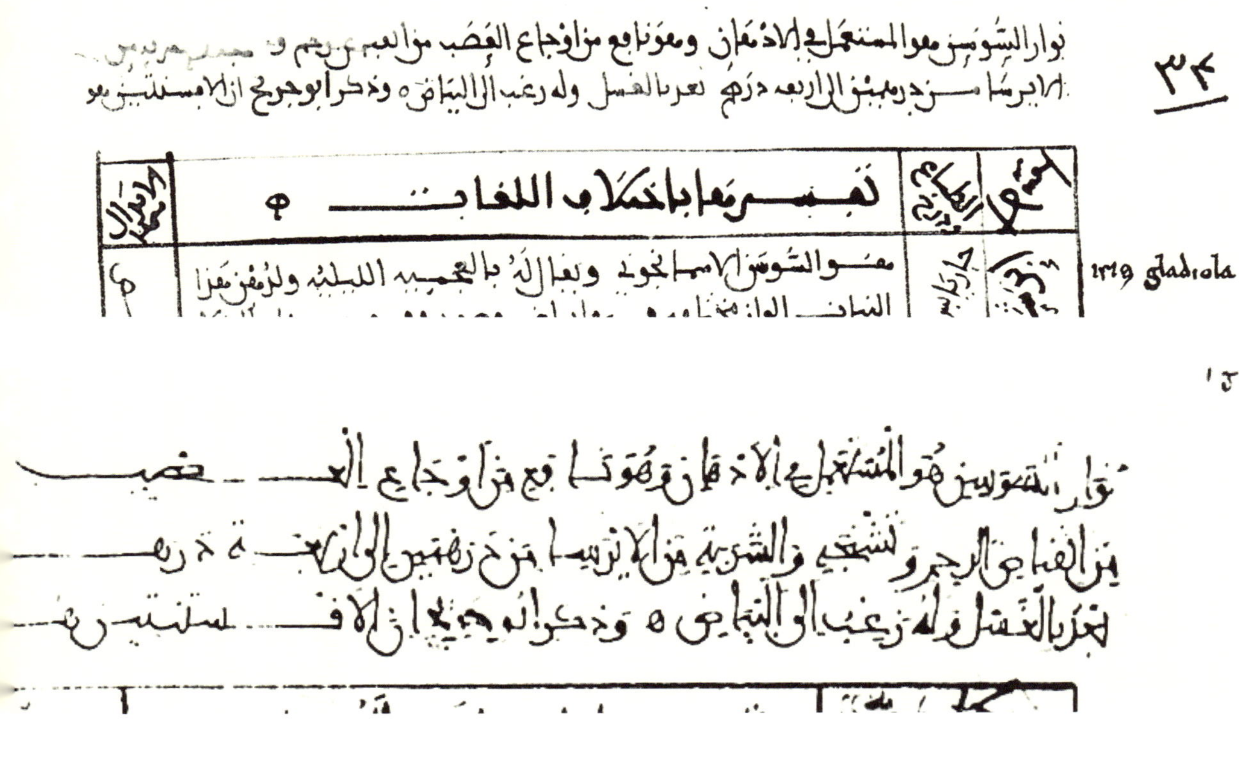

Fig. 10.
Comparison of the sequence of writing in the Arcadian Library manuscript, pp. 34–5 and the same sequence in the Madrid, Biblioteca Nacional, MS ar. 5009, fols. 18b–19a

أبهال: إضراره بالقلب من غير الأم.

Sabina :[24] *from another source, it is bad for the heart.*

This formula (من غير الأم) is missing in all the other manuscripts, with a single exception of the first notice of the Tables on berberis (أميرباريس) to indicate the Berber synonym, which is found in the other MSS as well as in M and A :

أميرباريس: وبالبربرية ارغز من غير الأم

Berbéris : In the Berber language is arghiz, from another source.

There are further elements that accentuate the parallelism between M and A :

~ these interpolations are often drawn up vertically in the margin[25] as we have shown in relation to the continuation of the text from the cells;

~ although they concern the effects of medicinal substances they are often placed under the rubric of the synonyms.[26]

In MS M, however, in contrast to MS A, these interpolations are sometimes completed by an indication of the correct dose (الشربة). [27]

Although these similarities have been established, there are nevertheless some differences between the two manuscripts which will allow us to be more specific about the nature of their connection.

Minor differences can be found in the Introduction. First of all, there are orthographic variants, mainly in the medical terminology, botanical terminology and proper names.[28] In MS M there are also some grammatical mistakes not reproduced in MS A, and *vice versa.*[29] Divergences also appear in the synonyms, particularly in the so-called *ʿajamiyya*, and only a study of these divergences made by specialists in the non-Arabic languages will decide which of the two manuscripts contains the more accurate transmission.

In the Introduction, all the manuscripts contain omissions, varying in quantity and importance, either peculiar to one of them or to a manuscript family. These omissions are rarer and generally identical in MSS M and A.[30] In addition to these shared omissions, however, MS A has omissions of its own. These include the absence of the mention of certain drugs[31] or an interruption in the author's

24. *Juniperus sabina* L.

25. E.g. M fol. 19a /A p. 35 ; M fol. 20a / A p. 37.

26. E.g. M fol. 29b / A p. 56 ; M fol. 32b / A p. 62 ; M fol. 35b / A p. 67 ; M, fol. 37b / A p. 72 ; M fol. 41b / A p. 80.

27. E.g. M fol. 18a / A p. 33 ; M fol. 19a / A p. 35.

28. A few examples : the intestines, M المعي / A المعاء ; the stomach, M المعدة / A المعيدة ; Aristotle, M أرسطاطاليس / A أرسططليس ; black nightshade, M عنب الثلب / A عينب الذيب ; gum of asafoetida, M حلتيت / A حتيت ; great basil, M باذورج / A بادروج.

29. E.g. M السيالة / A السائلة ; M درجة الأولى / A درجة الأول .

30. E.g. in the list of hot substances in the third degree, ginger (زنجبيل) is omitted in the two manuscripts (M fol. 6b / A p. 10).

31. E.g. M fol. 15a / A p. 37 (list of the substances which increase the flesh) : رماد (ash) حلزون (snail).

argument, and range from a single word to several lines.[32] This proves that MS A cannot have been the sole exemplar of MS M, particularly since MS A also includes two references to Galen and to Hippocrates in the Introduction, which are not in any other manuscript (p. 7, lines 12–14 and 15–16). Furthermore, there are lacunae and mistakes in the Tables in MS M, which while not extensive, are absent from MS A.[33]

THE UPPER AND LOWER MARGINS

The most significant comparative element between the two manuscripts is the manner of presentation and the drawing up of the additions to the text above and below the Tables. As Ibn Baklarish puts it: 'At the top and bottom of the table, I have added a complementary paragraph on each simple ... The table should be read from top to bottom; then the upper and lower sections should be read consecutively, as they constitute one inseparable unit.'[34] In the various copies I have seen this manner of presentation is respected irregularly. We should indeed read the first line of the right-hand page, continue with the first line of the left-hand page, return to the second line of the right-hand page, and so on, and then proceed to the part below the table as indicated in Figure 10.

If we compare MS M with MS A, certain features emerge. The text in the upper and lower margins of pp. 32 to 41 of MS A (which correspond to fols. 17b to 22a of MS M), makes no sense. At the end of the line the copyist does not go on to the other page, but regards each page as a unit and fills in the free space at the end of each line with the first words of the line below, as we see from his use of smaller characters [Fig. 10]. From p. 42 onwards, however, obviously realizing his mistake, the scribe restores the correct arrangement. When one compares these pages to the corresponding pages in MS M, one finds that each line of the right-hand and the left-hand pages begins and ends with the same words as that of MS A. The free space at the end of the line remains blank [Fig. 11]. In the Tables, the content of each line of the upper and lower margins is thus always identical in the two manuscripts and the scribe would then extend his writing to fill each line. This comparison shows that MS M cannot have been copied directly from MS A, but that the scribes of both MSS were constrained by the fixed line content of a certain model; and indeed the scribe of M in other places extends his handwriting (43b, 35a, 35b), puts the excess words in the edges of the margins (65a, 83a, 84a), or simply goes beyond the written surface (40a, 76a) in order to keep the right number of words on each double page. We must therefore assume that these two MSS have a common source, whose fixed line content each one preserves in a different way, thus implying a lost intermediary.

THE IMPORTANCE OF THE ARCADIAN LIBRARY MANUSCRIPT

The Arcadian manuscript is complete, the leaves are arranged in the right order (the ones listing of the simple drugs according to their secondary qualities situated after

32. E.g. M fol. 7a / A p. 12:
فوجدت على ما تقدّم لي فيها من القول و هو المأخوذ من تأثيرها و أفعالها في الأبدان المعتدلة
33. E.g. M fol. 16a gives تقى instead of نفتح (A p. 28, l. 8); M fol. 21a طبخ instead of نضج A p. 39 l. 19; M fol. 24a دم الطمث instead of قطع الطمث A p. 47, l. 6.
34. M fol. 4b.

Fig. 11.
Comparison of the contents of lines in the Arcadian Library manuscript, p. 42 and the Madrid, Biblioteca Nacional, MS ar. 5009, fol. 22b

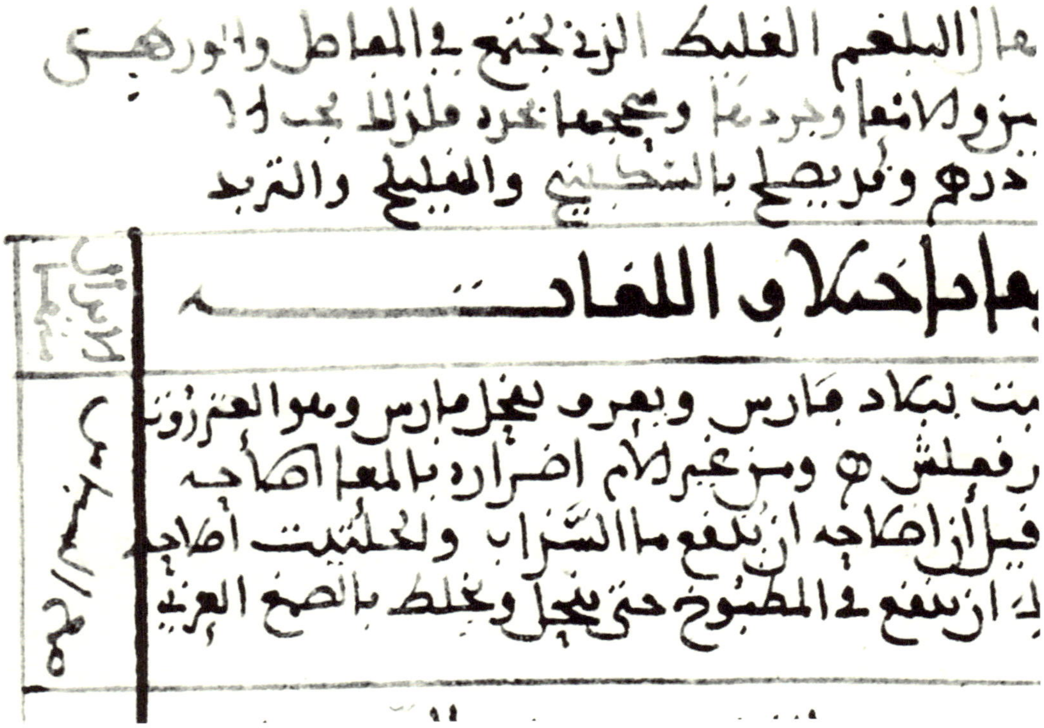

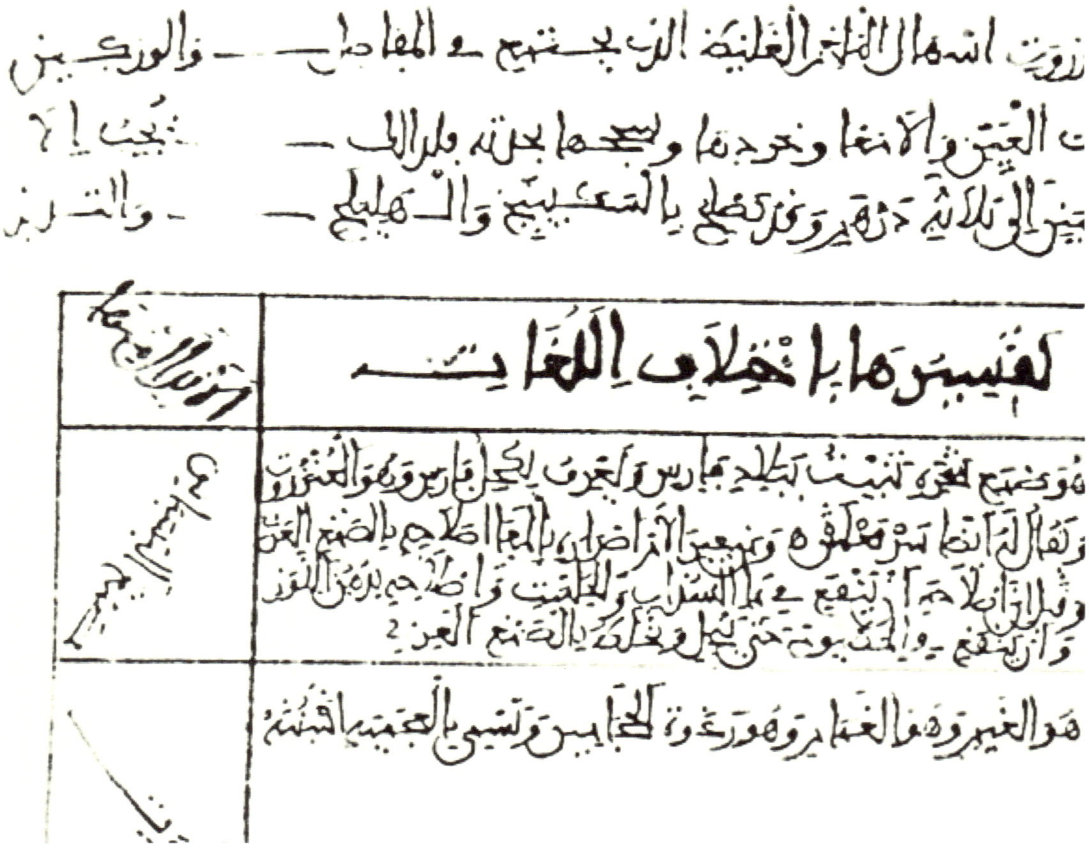

the colophon do not belong to the text),[35] and the handwriting is careful, quite easy to read, and usually furnished with the diacritical points even of the short vowels.

Damp stains have weakened the supports of the leaves of the Introduction, sometimes making it hard to read them. Similarly, the lower part of the last pages is damaged, so that from p. 114 it is increasingly difficult to read the lower margins, and it finally becomes impossible. This obviously limits the usefulness of A, particularly as the basis of an edition, although the damaged part only represents a small proportion of the whole text.

I cannot judge the value of the synonymic contribution represented by MS A; this is a matter for specialists. And yet, if the time and place of transmission influence the reliability of the elements transmitted, we must agree, in the case of this early copy, that it is less subject than later copies to the modernization of vocabulary and introduction of new synonyms and quotations from more recent authors.

The copy is anonymous and the place where it was made is not specified either. The guard leaves bear medical prescriptions in Arabic and perhaps a mark of ownership, too faint to be interpreted. The two handwritings of the marginalia and final pages, in Latin script, show that the manuscript circulated among Christians. Since the two copies M and A were based on the same model and MS M was copied in al-Andalus, where, judging from the mark of ownership of Yahuda Ibn Yaqar, it was still to be found in 1215, it is more than likely that MS A is of Andalusian origin too.

To conclude: the points emerging from this study show that the manuscript tradition of the *Kitāb al-Mustaʿīnī* followed two separate paths: one in al-Andalus, the other in the Maghreb.[36] Since there are no intermediate links it is not possible to go any further in the analysis of this transmission. Thanks to the manuscript bought by the Arcadian Library, we can say that it was in al-Andalus at a very early period, particularly if, as is likely, MS A and MS M are based on the same earlier exemplar. We cannot, however, date the beginning of the diffusion of the text in the Maghreb. MS 1652 of the Qarawiyyin Library might prove that it was present there earlier than the copies at our disposal lead us to believe.

On the other hand it is noteworthy that the 'Tables of simple medicines' of Ibn Baklarish were widely used in Muslim, Jewish and Christian communities and that the work was prized from the twelfth century until the nineteenth century (when it is often referred to in the medical manual *Ḍiyāʾ al-nibrās* compiled by the physician ʿAbd al-Salam al-ʿAlami).[37]

The copy the Arcadian Library has made accessible to scholars must be taken into consideration and play a major role, as a testimony, in any critical edition of the work. There is no doubt, moreover, that, besides its use for an edition, the study of the synonymic forms transmitted by the copyist and of the Latin marginalia will enrich the lexicographical domain.

35. MS A pp. 275–8.
36. The manuscript in Hyderabad could suggest that its diffusion was more extensive than has been thought, but its origin is as yet unknown.
37. ʿAbd al-Salam al-ʿAlami was born in Fez in 1830 and died in 1905. He studied the medicine in Cairo. The complete title of his book of *materia medica* is ضياء النبراس في حل مفردات الأنطاكي بلغة فاس . See: *ʿAbd al-Salām Ibn M. al-ʿĀlamī*, Rabat 1986.

JUAN CARLOS VILLAVERDE AMIEVA

TOWARDS THE STUDY OF THE ROMANCE LANGUAGES IN THE *KITĀB AL-MUSTAʿĪNĪ*

The treatise on simple medicaments entitled *Kitāb al-Mustaʿīnī*, apparently composed in Almeria by the Jew Ibn Baklarish (eleventh–twelfth centuries),[1] is one of the most remarkable works to emerge from the abundant production of repertories on medicine in al-Andalus. It is consequently surprising to find how seldom the author is mentioned in later treatises.[2] This hardly corresponds to the success and diffusion of his work in al-Andalus and the Maghreb, attested by a good dozen surviving manuscript copies, to which we can now add the codex recently acquired by the Arcadian Library in London.

Although Ibn Baklarish has not been entirely neglected by historians of Arabo-Islamic medicine and pharmacology,[3] it is only lately that specialists have drawn attention to the scientific value of his work,[4] and only in our own day that a complete edition and translation of this remarkable treatise has been attempted.[5]

The linguistic interest of the Kitāb al-Mustaʿīnī

The importance of the *Kitāb al-Mustaʿīnī* for medieval Arabic lexicography, on the other hand, has been fully acknowledged ever since the mid-nineteenth century. It was then that Reinhardt Dozy profitably consulted the codices in Leiden and Naples

1. Cf. Ana Labarta, 'El prólogo de *al-Kitāb al-Mustaʿīnī de Ibn Buklāriš* (texto árabe y traducción anotada)' in Juan Vernet (ed.): *Estudios sobre historia de la ciencia árabe*, Barcelona 1980, pp. 181–316, esp. p. 183.
2. If we except a single late mention of Ibn Baklarish (see n. 81 below), I have only found the *Kitāb al-Mustaʿīnī* quoted by the physician ʿAbd al-Ghani b. Abi Sarhan b. Masʿud al-Zamuri in a work which contains a chapter entitled *Sharḥ adwiya bi-l-lisān al-yūnānī wa-l-suriyānī wa-l-fārisī wa-l-ʿajamī wa-ghayr dhālika* ... (MS Rabat, Al-Khizana al-ʿAmma (General Library), D 1363, fols. 186b–200b). This Moroccan physician is the copyist of the manuscript of the *ʿUmdat al-ṭabīb*, completed, for his personal use, in Fez in 1587, and purchased by Gayangos in Morocco in the nineteenth century. It is now in the library of the Real Academia de la Historia in Madrid (cf. M. Asín Palacios, *Glosario de voces romances registradas por un botánico anónimo hispano-musulmán (siglos XI–XII)*, Madrid–Granada 1943, p. xi).
3. The the *Kitāb al-Mustaʿīnī* is included in the list of medical texts 'to be given priority in publication' in 1935, in the project of the *Corpus medicorum arabicorum* of the Académie Internationale d'Histoire des Sciences; cf. Aldo Mieli, *La science arabe et son rôle dans l'évolution scientifique mondiale*, Leiden 1966, p. 282.
4. To the bibliographical references collected in my 'Sobre el estudio del mozárabe en fuentes árabes: a propósito de Ibn Buklāriš' in: *Homenaje a Álvaro Galmés de Fuentes*, III, Madrid and Oviedo 1987, pp. 703–21 (at p. 705) should be added Martin Levey, 'The Pharmacological Table of Ibn Biklarish', *Journal of the History of Medicine*, 26, 1971, pp. 413–21; Albert Dietrich, 'Ibn Buklārish', *Encyclopedia of Islam,* new edition, Suppl., 5–6, pp. 383–4; M. al-ʿArabi al-Khattabi, 'Kitāb al-adwiya al-mufrada al-musammā bi-l-Mustaʿīnī ta'līf Yūnis b. Isḥāq Buklārish', in his book *Al-aghdhiya wa-l-adwiya ʿinda mu'allifī al-gharb al-islāmī. Madkhal wa-nuṣūṣ*, Beirut 1990, pp. 305–35; al-Faruq ʿUmar al-ʿAsli, 'Kitāb al-Mustaʿīnī fi l-ṭibb li-Ibn Buklārish', *Al-Ṣaydalī* (Tunis), 40, 1991, pp. 52–4; 41, 1991, pp. 56–9, 42, 1991, pp. 46–51 and 44, 1992, pp. 49–51; I. Garijo, 'Ibn Buklāriš' in: *Enciclopedia de al-Andalus. Diccionario de autores y obras andalusíes*, I, Granada 2002, pp. 666–7, and, above all, Joëlle Ricordel's doctoral thesis mentioned in the next note.
5. Joëlle Ricordel is the author of a fundamental work: 'Les Tables des medicaments simples d'Isḥāḳ ibn Biklāris͟h. Édition, traduction française et analyse (des lettres alif à zāy), 3 vols., November 2004, Université Paris VII-Denis Diderot' (hereafter *Al-Mustaʿīnī*). I would like to thank Dr Ricordel for supplying me with a copy of her thesis.

for his *Supplément,*[6] and that Francisco Javier Simonet, in his turn, used the Romance material in the work for his own celebrated *Glosario,*[7] in which Ibn Baklarish holds a privileged position.

The *Kitāb al-Mustaʿīnī* consists of an Introduction followed by the repertory of the simple medicaments themselves, ordered alphabetically and arranged synoptically by way of tables (*jadwal*)[8] spread over two pages and divided into five columns. For each medicament we are given: (1) its names (*al-asmāʾ*), (2) its nature and degree (*al-ṭibāʿ wa-l-daraj*), (3) its synonyms in different languages (*tafsīru-hā bi-khtilāf al-lughāt*), (4) its substitutes (*al-abdāl min-hā*), and (5) its uses, properties and modes of employment (*manāfiʿu-hā wa-khawāṣṣu-hā wa-wujūh istiʿmāli-hā*).

Apart from this formal presentation, the author himself informs us in his Introduction of the compilatory nature of his work ('what I have quoted, taken, united and presented'). He emphasizes the synthetic character of his method ('to unite what is separated, to sum up what is prolix, and to elucidate difficulties'), and does not hesitate to boast of the result: 'My work has these three qualities and I have never found in any other earlier book on simple medicaments what I have united in mine.'[9] In accordance with this compilatory purpose, one of the author's objectives was to assemble synonyms to which, as we saw, he devoted the third column of the *jadwal*. This is what he says in his Introduction: 'For each medicament I have reunited all the names I have found dispersed in numerous books,' and he justifies the compilation:

because I have seen that it was necessary on account of the perplexity in people's minds when faced by an unknown work which, moreover, may have been composed negligently by an author ignorant of the particular substance he was writing about.

First, however, he specified the various languages from which the synonyms included in the work are taken: 'I have given the names [of each medicament], both foreign and current in the various languages—Syriac, Persian, *yūnāniyya* [classical Greek], Arabic, *rūmiyya* [Byzantine Greek] and popular *ʿajamiyya*.'[10]

This last term refers to the Romance language of al-Andalus, for the knowledge of which these treatises on simple medicaments are the principal sources.[11] Indeed, in the absence of texts or testimonies closer to the Romance-Andalusi linguistic

6. Reinhardt P. Dozy, *Supplément aux dictionnaires arabes*, 2 vols., Leiden 1881. We read in an autograph note at the end of the Leiden manuscript that Dozy managed to borrow the Neapolitan codex for some time thanks to the mediation of Michele Amari.

7. Francisco Javier Simonet, *Glosario de voces ibéricas y latinas usadas entre los mozárabes*, Madrid 1888 (with various reissues in facsimile: Amsterdam, 1967; in smaller format, Beirut 1975, and in 2 vols. Madrid, 1981). Simonet examined the codex of the Biblioteca Nacional of Madrid, which he describes as 'toledano' because of its provenance, and he also used excerpts from the manuscripts in Leiden and Naples which he obtained from Dozy.

8. See a detailed discussion of the *jadwal* as a genre in the presentation of medical texts, and, above all, of the tables of the *Mustaʿīnī*, in Ricordel, *Al-Mustaʿīnī*, I, pp. 136–69.

9. From the Spanish translation by Labarta, 'El prólogo', p. 189.

10. From the Spanish translation by Labarta, 'El prólogo', p. 190. Besides these linguistic varieties the author occasionally also includes terms in other languages, including Coptic, Nabataean, Hebrew, etc. It is odd that there should be no specific mention of Berber, since the work contains almost thirty words in that language which have been studied by Henri P. J. Renaud, 'Trois études d'histoire de la médicine arabe en Occident: I. Le Mustaʿīnī d'Ibn Beklareš', *Hespéris*, 10, 1930, pp. 143–6. There are also a few Latin terms to which we shall return later.

reality, the words of the *ʿajamiyya* collected in these medical texts provide the most immediate and direct information available. Among them Ibn Baklarish's pharmacopoeia has held a place of distinction ever since Simonet drew attention to it in this connection. Around 200 lexical attestations of the *ʿajamiyya* which he collected from the three manuscripts then known, and which he recorded in his *Glosario* under the heading 'nombres españoles', justified Ibn Baklarish's primacy[12] among the Andalusi writers.[13]

After the publication of Simonet's work the Romance attestations of the *Kitāb al-Mustaʿīnī* were exploited exhaustively by Hispanists. We see this above all in the two most influential works on the linguistic history of the Ibero-Romance domain: the *Orígenes del español* by Menéndez Pidal[14] and the *Diccionario etimológico* by Corominas,[15] in the pages of which the name of Ibn Baklarish appears repeatedly.

The work of Simonet contains much valuable, albeit methodologically superseded, information, but it lacks the critical perspective necessary for the utilization of the Andalusi pharmacological sources, and, most particularly, of Ibn Baklarish. Its limitations and lacunae have led to a distorted perception and often to an erroneous appreciation of the material assembled. The aforementioned works by Menéndez Pidal and Corominas are consequently full of incorrect interpretations, and, in their wake, the same absurdities have been repeated by nearly all those scholars who, in

11. For the traditional classification of the sources of the Romance language of al-Andalus commonly accepted by Romanists, see Álvaro Galmés de Fuentes, *Dialectología mozárabe*, Madrid 1983, pp. 17–25, and my own reservations about this typology in a review article in *Aljamía*, 9, 1997, pp. 143–4.

12. Today this quantitative primacy of Ibn Baklarish seems less obvious. We have only to think of over 700 Romance terms used by the so-called 'anónimo sevillano', regarded as by far the most copious source for the study of Andalusi Romance ever since Asín Palacios made known an extract from it (in the *Glosario de voces romances*, n. 2 above). The work was published by M. al-ʿArabi al-Khattabi who attributed its authorship to the Sevillian agronomist Abu l-Khayr (*ʿUmdat al-ṭabīb fī maʿrifat al-nabāt li-Abī l-Khayr al-Ishbīlī*, 2 vols., Rabat 1990; new edition, Beirut 1995). The edition of al-Khattabi's Arabic text has been superseded by the more recent one edited by J. Bustamante, F. Corriente and M. Tilmatine: Abul̲hayr Al'išbīlī, *Kitābu ʿumdati ṭṭabīb fī maʿrifati nnabāt likulli labīb (Libro base del médico para el conocimiento de la botánica por todo experto)*, I, Madrid 2004. Federico Corriente, in his turn, recently provided a revision and re-examination of the Romance words in the work: 'El romandalusí reflejado por el glosario botánico de Abulxayr', *Estudios de dialectología norteafricana y andalusí*, 5, 2001, pp. 93–241.

13. The list of the botanical-pharmacological works relevant to the *ʿajamiyya* of al-Andalus is far longer than the one provided in his own day by Simonet. Some time ago, in order to enlarge the research project needed to apply for the lectureship in Arabic at the University of Oviedo (October 1991), I drew up a detailed catalogue of authors and works—Andalusi, but at the same time Maghribi and even Oriental (with an indication of the whereabouts of the manuscripts)—which exceeded thirty entries. The updating of the project has allowed us to increase this number considerably. The catalogue, albeit unpublished, is not altogether unknown, and has been used by certain colleagues such as Álvaro Galmés de Fuentes (*Las jarchas mozárabes. Forma y significado*, Barcelona 1994, pp. 87–8) and, above all, by Hans-Josef Niederehe in his *Bibliografía cronológica de la lingüística, la gramática y la lexicografía del español desde los comienzos hasta el año 1600*, Amsterdam–Philadelphia 1995. All but two of the first 27 entries of his work are taken from the catalogue in question (see J. C. Busto's review of Niederehe's work in *Aljamía*, 12, 2000, pp. 210–12).

14. Ramón Menéndez Pidal, *Orígenes del español. Estudio lingüístico de la Península Ibérica hasta el siglo XI*, 3rd edition, Madrid 1950 (1st edition, 1926).

15. Juan Corominas, *Diccionario crítico-etimológico de la lengua castellana*, 4 vols., Madrid–Berne 1958; also the 2nd edition, *Diccionario etimológico castellano e hispánico*, 6 vols., Madrid 1980–91 (hereafter *DCECH*); as well as Joan Coromines, *Diccionari etimològic i complementari de la llengua catalana*, 9 vols., Barcelona 1983–91 (hereafter *DECLlC*). Corominas quotes Ibn Baklarish systematically in his Castilian dictionary as an Aragonese author, and goes even further in his *Diccionari* where he actually refers to him as 'catalano-aragonès' (IX, p. 275 *a*).

one way or another, have studied Andalusi Romance.

We have only to recall the erroneous premise—a veritable topos amongst these scholars—that Ibn Baklarish came from Saragossa and that the Romance attestations in the *Kitāb al-Musta'īnī* were thus of Saragossan Mozarabic—something which is very far from being certain. I need only refer to what I said elsewhere, when I drew attention to certain critical requirements essential to the study of the Romance words in Ibn Baklarish, and above all to the necessary contextualization of the work if we are to provide a correct assessment of its attestations.

We must never forget, for example, the question of the sources used by authors like Ibn Baklarish, so important for determining the origin, transmission and value of the attestations of the *'ajamiyya* in their works.[16] As Ana Labarta writes, it is clear that the *Musta'īnī* is a pure product of book learning. Ibn Baklarish never mentions his travels, observations, or experiences, but simply compiles quotations from an extremely large number of different authors, Greek as well as Arab, and eastern as well as western.[17]

Labarta's words acquire a special significance when applied to the numerous synonyms of simple medicaments collected by the author, and above all to those of the *'ajamiyya* of al-Andalus. Ibn Baklarish does indeed cite a number of his Andalusi predecessors. These are the Cordovan Ibn Juljul (d. *c.* 994),[18] the Jew from Lucena Ibn Janah (d. *c.* 1040 in Saragossa),[19] the Toledan Ibn Wafid (d. 1067)[20] and, above all, the Cordovan al-Zahrawi (d. *c.* 1010).[21] It was from them that Ibn Baklarish derived, directly or indirectly, the words of the *'ajamiyya* of al-Andalus which appear in his work[22]—above all from al-Zahrawi, to whom he seems to owe far more than the good thirty quotations in the *Kitāb al-Musta'īnī*. The coincidences between the two are striking, as I will point out in due course.

This dependency of Ibn Baklarish on earlier authors allows us to draw certain pro-

16. See Carmen Barceló, 'Romance Lexicon in Pharmacological Treatises Written in Muslim Spain: its Origin and Transmission', *Journal for the History of Arabic Science*, 12, 2001, pp. 111–30, and also 'Mozárabes de Valencia y "lengua mozárabe"', *Revista de Filología Española*, 77, 1997, pp. 253–79.

17. See Ana Labarta, 'La farmacología de Ibn Buklāriš: sus fuentes' in: *Actas del IV Coloquio Hispano-Tunecino (Palma de Mallorca, 1979)*, Madrid 1983, p. 164, and p. 23 above. On Ibn Baklarish's sources see also Ricordel, *Al-Musta'īnī*, I, pp. 30–49.

18. Ibn Baklarish was to use this author's *Tafsīr asmā' al-adwiya min kitāb Diyusqūrīdūs*, ed. and transl. Ildefonso Garijo, Córdoba 1992, and, presumably, another lost work of his, the *Kitāb al-nabāt*, quoted with this title by al-Idrisi (1100–66), as one of the sources of his compilation of simple medicaments. It is from this work by Ibn Juljul that many of the passages in his name are taken which appear in later authors such as Ibn al-Baytar (d. 1248) and, of course, Ibn Samajun (tenth–eleventh century).

19. He used Ibn Janah's *Kitāb al-talkhīṣ*, which has since been lost. It contained explanations of the names of the medicaments.

20. He undoubtedly used his *Kitāb al-adwiya al-mufrada*, ed. and Spanish trans. Luisa Fernanda Aguirre de Cárcer, 2 vols., Madrid 1995. For the importance of this work for Andalusi Romance and, above all, for its translations into Latin, Hebrew and various Romance languages, see my review in *Aljamía*, 9, 1997, pp. 111–18, where I identified it as the Arabic original of the influential *Liber aggregatus in medicinis simplicibus*, translated by Abraham of Tortosa and Simon of Genoa and wrongly attributed to Serapion.

21. For synonyms, and above all for those of the *'ajamiyya* of al-Andalus, Ibn Baklarish used the first chapter of the *maqāla* XXIX of al-Zahrawi's *Kitāb al-taṣrīf*, of the title of which (*Tasmiyat al-'aqāqīr bi-khtilāf al-lughāt*) there seems to be an echo in the epigraph taken by Ibn Baklarish for the table of synonyms.

22. See my study 'Sobre el estudio del mozárabe', pp. 714ff. Besides the authors mentioned above I included another one who is also quoted in the *Kitāb al-Musta'īnī*, Ibn al-Jazzar (d. 1004) from Qayrawan, thus making the same mistake as Simonet, who had been led by Dozy (*Glosario*, pp. CXLII–CXLIII) to regard the Tunisian

visional conclusions, to establish the author's place with respect to his sources as a whole, and at the same time to give a finer nuance to the testimonial value of his Romance material hitherto unanimously regarded as evidence of a contemporary linguistic reality.

But apart from such observations, which might seem to restrict the importance of the work of Ibn Baklarish, the *Kitāb al-Mustaʿīnī* has an extraordinary added value on account of the variant readings which the terms of the *ʿajamiyya* present in some of the surviving codices. Even if this textual variation has been known ever since Simonet, one of the weak points in the interpretation of the work, as we shall see, is not to have taken into sufficient account the origin and the date of these variants, resulting from the intervention of copyists (and of eventual readers and users) of the different manuscripts, and above all to have overlooked the linguistic attribution of the novel readings.

The differences between the Romance words in the manuscripts of Madrid, Naples and Leiden were brought to light by Simonet, as we see in his *Glosario*. Menéndez Pidal too drew attention to the range of these textual variations which —contrary to what has sometimes been claimed—can on no account be reduced to mere dialectal variants of Andalusi Romance.[23] But Simonet's inadequate transcriptions, erroneous interpretations, and, above all, defective presentation of the material—the neglect of relevant aspects such as the indication of the manuscript in question—would frequently mislead students of the material and give rise to striking absurdities, particularly in the linguistic attribution of the words. Insufficient account was taken of the fact that the variants were merely the work of copyists of a later date, and could never be imputed to the original text of Ibn Baklarish.

Furthermore, we now know many things which were unknown in Simonet's day. We are better placed to contextualize the linguistic testimonies of the *Kitāb al-Mustaʿīnī* adequately, and, more important still, we have a far larger range of manuscripts at our disposal than the three known in the nineteenth century.

The Manuscripts of the Kitāb al-Mustaʿīnī

Let us now turn to the manuscripts. I shall here give a succinct description of them, drawing attention to certain data of interest to our subject and overlooking others which are less relevant.[24]

The known manuscripts of the *Kitāb al-Mustaʿīnī* are the following:

~ A. Manuscript of the Arcadian Library in London, dated 524 A.H. / 1130 A.D. It

writer as the author of two fragments contained in MS ar. 887 in the Escorial. This attribution, however, was already questioned in the catalogue by Derenbourg and Renaud (*Les manuscrits arabes de l'Escurial*, Paris 1941, II, fasc. 2, p. 99), and was corrected by me in the catalogue of sources for the Romance language in al-Andalus (n. 13 above), where I took the opportunity to include these two fragments of unknown authorship.

23. See my study 'Sobre el estudio del mozárabe', pp. 714ff. We shall return to the matter in greater detail later.

24. For a detailed description of the manuscripts see Ricordel, *Al-Mustaʿīnī*, II, pp. 185–205.

contains certain Latin annotations in a hand which, together with other circumstances of its composition, suggest that it could have been made in the Crown of Castile, perhaps in Toledo.[25] It is the earliest of the surviving copies, made within a few decades of the original.

~ M. MS ar. 5009 of the Biblioteca Nacional in Madrid. The frequent annotations show that the codex passed through various hands and, although it is undated, we know that one of its owners was Yahuda Ibn Yaqar (fl. 1215 in Barcelona).[26]

~ C. A manuscript copied in Córdoba 663 A.H. / 1265 A.D., which has not survived but from which the Naples manuscript was made. We know of its existence and date from the colophon.

~ Q. MS 1652 of the Library of the Qarawiyyin Mosque in Fez (Morocco), in two volumes, badly damaged, apparently undated but probably attributable to the medieval period (*c.* fourteenth century).[27]

~ La. The ancient part of Cod. Or. 15 of Leiden University Library, acquired by the Dutch Arabist Jacobus Golius during his diplomatic mission in Morocco (1622–4). Although it is not dated, the copy is medieval. For our purpose this early part of the manuscript must be separated from the modern part which completes it and will be discussed below.

~ N. MS III-F-65 of the Biblioteca Nazionale in Naples, a copy completed in Almería in 888 A.H. /1482 A.D. and taken from the above-mentioned Cordovan manuscript.

~ R1. MS D 2960 of the Khizana al-ʿAmma (General Library) of Rabat, dated 995 A.H. / 1586 A.D.

~ D. MS Ar. 4506 of the Chester Beatty Library, Dublin, copied in maghribi script, not dated, but attributable to the sixteenth century.[28]

~ Lm. The modern part of Cod. Or. 15 of Leiden University Library, made in about 1624, in the hand of the Morisco Ahmad b. Qasim al-Hajari al-Andalusi (alias Bejarano) to complete the defective, damaged, or non-existent passages in Ms La and intended for the Dutch orientalist Jacobus Golius.[29]

~ H. MS 763 in the Ḥasaniyya Library in the Royal Palace of Rabat, dated 1203 A.H. / 1788–9 A.D.

25. We shall return to this later.

26. Pieter Sjoerd van Koningsveld, 'Andalusian-Arabic Manuscripts from Christian Spain: a Comparative Intercultural Approach', *Israel Oriental Studies*, 12, 1992, pp. 75–110 (see p. 101).

27. According to Van Koningsveld, ibid. I have not been able to consult this manuscript.

28. A. J. Arberry (*The Chester Beatty Library. A Handlist of the Arabic Manuscripts*, VI, Dublin, 1963) describes the manuscript succinctly: '153 folios, 27.3 x 18.6 cm., clear scholar's maghribi script, undated, but 10/16th century' (I am grateful to Dr Elaine Wright, Curator of the Islam collections of the Chester Beatty Library, for her care in finding for me the correct number of the manuscript and for sending me a copy of the catalogue entry). I have not been able to examine this manuscript, to which I found a reference only after this article had already been written.

29. The identification of al-Hajari as the author of the modern part of this manuscript is due to Gerard Wiegers (*A learned Muslim Acquaintance of Erpenius and Golius: Aḥmad b. Ḳāsim al-Andalusī and Arabic Studies in The Netherlands*, Leiden 1988, pp. 64–8), to which I had already drawn attention (see my review article in *Aljamía*, 3, 1990, pp. 62–3). New information about the relations between the Morisco Ahmad ben Qasim and Jacobus Golius, with interesting new material about the Leiden manuscript, is provided by Jan Just Witkam in this volume (pp. 75–94), whom I thank for having allowed me to consult his original contribution. We now know that al-Hajari used two manuscripts (to which I shall refer as Y and Y′) in preparing the copy intended for Golius.

~ T. MS 3575 of the National Library in Tunis, an undated copy acquired in 1963 by the bookseller al-ʿAsli, whose family subsequently presented it to the Tunisian library.
~ R2. MS D 55 at the Khizana al-ʿAmma (General Library) in Rabat, copied in 1309 A.H. / 1891 A.D.
~ R3. MS D 2976 at the Khizana al-ʿAmma (General Library) in Rabat, undated and closely related to the previous entry.[30]

Besides these complete copies there are two other fragmentary manuscripts which are irrelevant to our purpose: MS ebreo 530/1 in the Vatican Library, written in Arabic in Hebrew characters, of Andalusi or Maghribi origin, and dating from the fourteenth century, which contains a part of the Introduction of the work;[31] and MS 589 of the Mauritanian Institute of Scientific Research in Nouackchott (Mauritania),[32] which only contains the Introduction. Mention has also been made of another manuscript of the *Kitāb al-Mustaʿīnī* in the Salar Jang Library in Hyderabad (India), the existence of which has not been confirmed.[33]

What we know about the various manuscripts provides us with some evidence, and a selective collation, limited almost exclusively to the Romance attestations, has allowed me to establish significant relationships between the different codices. This will ultimately enable me to contextualize the linguistic attestations of the work in the double perspective which interests us here: on the one hand to determine the words of the *ʿajamiyya* of al-Andalus indeed included by Ibn Baklarish in his work; and on the other, by way of the temporal intervals between the manuscripts and their additions and modifications, to establish the date of the new attestations, to localize their various geographical origins and to identify the linguistic attribution of the new Romance words with which copyists and annotators, over nearly 800 years, in al-Andalus, in Christian Spain and in the Maghreb, continued to enrich the textual transmission of the *Kitāb al-Mustaʿīnī*.

Collations of the known manuscripts[34] do not exhaust all the possibilities of comparison. Nevertheless, partial and selective though they may be, such collations suffice to bring us closer to our specific objective of studying the Romance words.

Let us now look at the relationships I have established between the manuscripts, which I shall illustrate with concrete examples when dealing with the variant readings in the *ʿajamiyya*. In the first place there can be no doubt that the London manuscript in the Arcadian Library (A), the earliest to survive (1130), is closely related to the Madrid manuscript (M), which can be dated as early as the twelfth century, but of which we only know the date *ante quem*. Together they both represent the version of the work closest to the original, where both the date and the

30. According to Ricordel, *Al-Mustaʿīnī*, I, pp. 191–2. I have not consulted this manuscript myself. My references to it are indirect and are taken from Ricordel's thesis, especially from the variants included in the critical apparatus of her edition.
31. Identified by Y. Tzvi Langermann, *The Jews and the Sciences in the Middle Ages*, Aldershot 1999, article I, addition at p. 54.
32. The Biblioteca Islámica Félix Pareja (Madrid) has a microfiche copy of this manuscript.
33. Cited in 'Corpus Medicorum Arabico-Hispanorum', *Awrāq*, 4, 1981, p. 87.
34. With the exception of Q, D and, in part, R3 which, as I have said, I have not been able to consult.

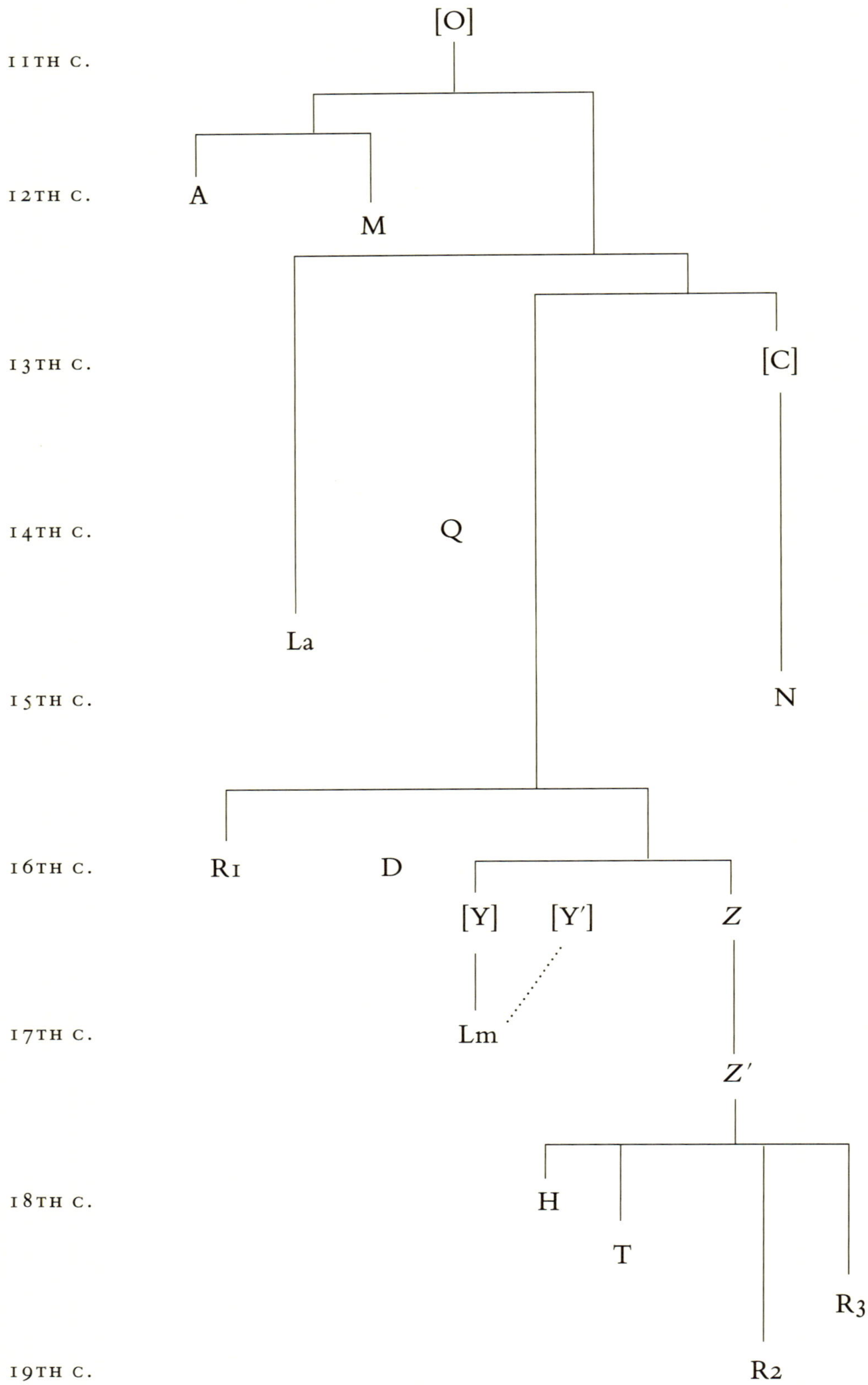

Fig. 12.
Proposal for a *stemma codicum* of the *Kitāb al-Mustaʿīnī* showing the relationships between the manuscripts according to their Romance testimonies (Note: In this *stemma*, R1 = Ricordel's R2, R2 = R4 and R3 = R1; see above, p. 33)

correction of the text are concerned. On the other hand the two share certain peculiarities and additions which demonstrate a close relationship. The peculiarities of each assure us that M cannot be a copy of A, while it also seems certain that none of the other known manuscripts descends from either of them.[35]

These circumstances lead me to postulate another branch close to the original from which La and the manuscript copied in Córdoba (C)—represented by the copy in Naples (N)—can be said to descend, since they both have certain common additions lacking in A and M. We also know that none of the manuscripts examined descend either from La or from N, while I have been able to establish that certain readings of N appear in all the Moroccan codices. This, together with the fact that La has certain characteristics lacking in N, but which do indeed appear to be incorporated in all the Moroccan manuscripts, implies a relationship between all the North African codices which would go back to a state earlier than N, supposedly related to C and implicitly to La.

Since I have been unable to examine MS Q, it obviously remains on the margin of my considerations, even if the antiquity attributed to it (*c.* fourteenth century), suggests that it might be of importance for establishing the connection between the Andalusi and the Maghrebi manuscripts. I shall simply situate it among the other manuscripts produced at the time in accordance with the dating given by Van Koningsveld, but without linking it to any other codex.

The Maghribi codices, in their turn, obviously belong to two groups, one represented by R1, close to the text circulated in the Iberian Peninsula, while all the others depend on a different branch which contains, among other interpolations, certain additions with information about al-Andalus, and particularly about Granada and its language.[36] This second group also consists of two branches: one represented by the manuscript Y (and implicitly by Y′), indicated respectively as the two manuscripts with which al-Hajari prepared Lm, and another, which I shall call *Z* (with a possible later phase, *Z′*) , from which descend H, T, R2 and R3. And even where these last four manuscripts are concerned certain connections could be established, of which I have given few details since they are of little relevance to my objective. T seems closer to H while R2 and R3 would seem to be very similar.[37] In the case of D, which has not been consulted, but which is certainly Maghribi, I have limited myself to placing it in its chronological context, without associating it with other manuscripts.

In view of all this, we can represent the relationship between the manuscripts in a *stemma codicum* [Fig. 12], keeping in mind that the exhaustive collation of the codices, not limited solely to the Romance material, would allow us to attain a greater accuracy in our judgement and a subtler vision of the ramifications of the derivations proposed here, and provide ever more details for the establishment of archetypes and subarchetypes. As I have observed, my only objective is to constitute connections and

35. See the detailed analysis by Joëlle Ricordel in this volume (pp. 27–41). I am very grateful to her for allowing me to see a copy of her article before publication, which informed me of the existence of the manuscript of the Chester Beatty Library (D).

36. See n. 79 below.

37. According to Ricordel (*Al-Mustaʿīnī*, I, p. 200) there are considerable correspondences between these two manuscripts, even in the marginal notes.

filiations between a number of codices sufficient for our exclusive objective of tracing attestations of the words in the *ʿajamiyya* with which the manuscript tradition of the *Kitāb al-Mustaʿīnī* has enriched itself. Nevertheless, I suspect that a detailed collation between the manuscripts not restricted to the concrete aspects prescribed by my own objective, would not modify, in general lines, the scheme I shall now set out.

The ʿAjamiyya of al-Andalus

Having presented the manuscripts and established the relationships between them, we must now examine the Romance material in the work. If we concentrate, in the first place, on the words of Andalusi Romance which Ibn Baklarish included in his treatise, we must immediately admit that the manuscript in the Arcadian Library is the best, not only because of its antiquity and its proximity to the original, but also because it generally furnishes us with the best readings.

Far from giving a detailed presentation of all the material of the *ʿajamiyya* of al-Andalus—something which I shall do elsewhere—I shall here limit myself to offering a few indications in order to determine the original readings of the work, bringing out, as I do so, the importance of the London manuscript, in which, after a rapid analysis, I have encountered certain novelties of the utmost interest.

The London manuscript often gives the words in the *ʿajamiyya* of al-Andalus either fully or adequately vocalized, and this facilitates their interpretation. Let us take some examples: فِيقُش [fīqush] (s.v. *tīn*), فُنْقُش [funqush] (s.v. *fuṭr*), ليتُوقَش [l·ytūqash] (s.v. *khass bustānī*), الليليُه [l·yl·ʸuʰ] (s.v. *ʾīrsā*[38]), مَالبَش [mālbash] (s.v. *khubbāzī*), and رُوطَه [rūṭaʰ] (s.v. *sadhab*), which we must interpret as *fíqos*, *fónqos*, *laytúqas*, *lílio*, *málbas* and *rúṭa* respectively.[39]

MS A thus comes to occupy a pre-eminent position which, from the point of view of this study, was previously occupied by the Madrid manuscript (M). The Madrid codex, which lacks a few folios, has some lacunae. It fails, for example, to attribute certain words to the *ʿajamiyya*, and, on occasion, it provides clearly erroneous readings. In the Andalusi-Romance expression *rábano gallisko*, which Ibn Baklarish gives in a quotation from Ibn Juljul, it thus offers بابنه [b·ʾb·n·ʰ] (s.v. *hazār*

38. MS ابرشا corrected by another hand to ايرسا.

39. This is not the place to give a detailed presentation either of the systems used in al-Andalus for representing Romance words in Arabic characters, or of the transliteration used by modern scholars. We limit ourselves to transcribing the Arabic text of the manuscripts, adding in square brackets transcriptions in Latin script, thus reflecting the principles of the system adopted by Andalusi authors (e.g., to represent the diphthongs, the final vowels, the accents etc.); we indicate the vocalization with raised points when it is not explicitly indicated. We have added in italics our proposals for the reading of the words, supplying the vowels that have not been specificied in the manuscripts and taking for granted certain accepted norms, such as the representation of Romance 's' with *shīn* and the mute palatal affricate (here transcribed as č) with *jīm* with *tashdīd*. Again we omit giving details in other cases, such as the phonetic value of Arabic velarized consonants in Romance words, which we transcribe as such. Note that we use the *hamza* sign (ʾ) to indicate an *alif* when it is a *mater lectionis* and the *fatḥa* is not expressly indicated. I have decided to omit repeated indications of the folio of the manuscript containing the words discussed. I shall simply quote the word under the entry of which the terms appear in the *ʿajamiyya* in the *Kitāb al-Mustaʿīnī*, generally in the table of synonyms. This will enable me to refer to various manuscripts indiscriminately and simultaneously.

jusān[40]) rather than the correct form رابنه [r·'b·n·^{h}], i.e. *rábano*, which we find in MS A. On other occasions, however, M provides better readings than A, above all in the correct notation of those diacritical points missing in some of the consonants in A.

In order to establish the original text we will take A as the base manuscript, with the assistance of M, but without forgetting the other ancient manuscripts (La, N), which occasionally give better readings than the two earliest ones. Thus, to give a single example, we find in La and N the reading بنجّاين [b·njj·'y·n] (s.v. *jāwars*) for the Andalusi-Romance word *pančáyin*, rather than the erroneous بلجاين [b·lj·'yin] given in both A and M.

Nor should we dismiss the contribution of later manuscripts in order to establish the original text, even where unequivocal readings in A are concerned. The following case is illustrative and reminds us of the caution that must be observed in choosing readings from the different manuscripts in order to establish the original forms of the *Kitāb al-Musta'īnī*. Under the entry *lisān al-'aṣāfīr* (describing the fruit of the ash-tree) the manuscripts give the following variants of the word in the *'ajamiyya*:

M	La	N	R1	HTR2
فراشته	فراشبه	فراشنة	فراشنه	فراشته

Judging from these forms it seems evident that R_{I} provides the best reading of the Andalusi-Romance word *frésno* [f·r·'shn·^{h}], which Ibn Baklarish originally included in the work and which, with varying fortunes, has been transmitted (and confirmed) by the majority of the codices. But, in contrast to this reading, MS A gives the form فرَخْشِنُه [f·rakhshinu^{h}], which I interpret as *fráẖsino* [Fig. 13], and which seems to document an archaic phase in the evolution of the Latin /ks/ group. It also makes us wonder whether this was indeed the form included in the original. Yet, despite what I said earlier about the preference accorded to the readings in MS A, and the archaicizing character of this derivative from the Latin *fraxinus*, I am inclined to think that this was not the form used by Ibn Baklarish. That it was not is suggested on the one hand by the unanimous testimony of all the other manuscripts (and especially M), and on the other by the fact that the developed form فراشنه [f·r·'shn·^{h}], i.e. *frésno*, already appears in al-Zahrawi,[41] from whom Ibn Baklarish generally took these words in the *'ajamiyya*. At the same time, moreover, the variant in A can have another explanation in the context of this manuscript.[42]

The derivation from A and M from the same archetype seems unquestionable, as we see from the presence of common errors such as بلا قه [b·l·'q·^{h}] (s.v. *dārshisha'ān*), as opposed, for example, to N, which gives the correct form يُلاقه [yul·'qa^{h}], i.e. *yuláqa*.

40. MS هزار حسان.
41. As I have observed in various manuscripts of his *Kitāb al-taṣrīf* (see, for example, MS 502 of the Beşirağa collection in the Süleymaniye Library of Istanbul, facsimile ed. F. Sezgin, Frankfurt-am-Main 1986, II, p. 429).
42. It would seem to me that the form *frakhsino* of MS A is a Latinizing modification of this word introduced by the copyist, who handled Latin with ease, as we shall see later when dealing with the Latin synonyms in the *Kitāb al-Musta'īnī*.

On other occasions the common errors are not limited to A and M, but appear in all the manuscripts. This is the case of the reading الاح بينطه [·l-·ḥ bynṭ^h], the *ʿajamiyya* synonym of the Arabic *yabrūḥ*, an error we find both in La and N, as well as in all the other codices, instead of the expected form الارجبلّيطة, whose full notation would be [al-arjjaballīṭa^t], i.e. *arča bellíṭa*, the well-known Andalusi-Romance term for the mandrake.[43] A similar case is that of the reading منابطة [m·n·ʾb·ṭ·^t], to be found in all the codices of the *Kitāb al-Mustaʿīnī* (s.v. *fawdhanj*),[44] rather than the expected نابطة [n·ʾb·ṭ·^t], i.e. *nébeṭa*. The unanimity of the readings in all the manuscripts suggests that the errors may proceed from the original.

The presence in the work of forms such as the two previous ones, as well as of other errors presumably made by Ibn Baklarish himself, lead us to question the probatory value of this author's attestations and, consequently, his effective knowledge of the *ʿajamiyya* of al-Andalus. To discuss this matter in detail would take us too far afield. For the time being we need only keep in mind what I said earlier about the compilatory and bookish character of the work and Ibn Baklarish's unquestionable debt to his predecessors.

This dependency on his sources must be kept in mind when assessing the *Kitāb al-Mustaʿīnī*, since it is largely a text that transmits a series of Romance words which, contrary to what one might think, do not refer to a contemporary period but are generally late testimonies of earlier linguistic realities. I emphasize this point since we often see from his sources that, at the turn of the eleventh and twelfth centuries, Ibn Baklarish offers us words of the *ʿajamiyya* collected from authors of the previous century who, in their turn, had taken them from authors of still earlier periods.[45]

Ibero-Romance varia

Yet all these observations and reservations, which might seem to relegate the work of Ibn Baklarish to a position of secondary importance, and allow us to classify him as the mere collector of attestations of the *ʿajamiyya* taken from his predecessors, do little to detract from the significance of the *Kitāb al-Mustaʿīnī*. On the contrary: owing to its complex textual transmission, Ibn Baklarish's work has progressively collected a rich, varied, and surprising store of Romance material, with numerous variant readings for the words of the *ʿajamiyya* resulting from the interpolations and additions of the copyists of the codices, while these same copyists (together with other readers and users of the manuscripts) enriched their margins with glosses concerning the simple medicaments. The manuscripts are an eloquent testimony of the circulation of this pharmacopoeia among Jews, Muslims and Christians, which

43. This word appears in the earliest authors (first half of the tenth century) who give the synonyms of the Andalusi *ʿajamiyya*, as Ibn Samajun recalls in his *Jāmiʿ* (s.v. *yabrūḥ*).

44. In this case outside the table of synonyms.

45. A few words of the *ʿajamiyya* which appear in these treatises of the eleventh century (and later) can ultimately be traced back to authors such as ʿImran b. Abi ʿUmar (who died in 932) or Yahya b. Ishaq (who lived at the beginning of the reign of ʿAbd al-Rahman III), the first two Andalusis to include systematically in their works the Romance terms for medicaments. Although the works have not survived, they are known from quotations in the *Jāmiʿ* of Ibn Samajun (tenth-eleventh centuries).

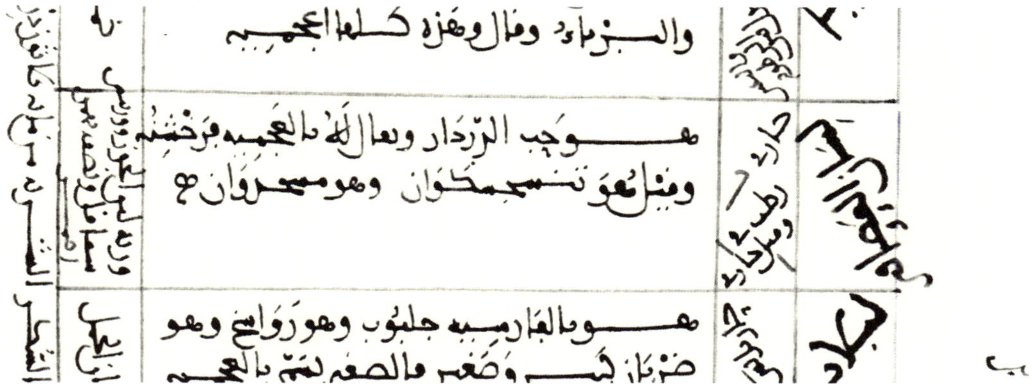

Fig. 13.
The Arcadian Library manuscript, p. 166

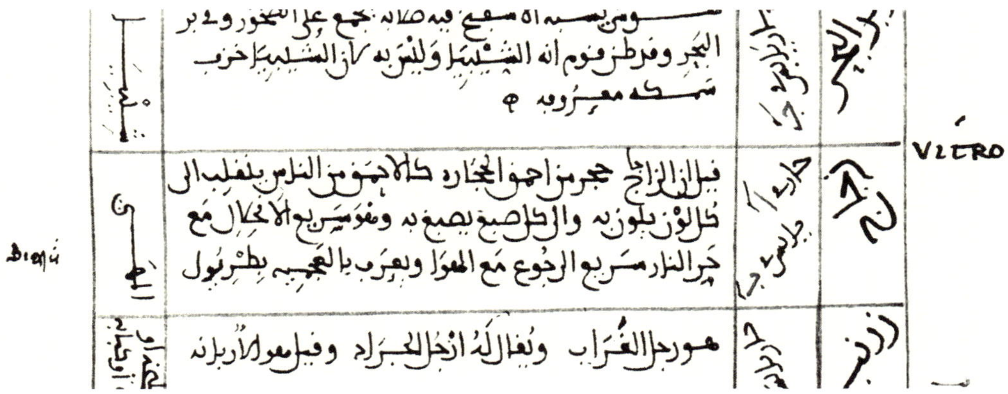

Fig. 14.
The Arcadian Library manuscript, p. 106

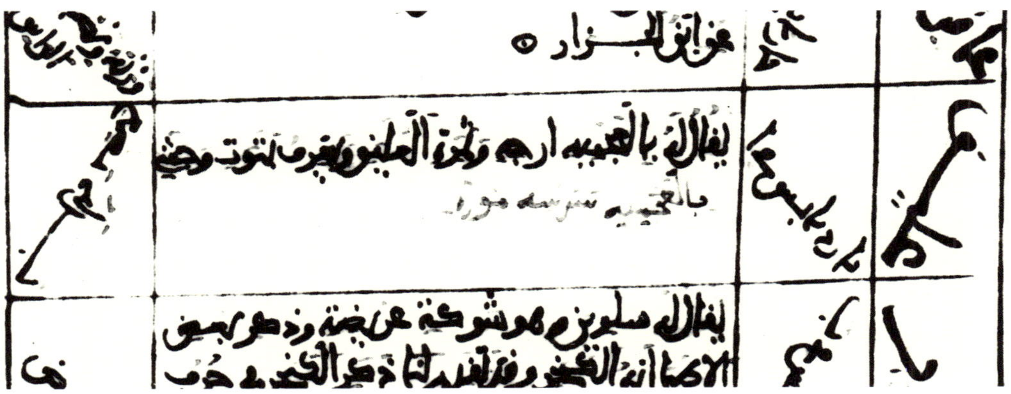

Fig. 15.
Madrid, Biblioteca Nacional, MS ar. 5009, fol. 107b

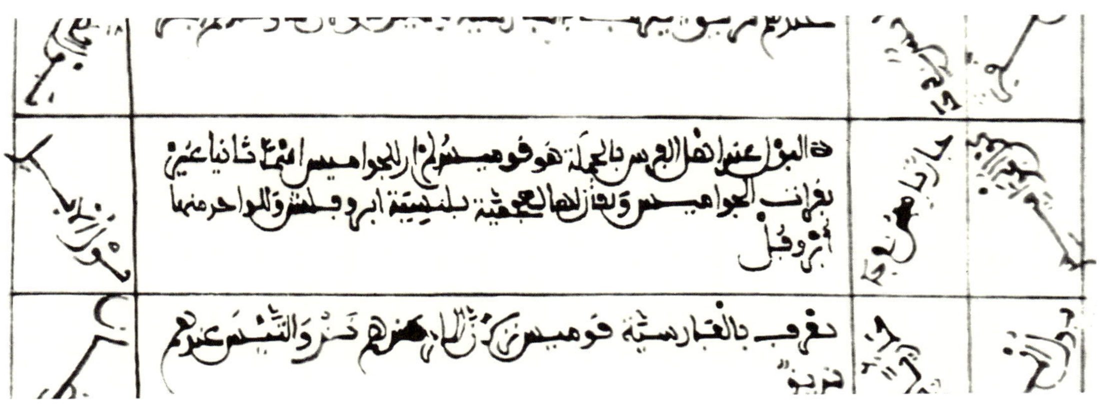

Fig. 16.
Naples, Biblioteca Nazionale, MS III-F-65, fol. 93

has given us an abundant medical lexical repertory in various varieties of Romance from the Iberian peninsula, and even from north of the Pyrenees.

We have already seen that, ever since Dozy and above all since Simonet, scholars have realized that the three codices of the work known at the time (M, La/m, N) offered variant readings of the Romance words. Simonet emphasized this in his *Glosario,* and Menéndez Pidal drew attention to these variants.[46] Yet Simonet's not always very rigorous presentation of this material, together with certain methodological deficiencies in the critical interpretation of the data, did not allow a proper assessment of the extent of these differences which, I should insist, can never be regarded as mere dialectal variants of the *ʿajamiyya* of al-Andalus.

The question is complex and the mere presentation of the manuscripts should already alert us to the chronological differences of the various attestations. The Romance material must be considered individually in each manuscript, but without losing sight of possible connections when the additions are not limited to a single codex.

Before passing on to an analysis of the interpolations we should first examine the case of a supposed addition which does not appear in A or in M. Its existence in the other manuscripts suggests two possible interpretations but does not allow us, for the time being, to incline towards either. Mss La and N give the form غرامِن [g·r·'min], i.e. *grámen*, as a word pertaining to the *ʿajamiyya* of the Sharq al-Andalus (s.v. *najm*). Since this attestation is not be found in either A or M, however, we do not know whether it is due to a lacuna in the archetype from which these two manuscripts proceed. If that were the case we should add the word to Ibn Baklarish's original material, although it was only transmitted subsequently by the other branch from which the other manuscripts descend. But the word *grámen* could also be an early interpolation introduced into the archetype from which La, C (whence it would pass on to N) and all the other manuscripts are derived. The question is by no means futile since this textual detail is related to the linguistic attribution and the date of the word. In the first case it would be a term peculiar to the east of al-Andalus, documented exclusively in Ibn Baklarish. Otherwise, if Ibn Baklarish had not included it in his work, we could still consider it Andalusi, but would have to postpone the date of its documentation. But there is also a third possibility, namely that the word was taken from the north-eastern Romance languages and was consequently closely related to its Aragonese (*agramen*) and Catalan (*agram*) congeners.[47]

THE MANUSCRIPT IN THE ARCADIAN LIBRARY

We must now proceed to consider the particular situation of the various manuscripts, starting with the Arcadian one which, even if copied within a few decades of the original by Ibn Baklarish, presents some interesting modifications.

As a romance synonym of the Arabic *zujāj*, the *Kitāb al-Mustaʿīnī* (s.v.) offers the form بِطْرِيُهْ [biṭri^{y}u^{h}], i.e. *bíṭrio*, as it appears in M and other manuscripts.[48] In contrast to these MS A apparently presents a form in the *ʿajamiyya* which is unequivocal: بِطْرِيُولْ [biṭri^{y}ūl], i.e. *biṭriol* [Fig. 14], an obvious Catalanism whose early documentation in this manuscript (1130) is somewhat disconcerting and

46. *Orígenes del Español*, § 82_2.

47. See Corominas, *DCECH*, s.v. *grama*.

enigmatic. On the one hand the precocious appearance of this form suggests a connection with the Catalan-Aragonese area, something which does not fit in with the execution of the manuscript, more typical of the Crown of Castile (presumably of Toledo). But even if this were so, the early occurrence of this Catalanism in Castile, documented here some time before its appearance in the Catalan area,[49] is no less surprising. It would also long precede the earliest Castilian testimonies known hitherto. On the other hand the marginal Latin gloss *vitro*[50] leaves no room for any doubt about the identity of the entry *zujāj*, the Romance synonym of which was presumably modified by the copyist of the manuscript as *biṭriol*, based on the form *biṭrio* which must have been in the original text he was copying.

A closer analysis of the manuscript allowed me to solve this apparent problem. I discovered that MS A must indeed have offered the reading بِطْرِيُه [biṭri^{y}u^h], but that this was modified subsequently, in an indeterminate period, in a hand different to that of the copyist and in which we also find other attestations in Arabic characters in the margins. This 'amender' of the manuscript changed the original form by placing, above the final *ḥā'*, a *wāw* (و) and adding a *lām* (ل) with a *sukūn*, which transformed an original بِطْرِيُه [biṭri^{y}u^h] into بِطْرِيُولْ [biṭri^{y}ūl]. He thus adopted the term *vidriol* which seemed to him more suitable.

This interpolation in the Arcadian manuscript raises two questions. First of all, it draws attention to the fact that the author of this emendation in the codex replaced the word *biṭrio* 'glass' with *biṭriol*, which obviously refers to another substance, namely vitriol. This could be due simply to the carelessness of the anonymous user of the manuscript who inadvertently modified the Romance synonym in the entry *zujāj* 'vidrio', instead of doing so in the corresponding table of the entry *zāj*, which is indeed vitriol and appears on the same page of the manuscript two entries higher. A second question, closely related to the date and the place where this emendation to the manuscript was made, remains unanswered. The ancestry of the word *biṭriol* is beyond a doubt, but are we dealing with the Catalan form *vidriol* or with a Catalanism in the Castilian area only documented in the fifteenth century?[51]

This question alerts us to the unusual aspects of Ibero-Romance which have passed down to us in the various manuscripts of the *Kitāb al-Mustaʿīnī*.

THE MANUSCRIPT IN THE BIBLIOTECA NACIONAL OF MADRID

MS M has a number of interventions and additions in a hand later than that of the copyist. These are from an indeterminate period (presumably late medieval) and can be related to the Toledan dialect of the time. At all events it seems clear that we are dealing with forms from the Castilian linguistic domain.

We can already detect this hand in the very first term in the *ʿajamiyya* in the work.

48. Like R_I which offers بطْرِيُهْ [b·ṭryu^h] *bíṭryo*. For the variants بطرقه [b·ṭr·q·^{h}] of L_a and بِذْرِيُه [bidri^{y}o^h] in N, see below.

49. The Catalan form *vidriol* was first documented by Ramon Llull, according to Coromines, *DECLlC*, s.v. *vidre*.

50. For the Latin glosses of the London manuscript see below.

51. Cf. Corominas, *DCECH*, s.v. *vidrio*, and Coromines, *DECLlC*, s.v. *vidre*. Earlier documentations of Catalanism in Castilian texts are given in M.ª Teresa Herrera (ed.), *Diccionario español de textos médicos antiguos*, I, Madrid 1996, s.v. *vitriolo* (hereafter *DETEMA*).

Under the entry *uqḥuwān* Ibn Baklarish gave a synonym of the *ʿajamiyya*: غشونش [gh·sh·wn·sh], modified in this manuscript to أقشونش [·qishūnish], a form which Simonet, aware of the correction in the manuscript, interpreted as *aquixonex* and identified with the early Castilian *quixones* (mod. *quijones*).[52]

Other interpolations in the same hand (with its characteristic small letters, also to be found in further additions to the Arabic text)[53] have no clear linguistic identity. These include قانطوشه [qānṭūsh·^{h}] (s.v. *usṭūkhūdūs*), which we must interpret as *qanṭóso*. The lack of a diphthong in this word (in contrast to the Castilian *cantueso*) suggests that it is a dialectalism which we could connect with forms peculiar to the peninsular west (cf. the Galician *cantoso* and Leonese *cantojo*).[54]

Interesting, too, is the form جوجوباش [j·wj·wb·'sh] (s.v. *ʿināb*), undoubtedly *jújubas*, a Latinism frequent in the jargon of the apothecaries of the late medieval period, of which Corominas could only find a late attestation in Laguna (in its variant *yuyubas*),[55] but which often occurs in the medical-botanical texts of the time.[56]

We can complete this group of additions to the Madrid manuscript with the words سرسه موره [s·rs·^{h} m·wr·^{h}], i.e. *çarça mora* [Fig. 15], a composite form documented in Castilian as from Alonso de Palencia and Nebrija at the end of the fifteenth century.[57]

THE LEIDEN MANUSCRIPT: EARLY PART (La)

The ancient part of the Leiden manuscript, which does not have any relevant peculiarities where additions and interpolations are concerned,[58] nevertheless contains certain interesting variants. Contrary to A and M, which give the anomalous form الوردس [al-wrds] as a Romance synonym of the Arabic *ward,* 'rose', La contains the expected form روشش [r·wsh·sh], i.e. *rosas*. Since we also encountered the form *rosas* in N (الرُوشَشْ [al-rūshash]), we are entitled to think that the two forms are derived from a common source, but in fact it would seem to be a case of independent correction in the two manuscripts. This emerges from the fact that, on the one hand, N retains the Arabic article in the Romance word, which does not appear in La, while, on the other, all the Moroccan manuscripts give the incorrect form (of the الوردس [al-wrds] type)—a continuation of the erroneous reading attested in A and M, which seems to proceed ultimately from Ibn Baklarish's original.

We also encounter other modifications in La, undoubtedly due to the copyist of Lm to whom we shall return later.

52. Simonet, *Glosario*, pp. 257–8. This Romance-Andalusi form, as well as its correction in MS M (which is discussed in Corominas, *DCECH*, s.v. *quijones*) and another form appearing in the *ʿUmdat al-ṭabīb* (edited in Corriente, 'El romandalusí', p. 114), merit a close re-examination which we cannot undertake here.

53. For example, s.v. *īrsā* ,'white lily'.

54. Cf. Corominas, *DCECH*, s.v. *cantueso*.

55. See Corominas, *DCECH*, s.v. *azufaifo*.

56. See Guido Mensching, *La sinonima delos nombres delas medeçinas griegos e latynos e arauigos*, Madrid, 1994, p. 260; *DETEMA*, s.v. *jujuba*.

57. Corominas, *DCECH*, s.v. *zarza*.

58. With the exception of occasional variants such as the aforesaid بطرقه [b·ṭr·q·^{h}], for بطريه [biṭri^{y}u^{h}], which may stem from a mere error in the interpretation of the final vowel *ḍamma* as if it were the dot of a consonant, which would give rise to *qāf*.

THE NAPLES MANUSCRIPT

But the most striking case of interventions by the copyist in a manuscript of the *Kitāb al-Mustaʿīnī* is to be found in the Naples manuscript (N), whose variant readings and exact date (1482) have been known ever since Simonet. Owing to the lack of an adequate contextualization, certain inaccuracies in the presentation of the material and, above all, methodological deficiencies in the interpretation of these attestations have misled students in respect to the interesting additions in this codex.

Besides unchanged words such as the ones that we can deduce to have been in C, its exemplar, Ms N provides us with interventions by the copyist of various types. In the first place there are cases of a new vocalization and pointing of the received consonantal *ductus*, which reveal certain interesting phonetic shades. Thus, for example, we have the form اِشْبَرِّقُش [ishbarighush] (s.v. *hilyawn*). The two *kasra* vowels suggest the reading *espárreqos*, which we might be able to connect with the forms of eastern Ibero-Romance (cf. Catalan *espàrrec*). Another case of this type could be the form بِشُّوطْ [bishshūṭ] (s.v. *māsh*) which must be interpreted as *pixóṭ*, without a diphthong. It would separate this new reading from the supposed Romance-Andalusi original of Ibn Baklarish—*pisawṭ*, with the diphthong /*áw*/.[59] Similarly, the copyist of this codex introduced other variant readings in the words of the ʿ*ajamiyya*, giving rise to certain allomorphs, the linguistic attribution of which will have to be determined. An example is the form without a diphthong *porqo* (بُرْ قُه [burqu^{h}], s.v. *zibl al-khinzīr*), which corrects the original diphthonged form of the Romance-Andalusi *puerqo* [bu^{w}ārqu^{h}] in A and M, and *puerko* [bu^{w}ārku^{h}] in La.

A highly revealing case of the intervention of the copyist in the text, which I have studied elsewhere,[60] is to be found in one of the Romance synonyms under the entry *ḥasak*. Ibn Baklarish has taken a composite form as the word in the ʿ*ajamiyya*, which we can interpret as *gallo čeqo* (on a *ductus* of the غاله جاقه type, whose full vocalization and pointing would be [ghāllu^{h} jāqu^{h}]). The author provides the translation, *dīk aʿmā*, i.e. 'blind cock', which appears in A, M and La. In contrast to the form mentioned, C (from which N was copied) must have given a variation in the representation of the stressed vowel of the second word, with *ī* instead of *ā*, i.e. غاله جيقه , and he might even have given *tāʾ marbūṭa* instead of the final *hāʾ*.[61] These circumstances could have led the copyist of N to give the reading غَالَه جيقَه [g·ʾla^{t} j·yqa^{t}], which, if we are to judge by the Arabic translation he offers, ʿ*afṣ ṣaghīr*, i.e. 'small gall-nut', instead of the original *dīk aʿmā* ('blind cock'), he interpreted as the Romance composite *gálla číqa*.

Besides all this there are eloquent cases in which the copyist of N adds synonyms of the ʿ*ajamiyya* in those entries of the *Kitāb al-Mustaʿīnī* which do not contain any synonym in Romance-Andalusi. For example, we have *qarne* (قرْ ن [q·rni], s.v. *laḥm al-khirbā*), *bino* (بِينُهْ [bīnu^{h}], s.v. *khamr ʿatīqa*), *qabalyo* (قَبَلْيُه [qabalyu^{h}], s.v. *zibl al-khayl*), *agila* (اغله [·gh·l·^{h}], s.v. *marārat al-ʿuqāb*), *agwa* (اغْوَة [aghwa^{t}], s.v.

59. Cf. Corominas, *DCECH*, s.v. *guisante*. MS N is the only one that vocalizes the consonantal *ductus* of this word.

60. 'Sobre el estudio del mozárabe', pp. 716–19, where I provide all the details of this revealing case.

61. This reading with a final *tāʾ marbūṭa* (غالة جيقة) is the one offered by all the Maghribi manuscripts which unanimously retain the translation *dīk aʿmā* ('blind cock').

mā'), and so on. In other cases, the copyist of N adds new Romance synonyms to the words of the *'ajamiyya* of al-Andalus which already appeared in the text of Ibn Baklarish. For the item *untura* (انتوره [·nt·wr·ʰ], s.v. *samn*), for example, he now adds *manṭeqa* (منطيقة [m·nt·yq·ʰ]), or after the word *pančáyin* (البَنجّاين [·l-bbanjj·'y·n], s.v. *jāwars*) he puts *pannizo* (بَنِز [bbanizᵘⁿ]). He places the word *plaṭa* (ابلاطة ['·bl·'ṭ·ᵗ], s.v. *fiḍḍa*) after *arzento* (ارزنْتُه [·rz·ntuʰ]), a modification, in its turn, of the original *aryento* (ارينْتُه [·ry·ntuʰ]), and, finally, he adds the word *raṭa* (الرَّاطة [raṭ·ᵗ] , s.v. *laḥm al-fār*) to the Romance-Andalusi *sorče* (شرجي [sh·rj·y]). So to what can we ascribe these new words contained in the manuscript? While their Castilian appearance can hardly be doubted, the very date of the codex must oblige us to exclude them from the early *'ajamiyya* of al-Andalus.[62]

But the linguistic information in this manuscript is even more abundant and the text itself gives other data of the utmost importance. Occasionally the copyist himself says specifically that the new words come from the *'ajamiyya* of Valencia. He does so, for example, in the case of *ṭápares* (طـابرش [ṭāb·r·sh]),[63] i.e. 'capers' (s.v. *aṣaf*). The same Valencian origin is indicated for the word *arjelaqa*, ارجلاقة [·rjilāqaʰ], added by the copyist to the aforesaid Romance-Andalusi plant name, *yuláqa*, as a synonym of the Arabic *dārishayshaʿān*. When it is mentioned again, outside the table of synonyms, we are told that, in the vernacular (Arabic) language of Valencia, people say *al-ʿajram,* and *arjelaqa* in its *'ajamiyya*. Similarly we encounter another word specifically indicated as being in Valencian Romance, with the added peculiarity of appearing in the plural and in the singular: under the entry *bawl al-jawāmīs,* 'the urine of buffalos', the manuscript specifies the fact that, in the Valencian *'ajamiyya*, the word is *brúfols* (أبْرُوفلش [·brūf·lshⁱ]), whose singular (lit. *ism al-wāḥid*) is *brúfol* (أبْرُوفُلْ [ᵘbrūful]) [Fig. 16].[64]

The Catalan origin of these words attested in Valencia appears beyond a doubt, and to them we can add still others not specifically indicated as being from the Valencian *'ajamiyya*, such as مَغرانش [magr.'nish] i.e., *magránes*. In this manuscript it substitutes the Romance-Andalusi form *marganeṭas* (مرغناطش [m·rg·n·'ṭ·sh]) included by Ibn Baklarish as a synonym for pomegranates (s.v. *rummān*).[65]

The precise localization of these words draws our attention to the Arabic (Andalusi)—Romance (Catalan) bilingualism of late medieval Valencia—a situation with which the copyist of the Neapolitan manuscript was obviously acquainted and of which he provides us, as we saw, with unequivocal evidence. And yet we know that

62. Most of these words added to N (dated 1482) are quoted in *DCECH* as Mozarabic forms, with the date 1106 which Corominas attributes to Ibn Baklarish.

63. Such is the reading of the manuscript which Simonet (*Glosario*, p. 530) vocalized arbitrarily as طَابَرَش [ṭābarash]. This is not the place to discuss whether this word is evidence for feminine plurals in *-es*, as claimed both by Álvaro Galmés de Fuentes (*Dialectología mozárabe*, Madrid 1983, pp. 36, 111 and 307) and Leopoldo Peñarroja Torrejón (*El mozárabe de Valencia*, Madrid 1990, p. 433), since the readings of both authors are unfounded. Moreover, as is now clear, even less can one suppose an autochthonous pre-Arab existence for the word, as do Menéndez Pidal (*Orígenes*, § 89_3) and Corominas (*DCECH*, s.v. *alcaparra*).

64. The copyist made a mistake and first wrote the text corresponding to the synonyms of the entry *bawl al-jawāmīs* in the box of *bawl al-khinzīr*, 'pig's urine', which he then changed and copied again in the right place.

65. Coromines (*DECLlC*, s.v. *magrana*) was wrong when he imagined Ibn Baklarish to be a sort of modern dialectologist, collecting these forms in Catalonia and Aragon in about 1111. Equally unlikely, as we shall see, is his claim that the variants in the different manuscripts were collected by Ibn Baklarish himself.

Valencia was a multilingual society in the late fifteenth century and that its linguistic Romance varieties were not limited to the language introduced by the Catalans. In this respect, too, the Castilian forms added by the copyist can be considered peculiar to Valencia.

Another separate group would be formed by certain words which we might call 'hybrid' and which cannot easily be reduced to the exclusive remnants of a single language. An example is the *porqo* mentioned above, whose lack of a diphthong reminds us of the Catalan *porc*, while the final vowel would seem, rather, to be a residue of Castilian.[66]

But we must continue since the interpretative possibilities of this word are by no means exhausted, and the significance of the manuscript does not end here. Of particular interest is the attestation we encounter in connection with the *qarn al-ayyil,* 'deer horn', for which the cell for synonyms is blank in all the codices of the *Kitāb al-Mustaʿīnī* (a feature which may be attributable to Ibn Baklarish's original), while N offers the following text:

قرْن الأَيِّل ... يقال له بالعجمية بَيْنَه دى سِربُه اعنى بَيْنَه قرن وسربه عندهم ايل وذالك بعجمية راغون من عَمل سَرقسطة وبلنسية

Deer Horn [qarn al-ayyil]... *comes from the* ʿajamiyya [*bayna*^{h} *d·y sirbu*^{h}], *since among them* [*bayna*^{h}] *it means 'horn' and* [*s·rb.*^{h}] *'deer', and this is the case in the* ʿajamiyya *of Aragon in the region of Saragossa and Valencia.*

Here *bayna de çerbo,* the first element of which was connected by Simonet with Catalan and Valencian,[67] may well have links—however problematic—with Aragonese territory, if we are to accept the express statement in the manuscript.

On the other hand the linguistic reference to the *ʿajamiyya* of Aragon, which would also include the regions of Saragossa and Valencia, should probably be understood as an allusion to two geographical areas of a political unity (the Crown of Aragon) rather than as an effective linguistic identity between the two territories, although it should not be excluded that this testimony indicates, in fact, the spread of the Aragonese language throughout Valencian lands. This suggestive passage, the interpretation of which cannot be treated exhaustively here, will have to be examined more attentively. However that may be, the connection of Saragossa with Valencia in this context is of the greatest interest, and opens up the possibility of introducing the Aragonese dialect as a third discordant linguistic factor in Romanic Valencia in the late fifteenth century, faithfully reflected in the attestations of the Neapolitan manuscript of the *Kitāb al-Mustaʿīnī* under examination.[68]

In this connection we should look at another case of the interpolation of two

66. We might have to connect the 'hybrid' words with analogous forms in certain Castilian-Aragonese dialects of the Valencian region which restore the final *-o* in words of Catalan origin: *grogo* (< Catalan *groc*), *alborzo* (< Catalan *arboç*), etc.: see Manuel Sanchis Guarner, 'Las hablas del Alto Mijares y de Fanzara (Provincia de Castellón)', *Boletín de la Real Academia Española*, 47, 1967, p. 204.

67. Simonet, *Glosario*, pp. 28–9. Note the spelling *yn* of the manuscript to represent the palatal nasal consonant. Coromines (*DECLlC*, s.v. *banya* and *cervo*) mentions the Catalan expression *banya de cervo* as a plant name (the form in N refers to the horn of the animal), taken from the dictionary of Alcover-Moll (s.v. *banya*).

words by the copyist of N. Simonet in his *Glosario* did not realize that both words were added exclusively in this codex, thereby seriously misleading later students. As a synonym of the Arabic *jubn* Ibn Baklarish included the form تري [t·r·y], indicating that it came from the *'ajamiyya*.[69] It is to be found in all the manuscripts (s.v. *jubn 'atīq*). N, however, adds two other synonyms, the readings of which are, respectively, قيجهْ [q·yju^h] and فرمَاجِّهْ [f·rmājji^h] [Fig. 17]. I must insist that both forms are in this manuscript since Simonet only pointed out the first.

In view of what has been said about this manuscript, there is no doubt that the second of these two words, which we must interpret as *formače*,[70] is peculiar to the Catalan of Valencia, while the other seems to be Castilian, even if, as we shall see, it might conceivably be Aragonese. In the initial syllable of the sequence [q·yju^h], we must dismiss the interpretation of an archaic descending diphthong /ai/, of the *qayžo* type, as proposed by Menéndez Pidal (who rejected the reading of Simonet, who offered in his *Glosario* the possibility of interpreting it without a diphthong).[71] Menéndez Pidal supposed that it was a word peculiar to the Mozarabs of Saragossa,[72] but his claim is quite untenable since, on the one hand, the mere date of this codex excludes such an attribution, and on the other, the word, as we shall see, does not present this supposed diphthong on which Menéndez Pidal based his argument. The reading of the manuscript cannot be doubted, and, since there is no *sukūn* above the letter *yā'*, this has the function of a *mater lectionis* to indicate a stressed vowel which, in this case, cannot be any other than /é/.[73] We are therefore dealing with the initial /ké-/ sequence, which has already evolved, rather than with the supposed archaic diphthong.

As for the second syllable of the word, it would seem clear that the *jīm* represents a voiced consonant—not a palatal one but the ancient apical alveolar /z/, the result of the voicing of an intervocal etymological /s/. We are dealing with an orthographic habit adopted in Andalusi manuscripts to represent the result of the Romance voicing of the intervocal Latin *s*, which is based on the use in Andalusi Arabic of the palatal *jīm* to represent certain Romance words with a voiced /z/, thus giving precedence

68. The attestations of this manuscript undoubtedly make an interesting contribution to the controversial linguistic history of Valencia; cf. Juan A. Frago Gracia, 'Castellano y aragonés en el Antiguo Reino de Valencia', in Federico Corriente *et al.*, *Las lenguas prevalencinas*, Alicante 1986, pp. 45–63, and Antoni Ferrando, 'La configuració lingüística del País Valencià després de la conquista jaumina', in the same volume, pp. 81–91. See also various pieces in Jordi Colomina i Castanyer, *Llengües en contacte als regnes de València i de Múrcia (segles XIII–XV)*, Alicante 1995.

69. Instead of *rūmiyya*. This is not the only case in which Ibn Baklarish attributes to the *'ajamiyya* words peculiar to Byzantine Greek.

70. The *jīm* with a *tashdīd* guarantees that the last consonant is voiceless, while the *kasra* allows us to interpret *-e*, whereas the *hā'* has a purely orthographic value before the final vowels of the Romance. On the other hand, the late date and the Catalan origin of the word allow us unhesitatingly to dispel the doubts about the interpretation of the word expressed by Menéndez Pidal (*Orígenes*, § 82_2 and 106_2) and Corominas (*DCECH*, s.v. *queso*, and *DECLlC*, s.v. *forma*).

71. Although the transcription with the spelling *ch* for the *jīm* was not very felicitous, the double possibility *quécho* or *quéicho* proposed by Simonet and, above all, the form of the word in Arabic characters, without a *sukūn* above the *yā'* (قيجه), suggest the reading without a diphthong.

72. *Orígenes del español*, § 18_2b.

73. In N there is a frequent representation of the Romance vowel /e/ by a *kasra*, provided with a *yā'* of prolongation when it is a stressed syllable, such as in the form *manṭeqa* [manṭ·yqat] signalled before.

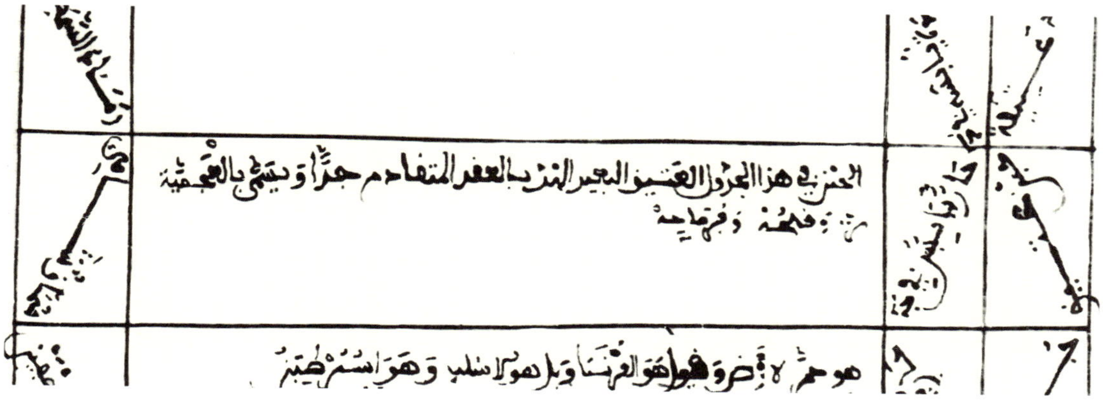

Fig. 17.
Naples, Biblioteca Nazionale, MS III-F-65, fol. 16

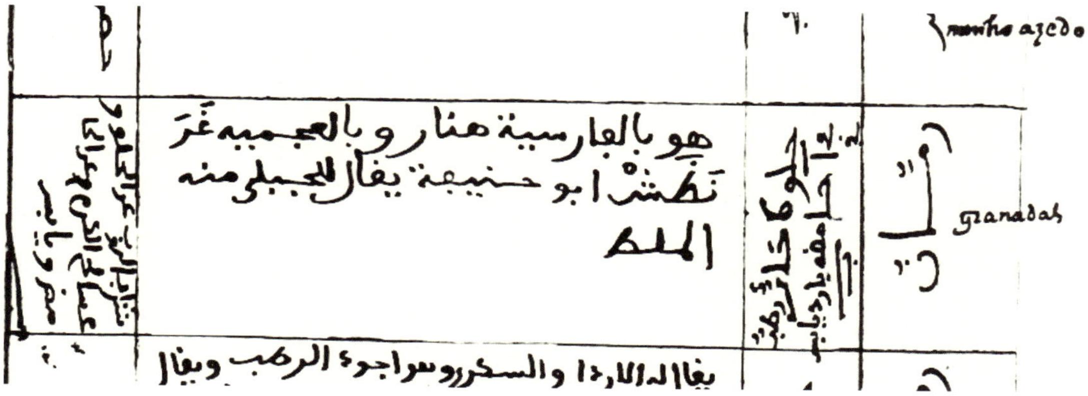

Fig. 18.
Leiden, University Library, Cod. Or. 15, fol. 103b

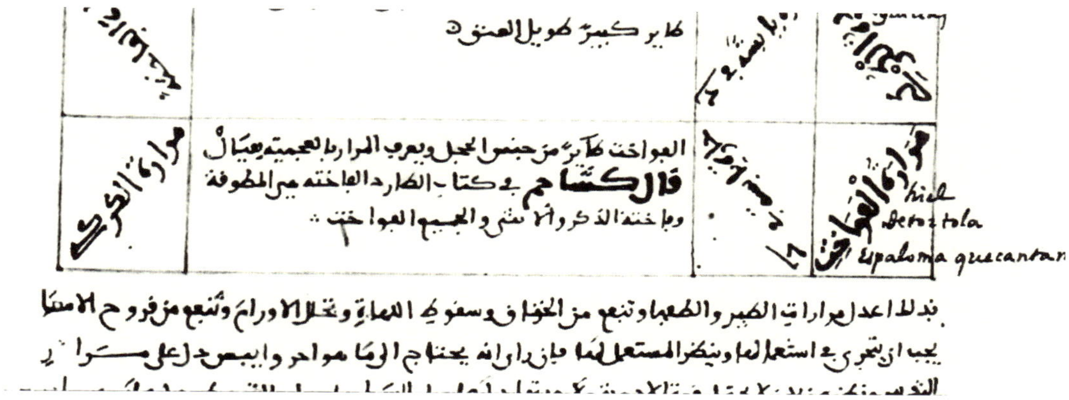

Fig. 19.
Leiden, University Library, Cod. Or. 15, fol. 78b

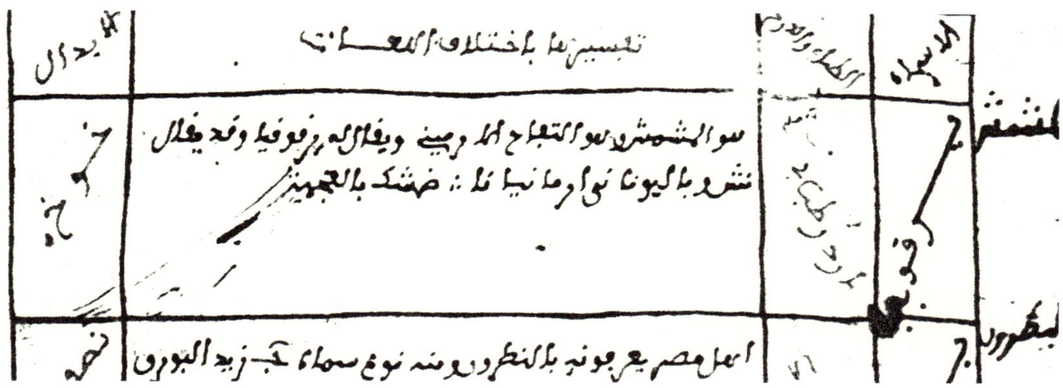

Fig. 20.
Tunis, National Library, MS 3575, fol. 28b

to the voice rather than to other aspects of the consonant.[74] Consequently, beneath the *qéjo* reading of this word, there definitely lies a /kézo/ Romance form, with an intervocal voiced consonant.[75]

So to what language should this word be attributed? We could suppose that it was a Castilian form, although, according to what we are now discovering about the manuscript, we cannot exclude the possibility of its being a genuinely Aragonese word.[76] We should remember that there were Aragonese-speaking enclaves in the Valencian region dating back to medieval times, and surviving in the face of the predominating Castilian. Some of these are characterized by their pronounced archaicism, such as the locality of Fanzara (Castellón) in whose dialect the ancient distinction between voiceless and voiced consonants still survives, as we see from words such as *quezo* (with a voiced /z/)[77] which must be connected with the form *qéjo* in MS N of the *Kitāb al-Mustaʿīnī*.

More examples could be provided, and new cases[78] added, to the rich collection of lexical novelties introduced by the copyist of N, but what we have seen so far will suffice to draw attention to the peculiarities and the immense interest of this codex.

THE MANUSCRIPT R1

If we now turn to the Maghribi manuscripts we will also find interpolations and new additions of interest, to be added to this complex panorama of the textual transmission of the work.

Although the manuscript R1 has few additions which are of interest to us, it nevertheless offers the first attestation of another word interpolated from the *ʿajamiyya*: *murtas* (مرتش [m·rt·sh], s.v. ās), which does not appear in the Andalusi manuscripts, but which has been adopted by all the North African copies, including Lm.

THE LEIDEN MANUSCRIPT: MODERN PART (Lm)

The clearly established authorship and date (*c.* 1624) of Lm allow us to situate the additions in the codex with some precision. We also know that, in order to complete the work of Ibn Baklarish, al-Hajari used a manuscript (Y), which he subsequently corrected from another manuscript (Y′). One of these (or both) had additions, presumably made in al-Andalus or, at all events, by someone who had lived in Granada, for we read in Lm that he came across certain plants there the names of

74. The matter was solved brilliantly some time ago by A. Alonso, 'Correspondencias arábigo-españolas en los sistemas de sibilantes', *Nueva Revista de Filología Hispánica*, 8, 1946, pp. 12–76, esp. pp. 48–53.

75. This is not the only case of the representation of a voiced /z/ with a *jīm* in N. In contrast to the other codices which give the word *resina* رشينه [r·sh.yn·h] as the Romance synonym of the Arabic *ṣamgh* (s.v. *ṣamgh al-ʾijjāṣ*), the N gives the reading رَجينه [rajīn·h], with a clear voicing of the intervocal consonant.

76. This manuscript thus confirms the Catalan-Aragonese duality *formatge/queso*, frequent in chancery documents of the Archivo de la Corona de Aragón, as was pointed out by Germán Colón ('Les relacions del lèxic aragonès medieval amb el lèxic català', included in his *Estudis de filologia catalana i romànica*, Valencia and Barcelona 1997, p. 175).

77. Cited by Frago Gracia, 'Castellano y aragonés en el Antiguo Reino de Valencia', p. 55 (who takes it from Sanchis Guarner, 'Las hablas del Alto Mijares y de Fanzara', p. 210).

78. I have not discussed an aspect of this manuscript which deserves closer examination in the future: namely, certain features of the spellings adopted by the copyist to represent Romance forms, such as the absence of emphatics (e.g. in the above-mentioned *bídrio*) and his rendering of the palatal series of consonants, with the digraph *yn* for the nasal (*bayna*) and *ly* for the lateral (*qabalyo*).

which he gives in Granadan Arabic.[79] These interpolated passages do not appear in R1, but undoubtedly figured in the subarchetype from which *Z* descends, since the other four Maghribi manuscripts all include the same attestations.

It is to this same source that we can probably trace certain additions in Lm, such as the word *çenço* سِينْسُه [s·ynsu^{h}], s.v. *afsintīn*), said to have been seen in a manuscript (*fī ba'ḍ al-nusakh*) which cited it as belonging to the *'ajamiyya* of Saragossa. At all events it is clear that this addition goes back to the source from which Y (Y′) and *Z* proceed, since it figures in Lm, H, T, R2 and R3.

On the other hand, it is obvious that, in the part of the manuscript which he reconstructed, al-Hajari modified the words of the *'ajamiyya*, modernizing them and adapting them to the forms proper to Castilian, a language which he knew as well as he knew Arabic. Thus the Romance-Andalusi form *marganeṭas*, originally in the work (s.v. *rummān*) and which, as we saw, was replaced in N by the Catalan word *magránes*, is now substituted in al-Hajari's hand by its Castilian form, *granaṭas* (غَرَنَطَشْ [g^{a}ranaṭash]) [Fig. 18].[80]

Nor did al-Hajari limit himself to altering the words of the *'ajamiyya* which he found in the manuscript he was copying. At times he also intervened in the ancient part (La). Just as we have seen other copyists do, al-Hajari occasionally provided a precise vocalization and pointing to the consonantal *ductus* of certain Castilian forms in the manuscript, such as أَشْبَرَّغُشْ ['ashbbarraghush], which should be read in the Castilian manner as *espárragos*. Another intervention in this ancient part of the manuscript is more subtle, but has hitherto been overlooked, despite the remarkable reading it presents. Ever since Simonet we know that the Leiden codex provided a variant *hiel*, with an aspiration and without a final vowel, in contrast to the other manuscripts (*fiele*, فيالى [f·^{y}·'l·y], s.v. *marārat al-fawākhit*). What was surprising was that this form did not appear in the modern part of the manuscript (as the Castilianism we might expect from al-Hajari), but in the ancient part, an innovation which was not consonant with the attestations of the early *'ajamiyya* included in La. Now, however, a close analysis of the manuscript shows that it was a later alteration of the original consonantal *ductus*, undoubtedly in the hand of al-Hajari, who, with a slight touch of the pen, transformed the initial *fā'* into *hā'*, vocalized the diphthong with a *kasra* and a *fatḥa,* and placed a *sukūn* above the final *lām*, which resulted in the form هِيَالْ [hi^{y}āl], i.e. *hiel* [Fig. 19], reflecting the aspiration typical of al-Hajari's Castilian, which was obviously unimaginable for the copyist of La.

OTHER MAGHRIBI MANUSCRIPTS

The more recent Maghribi manuscripts also present certain additions of interest which complete this panorama of the various elements of the *'ajamiyya* in the *Kitāb al-Musta'īnī*. A consultation of the codices H, T, R2 and R3 reveals another trail of Romance words. Since they figure in H, the earliest in this group of manuscripts, they must have been introduced before the end of the eighteenth century. On the

79. He says, for example, that he saw the white lily (s.v. *īrsā*) in Granada where it was called *lúlu* (لُولُه). This is a Romanicism of Granadan Arabic familiar to us from other sources (see Federico Corriente, *A Dictionary of Andalusi Arabic*, Leiden 1997, p. 488).

80. We are left wondering whether we should read [g^{a}ranaẓash], with the voiceless consonant ظ, since the manuscript seems to have a point between the supposed ط and its vowel.

other hand, we apparently have to establish two different groups of new Romance terms collected in these manuscripts since, although they appear in all the codices, we do not know if they were introduced simultaneously or whether—and this is more likely—they proceed from different sources. I have consequently posited two phases (*Z* and *Z* ′) in the filiation of this group of codices. We shall see in any case that they belong to clearly differentiated linguistic strata.

A first group is constituted by a few words taken from ancient treatises which, in view of the period, must be considered late bookish echoes of the Andalusi *ʿajamiyya.*[81] It is in this small group that we can place such examples as the composite expression *yerba foqo* (يربه فوقه [y·rb·^{h} f·wq·^{h}], s.v. *yāsimīn*), indicated as belonging to the *ʿajamiyya,* and its translation (*ʿushbat al-nār* 'grass of fire'), which is the Romance-Andalusi synonym of 'jasmine' known to us from other sources.[82]

But besides words such as these we find another group of words attributed unanimously in H, T, R2 and R3 to the *ʿajamiyya*, and which must be considered apart. They are: *plom* (بلوم [b·l·wm], s.v. *asrab*), *ḍamasq* (ضمشك [*ḍ·m·shq*], s.v. *barqūq*) [Fig. 20], *nabos* (نابوس [n·ʾb·ws], s.v. *būshād*), *cabras* (كبرس [k·br·as], s.v. *baʿr al-māʿiz*), *berehenas* (برهنش [b·r·h·n·sh] s.v. *badanjaān*), *fabas* (فابص [f·ʾb·ṣ], s.v. *baqillā*), *çebolyas* (سبوليس [s.b.wly.s] s.v. *baṣal*).[83] There is no doubt that these are Hispanic words, but not Andalusi ones. They appear, rather, to be modern Spanish. In their transliteration in Arabic characters we see certain novelties like, for example, the manner of representing the consonant /s/, with vacillations between *sīn*, *shīn* and *ṣād*, which shows us that we are dealing with a system different from the usual one in al-Andalus, and which at the same time reflects the regular adaptation of modern Hispanicisms in the Moroccan dialect with the soft consonants *ṣād* and *ḍād* and the adoption of the Spanish /s/ and /d/. On the other hand, the word *berehenas* reveals traces of modern Spanish, as does the softening of the ancient palatal, while the fact that this is not be represented by *khāʾ*, but by *hāʾ*, seems to indicate an aspirated pronunciation [Fig. 21]. All this, together with the lisp apparently presented in the word *çebolyas*, might indicate that these forms belong to the modern Andalusian dialect. This would be confirmed by the lexical evidence of the word *ḍamasq*, as a Hispanic synonym of the Arabic *barqūq*, since we know that *damasco* is the modern term for 'apricot' in Cadiz and elsewhere in Andalusia.[84]

81. This bookish practice of accumulating synonyms of the Romance of al-Andalus continued until recently. Renaud for example ('Trois études', p. 149), pointed out certain references to Ibn Baklarish in the treatise entitled *Ḍiyāʾ al-nibrās*..., completed in 1318 A.H. (lithograph edition, Fez 1900), by ʿAbd al-Salam Muhammad al-ʿAlami, in which I have found various words from the *ʿajamiyya* of al-Andalus (new edition, Rabat, *c.* 1986, pp. 27, 50), and some others without any mention of their attribution. And we also find synonyms of the simples in the old *ʿajamiyya* of al-Andalus in even more recent works, such as the *Tafsīr mufradāt al-Anṭakī bi-l-lahja al-tūnisiyya*, by the Tunisian Muhammad Mahfuz (1923–88), ed. Ibrahim ben Mrad, Beirut 1996.

82. See Asín Palacios, *Glosario*, 649°.

83. I am not sure whether the form *mustaza* (مستز [m·st·z], s.v. *khardal*), which figures as a word from the *ʿajamiyya* in this entire group of codices, belongs here. It could be an addition with a different provenance.

84. Cf. Corominas, *DCECH*, s.v. *damasco*.

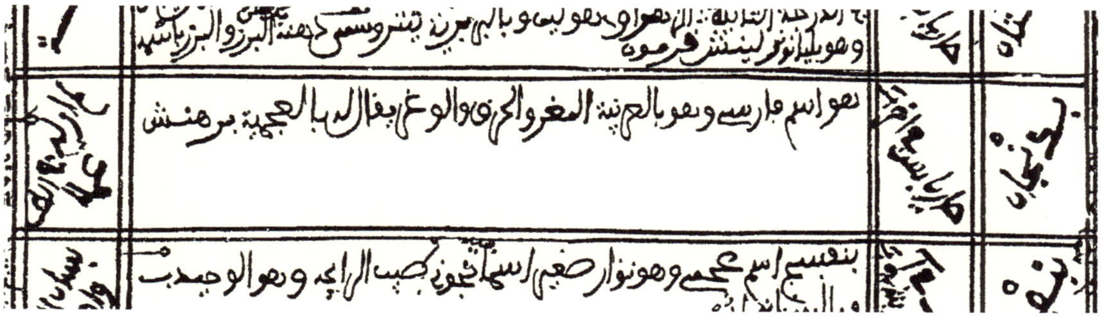

Fig. 21.
Rabat, Ḥasaniyya Library in the Royal Palace, MS 763, fol. 23b

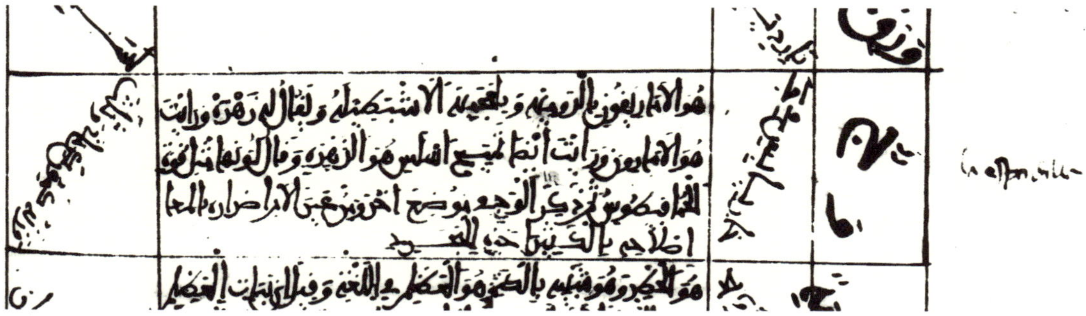

Fig. 22.
Madrid, Biblioteca Nacional, MS ar. 5009, fol. 50b

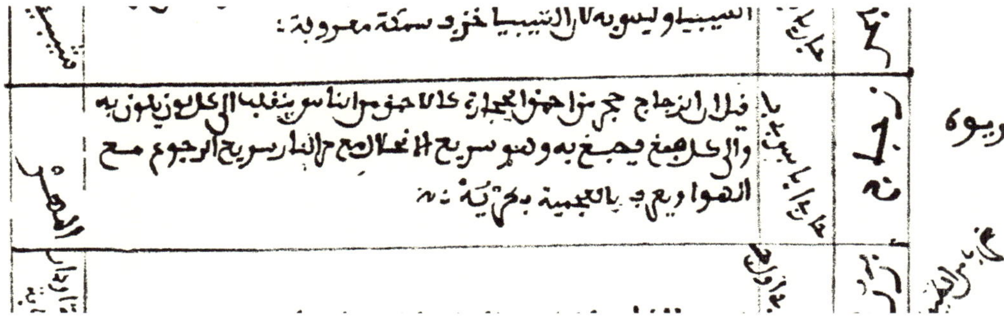

Fig. 23.
Rabat, General Library, MS D 2960, p. 113

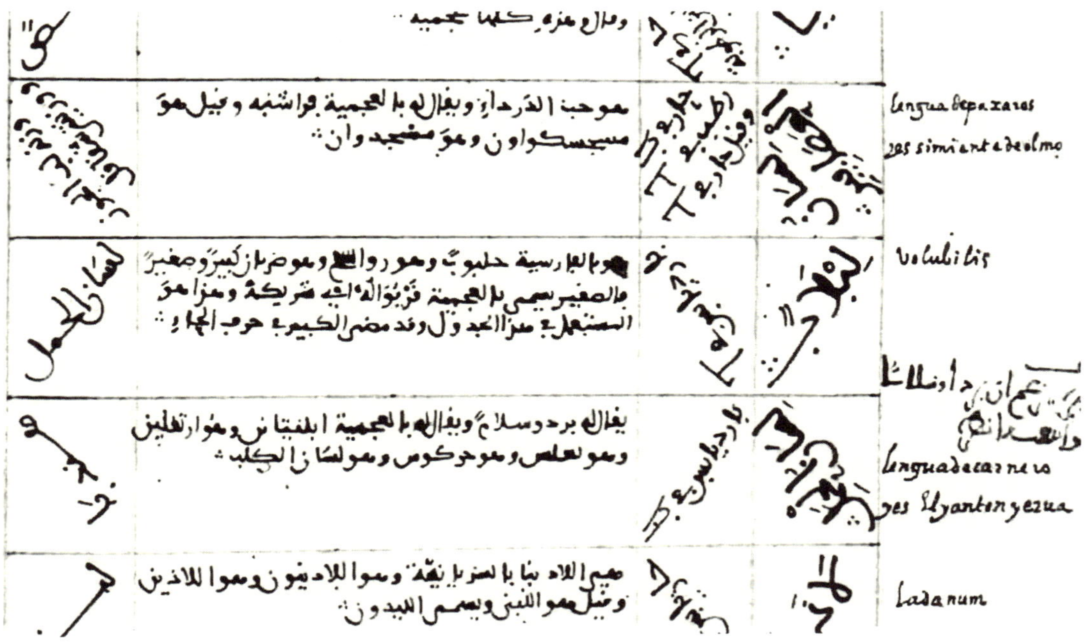

Fig. 24.
Leiden, University Library, Cod. Or. 15, fol. 68b

We thus see how the copyists (and perhaps readers) of the various manuscripts of the *Kitāb al-Mustaʿīnī* modified and adapted terms of the *ʿajamiyya* of al-Andalus in the original text of Ibn Baklarish, while enriching the Romance synonyms with new words from various parts of the Ibero-Romance linguistic area.

Marginalia

But the interest of the various manuscripts of the *Kitāb al-Mustaʿīnī* for the Hispanic Romance languages goes further still. The copyists and readers (as well as other occasional users) also left evidence of their consultation of these codices with glosses and other marginal notes concerning the names of the *materia medica*. These *marginalia* allow us to discover new Ibero-Romance linguistic varieties and add further lexicographical material to be added to the rich harvest we have reaped so far.

Although it should come first because of its date, I shall leave the case of the Arcadian manuscript to the end, in the form of an epilogue. Where the Latin synonyms in the work of Ibn Baklarish are concerned, this manuscript provides the most fascinating perspectives and its glosses introduce us to the area of middle Latinity which will provide still more new Romance words.

Let us start with the Madrid manuscript (M). In its margins, besides various annotations in Arabic and Hebrew, it provides frequent glosses in Latin script with the names of the medicaments in Castilian. These were already referred to by Simonet who observed, for example, that the word *qurrat al-ʿayn* is glossed by the expression *cunylla del agua*.[85] To this we can add forms such as *espadilla* [Fig. 22], which we read in the margin of the Arabic entry *wajj*, *poleo* for the Arabic *miskitrāmashīr*, or *fueya de la rosa*, as a gloss to the entry *ward*, 'rose'. In the last case we should note that the word *fueya* has a diphthongization of a short *o* before the *yod* and the resulting /y/ for the Latin group *-lj-*. This alerts us as to certain dialectal shades assumed by some of these unequivocally Castilian forms, whose geographical location must still be determined, but which, in tune with the provenance of this codex, we can regard as coming from the late medieval dialect of Toledo.

R1, in its turn, also provides frequent marginal notes. They are generally Arabic synonyms of the *materia medica*, but there are also a few other indications both by the copyist himself and in other hands. For our purpose it is worth pausing at the form *biṭriō* (بطريوه [b·ṭr.yū^{h}], in the margin of the entry *zujāj*) [Fig. 23] which hardly allows us to do more than establish its existence, although its particular spelling could suggest the intention of emphasizing the /o/ sound (and not /u/) of the final vowel.

The marginal glosses of the Leiden manuscript are especially interesting. We know that they are the work of al-Hajari,[86] and we now also have the testimony of al-Hajari himself who, in a letter of 2 February 1624, informed Golius that he had personally translated 'most of the names of the *materia medica* into Romance (*bi-l-ʿajamiyya*).'[87] These are the marginal notes we find in both the ancient (La) and the

85. Simonet, *Glosario*, p. 146.

86. Cf. Wiegers, *A Learned Muslim Acquaintance of Erpenius and Golius*, p. 66.

87. See the text of the letter in Jan Just Witkam's essay in the volume, pp. 78–9 below.

modern part (Lm) of the Leiden codex.

Most of al-Hajari's marginal notes consist of a simple gloss in Castilian on the Arabic names of the simples, placed next to the entry:

قشرَ اصل الرازيانج : *cortezas de raíces*
زَعْـرُورٌ : *níspolas*
بقْلة حمقـا : *uerdolaga*
جَاوَرْسٌ : *panizo*
ايرسا : *lirio azul*
افسِـنْـتين : *asensos*
شاه بلوط : *castañas*

On one occasion he states explicitly:

بَرْقُوقٌ : *en la lengua española albaricoques*

In some case the gloss gives the Latin name:

اقحوان : *parthenium*
لُـبِـيَا : *faseoli*
قرة الـعين : *pupilla oculi*

But the most frequent cases are those which contain both the Latin and the Spanish term:

فُـطْر : *fungi hongos*
تِينٌ : *higos ficus*
خَرْدَل : *sinapi mostaza*
حِمِّصٌ : *garuanços cicer*
أرْنَـبٌ : *liebre lepus*
سَفَرْجَلٌ : *cotonium membrillos*
سُوسٌ : *liquiritia oroçuç*

And there are also cases when the synonym is given not only in Spanish but also in French:

قَصْـدِيرٌ : *estaño eteyn.*

Sometimes we have a literal translation of the Arabic names as well as their Spanish equivalent:

لِسَانُ الـعَصَـافِير : *lengua de páxaros y es simiente de olmo*
لِسَانُ الـحَمَل : *lengua de carnero y es el yantén yerua* [Fig. 24].

Elsewhere the gloss is accompanied by a supplementary explanation:

سَدْرٌ : *árbol que haze nabac que es en Berbería*
عُلَّيْقٌ : *çarça que haze moras silvestres*
اشنه : *usna: muscus arboris que se cría en las enzinas y nogales*
إثْمدٌ : *alcohol con que alcoholan los ojos*
بَرْدِي : *entiendo que es enea*

When he does not seem to know an equivalent term in Castilian or Latin, al-Hajari simply gives the transliteration of the Arabic names in his gloss:

قُلْبٌ : *culbun*
حَنْدَقُوقَا : *handacuca*
يَنْبُوتٌ : *yambut,* etc.

We should also note that in this last example the transcription in Roman characters of the Arabic word reflects Hispanic orthographical habits (with an *m* before a *b*), while the gloss given above for *lisān al-ḥamal* is a clear and early case of *yeísmo* (*es el yantén* for *llantén*).

Finally, these glosses reveal another aspect of the many-sided and elusive personality of al-Hajari. He now emerges as versed in pharmacopea and able to translate into various languages the technical terms peculiar to the medical lexicon.[88]

We must complete this panorama of *marginalia* with R2, whose margins are full of notes by the copyist himself. He gives various textual indications and makes frequent comparisons between the *Kitāb al-Mustaʿīnī* and other treatises on *materia medica*, such as the *Tadhkira* by al-Antaki and, above all, the *Taṣrīf* by al-Zahrawi who, as I observed earlier, is Ibn Baklarish's main source for the synonyms of the names of the *materia medica* and, above all, for the *ʿajamiyya* of al-Andalus.

Of all the notes in this manuscript, we should observe one passage in particular in the margin of the entry *khardal*. Here the copyist transcribes an anonymous attestation (*dhakara baʿḍu-hum*) of a term 'in the Spanish language' (*bi-lisān al-isbanyūl*), namely, مصْطَزَّة [m·ṣṭazz·ᵗ], i.e. *moṣṭazza* [Fig. 25]. This is a modern attestation, in tune with the late date of the manuscript (1891), which reveals a system of Romance transliteration different from the one used in al-Andalus. It uses, rather, the soft consonants *ṭa'* and *ṣād* for the Hispanic consonants /t/ and /s/, according to the adoption of Hispanicisms in the modern Moroccan dialect to which I alluded earlier. On the other hand the representation of the last consonant with *zāy* seems to indicate that we are faced with a voiced sibilant, like the one in the medieval Hispanic system, and consequently neither interdentalized nor pronounced with a lisp. This would seem to contradict the 'modernity' of a word expressly described as Spanish. The explicit addition of the *tashdīd* above the *zāy*, however, suggests that this word *mostazza,* in a Moroccan manuscript of the late nineteenth century, could

88. This polyglottism, surprising in the case of pharmaceutical Latin, seems to indicate that al-Hajari was familiar with the medicine practised in Christian Spain, a circumstance which should perhaps be connected with a passage in his autobiography where he refers to his supposed studies in Madrid with a Morisco doctor from Valencia who taught him to read Arabic. The episode is substantiated and discussed by Luis F. Bernabé Pons, 'Una nota sobre Aḥmad ibn Qāsim al-Ḥaŷarī Bejarano', *Sharq al-Andalus*, 13, 1996, pp. 123–8 (esp. p. 126).

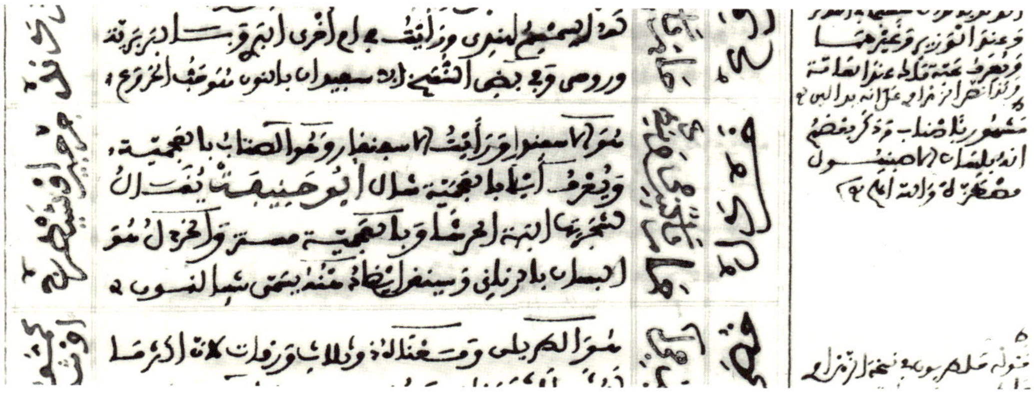

Fig. 25.
Rabat, General Library, MS D 55, p. 359

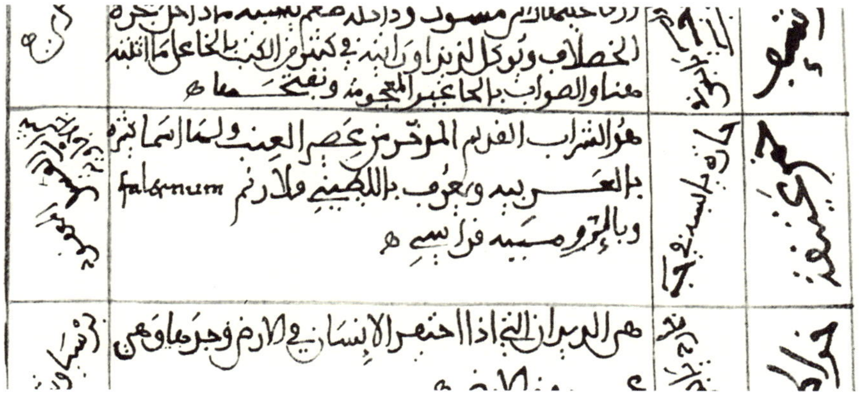

Fig. 26.
The Arcadian Library manuscript, p. 258

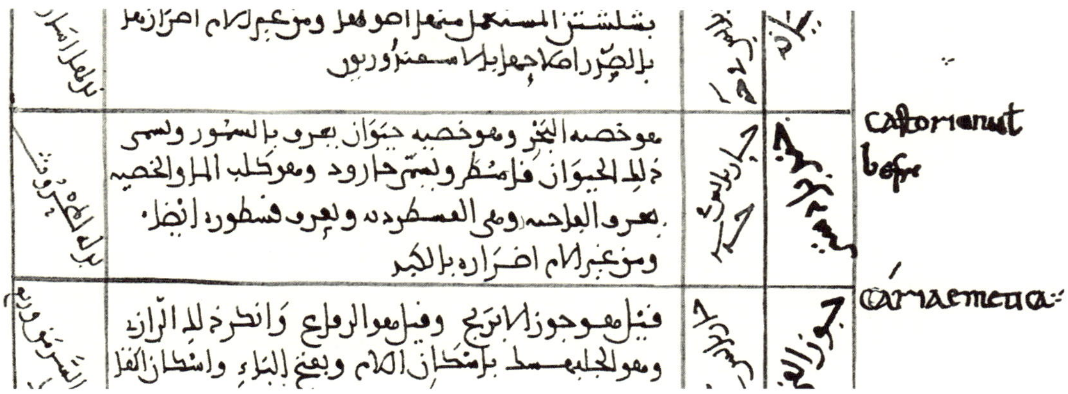

Fig. 27.
The Arcadian Library manuscript, p. 72

be taken from the *haketía* or Judaeo-Spanish of Morocco, in which we know that it was pronounced with a double voiced consonant.[89]

Latin epilogue: the manuscript in the Arcadian Library

To end this survey of the marginal notes by copyists and users of the various manuscripts of the *Kitāb al-Mustaʿīnī* we must return to our starting point, the earliest surviving testimony of the work, the manuscript in the Arcadian Library. I have deliberately postponed a consideration of its Latin glosses in order to consider them in the context of a different linguistic area occasionally present in the work of Ibn Baklarish. They take us to the Latin of the Middle Ages which, in this manuscript, reveals interesting connections with Romance.

We should bear in mind that, besides the languages already mentioned, Ibn Baklarish also considered Latin. He provides a number of synonyms of medicinal substances in the language. Although this is not altogether exceptional for the period, it certainly cannot be considered habitual among Andalusi writers on *materia medica*. We do not know the source from which Ibn Baklarish derived these words. All we can say for sure is that the *Kitāb al-Mustaʿīnī* contains certain examples indicated as coming from the Latin language (*laṭīniyya*),[90] and the readings of which have been transmitted by the different codices with varied fortunes. They are as follows: وير [w·yr] (s.v. *bawl al-insān* 'human urine'), شانقم د قانم [sh·ʾnq·m d· q·ʾn·m] (s.v. *damm al-kalb,* 'dog's blood', تريدقوم [tr·yd·q·wm] (s.v. *ḥinṭa,* 'wheat'), ملازيم [m·l·ʾz·ʸ·m] (s.v. *khamr ʿatīqa,* 'old wine') and فرمينتم [f·rm·ynt·m] (s.v. *khamīr*, 'yeast').[91] Here we can recognize, respectively, the Latin words or Latinized expressions *vir*, *sanguinem de canem*, *triticum*, *mellaceum* and *fermentum*.

In the case of these words the Arcadian manuscript presents some peculiarities of the greatest interest. First, however, certain points should be kept in mind. In the absence of the full codicological study required by this remarkable manuscript, we should remember that it was copied in a cultivated Hispanic ambience of the first third of the twelfth century, where both Arabic and Latin were the languages of the educated, while Romance Castilian was the spoken vernacular. This, as we shall see, seems to point to a particular place in the Crown of Castile, namely to Mozarabic Toledo, from which other comparable manuscripts originated.[92]

89. See Corominas, *DCECH*, s.v. *mostaza*.
90. Under the attribution to *laṭīniyya* the earliest medical treatises of al-Andalus (tenth century) provide a certain amount of lexical material which can on no account be regarded as Latin, but is unequivocally Romance. The specification *laṭīnī ʿāmmī,* which we sometimes find in Ibn Juljul, should consequently be understood as applying to a popular language in everyday use. The term *ʿajamiyya* referring to Romance becomes general after al-Zahrawi and is to be found in all later authors. Nevertheless they still contain sporadic traces of the earlier term, as we see in Ibn Baklarish himself when, for example, he ascribes to *laṭīnī* the Romance words *yedqo* and *sabúqo* (s.v. *ḥamā aqṭī*), or in Ibn al-Baytar's statement (thirteenth century) that 'Latin is the *ʿajamiyya* of al-Andalus' (*al-laṭīniyya wa-hiya ʿajamiyyat al-Andalus*), repeated in his *Kitāb al-Jāmiʿ*.
91. The forms transcribed here are from M. I have corrected the second word according to the other manuscripts.
92. See Pieter Sjoerd van Koningsveld, *The Latin–Arabic Glossary of the Leiden University Library. A Contribution to the Study of Mozarabic Manuscripts and Literature*, Leiden 1997.

Furthermore, it is not unlikely that the marginal notes in this manuscript which gloss, in Latin, in a carefully executed Carolingian script with some traces of uncial, the names of the medicaments, were written at the same time as the Arabic text. This needs to be confirmed. What is beyond doubt is that certain Latin annotations, not in the margin but in the work itself, were written simultaneously with the Arabic and presumably by a single copyist. This copyist, moreover, being equally versed in both languages and alphabets, made some changes in the Latin words which give rise to curious variants in both the Arabic and the Latin script, to which we shall now turn.

In the entry *damm al-kalb* the copyist slightly altered the reading contained in the other manuscripts, and gives شانْقون دِ قان [shānqwin di qān], which we can interpret as *sanqwin de qan*.[93] Beneath this expression, furthermore, he wrote its equivalent, *sanguinis canis* [see Fig. 1], in a round Visigothic hand. But the conclusive evidence that these glosses in Latin script were written at the same time as the manuscript in Arabic is provided by other cases. In the entry *ḥinṭa,* for example, the copyist wrote in a Visigothic script the Latin word *triticum*, after saying that the synonym was *bi-l-laṭīniyya*, and not in Arabic script as it probably was in the original. And the Arabic text continues in the same line immediately after the Latin word.

No less interesting is the fact that, on other occasions, the copyist replaced the Latin term in Arabic script of the original with another word also in Arabic script. This is the case of the Latin synonym for 'man' (s.v. *bawl al-insān*), of which, as we saw, M gives the original form *wīr*, but which this copyist replaced by برُون [b·rūn], i.e. *baron*, with a strange lexical preference for this Germanicism, albeit a Romance one, as opposed to the classical Latin form *vir*.

The copyist also made an eloquent correction of other terms, as, for example, in the case of the Latin synonym of the Arabic *khamr ʿatīqa,* 'old wine', where he does not hesitate to change the original consonantal *ductus* (ملازيم) to فلارنم [f·l·ʾrn·m] [Fig. 26]. He glosses it in the same line and in Latin characters with the word *falernum*, thus acknowledging the fame of the *vina falerna* in the Spain of the first third of the twelfth century.[94]

On yet other occasions the copyist glosses other words inside the table of the synonyms, which are not truly Latin but whose ancestry he recognizes. Thus, next to the word بشتِناقة [b·shtināqa^{t}], but without any specific attribution, he notes in Latin script *pastinaca*. Similarly, above the word of the *ʿajamiyya* فيالى [fi^{y}el·y], i.e. *fiele*, he puts the Latin term *feli*.

And he goes further still, since he sometimes actually replaces the word of the *ʿajamiyya* included in the work with a Latin form in Roman characters. This happens, for example, in the case of the form بنترونقة [b·ntr·wn·qa^{t}], which Ibn Baklarish records as proper to the *ʿajamiyya* of Saragossa (s.v. *kamādaryūs*), and which the copyist replaces by the Latin word *bettonica,* written in a Visigothic script.

93. Judging from the preposition and the form *qan* I would say that we are dealing, rather, with Romance words, while the first element of this composite expression seems to contain the nominative variant *sanguen* rather than *sanguis*.

94. On the same folio we find, for the entry *khamīr,* its Latin synonym in Arabic characters (فرْمنْتم) and, immediately afterwards, the same word in Latin characters (*furmentu*) [see Fig. 2], a variant of the Hispanic Latin (as opposed to the classical *fermentum*) postulated by various Ibero-Romance terms for yeast (e.g. Asturian *formientu*).

This promiscuity of Latin and Romance can also be found in the marginal glosses. Numerous entries of A are glossed in Latin in the margin and written in a carefully executed Carolingian script with traces of uncial and with the same ink used in the entries of the Arabic text to label the names of the medicaments.[95]

We cannot go into any further detail concerning these Latin terms (which are often of Greek origin), but it is interesting to note that they are sometimes Latinized Romance forms. An example is the gloss *castaniola*, in the margin of the entry *baṣl al-dhabir*, which must be connected with the word *qastanyuela* (قشتنواله [q·shtany·^{w}·ʾla^{t}]) from the *ʿajamiyya* of Saragossa offered in the text itself. Other glosses are entirely in Romance, such as *sarça*, in the margin of the Arabic *ʿullayq*, or *rata,* connected with *laḥm al-fār*, or, finally, cases such as that of the *castoreum* (s.v. *jundābustur*), glossed by a Latin form and a Romance synonym: *castorion vel befre* [Fig. 27], all early attestations (1130?) of Hispanic words for which Corominas gave later attestations in the Castilian domain. He found *sarça* in a document of North Castile dating from 1132, *rata* in the mid-thirteenth century in the translation of *Calila e Dimna*, and *befre* attested only very late, in 1606.[96]

Conclusion

In these pages I have concentrated on the work of Ibn Baklarish as a source for the study of the *ʿajamiyya* of al-Andalus. I have also tried to define the value of his attestations in the broader framework of Andalusi sources of a medical-botanical character. At the same time, the inventory of the various manuscripts of the *Kitāb al-Mustaʿīnī* and the filiation of its complex textual transmission have allowed me to contextualize the additions with which copyists and readers modified the text and enriched the margins of the various codices of the work, the detailed consideration of which has revealed a varied and surprising multilingual panorama which was hitherto unknown. And if, from the point of view of linguistic geography, the analysis of these codices has produced a survey of a considerable variety of Ibero-Romance languages (as much in al-Andalus as in Christian Spain and even in the Maghreb), from a chronological perspective the Romance attestations of these manuscripts cover a period which stretches from the early Middle Ages to the dawn of the twentieth century.

The manuscript of the Arcadian Library, which has now come to light in the dawn of the twenty-first century, not only marks the highest point of this temporal horizon (with its extremely early date), but it has also revealed an unsuspected range of Ibero-Romance variation. With its curious orthographic and linguistic promiscuity, it has taken us from Arabic to Romance, or *vice versa*, and from both to the area of Hispanic Middle Latin.

95. Together with this there are other marginal notes which are later and in another hand, and which, on some occasions, gloss these first ones. In the margin of the Arabic entry *anjura* ('nettle'), for example, we get *aqalifi*, which is later glossed as: *id est ortica* (that is, 'urtica'). The entry *asrab* ('lead') is glossed successively in both hands: *sirico .i. plunbi*, etc.

96. Corominas, *DCECH*, s.v. *zarza*, *rata* and *befre*. Fifteenth-century attestations of the last word appear in *DETEMA* (s.v.)

JAN JUST WITKAM

THE LEIDEN MANUSCRIPT OF THE *KITĀB AL-MUSTAʿĪNĪ*

Introduction

The Leiden copy of the tabular pharmacopoeia, the *Kitāb al-Mustaʿīnī* by Yusuf b. Ishaq Ibn Baklarish al-Isra'ili (*c.* 500/1106), is one of the oldest Oriental possessions of Leiden University Library.[1] It is associated with Jacobus Golius (1596–1667), who acquired the manuscript while participating in a diplomatic mission to Morocco in 1622–4, before his dazzling scholarly and academic career had even started. In 1629 the manuscript was incorporated in the Library, together with the other manuscripts which Golius had collected by that time, not only in North Africa, but above all in Aleppo and Constantinople.

The sudden influx of more than 200 Oriental manuscript volumes[2] in the Library made it necessary to organize these materials. The University librarian decided to create an Oriental manuscripts section and to place the new arrivals together, with a separate system of class-marks. These are the well-known Cod. Or. numbers of Leiden University Library, a system which is in use to this day.[3] That moment in 1629 can be regarded as the foundation of the Oriental collection within the Leiden Library. Oriental manuscripts had already been available in Leiden, albeit in small numbers, but it was the sheer bulk of Golius' acquisitions which made this novel approach necessary. The Golius manuscripts were simply and roughly arranged according to their size, and then numbered from Cod. Or. 1 onwards. Since the binding of the *Kitāb al-Mustaʿīnī* is of considerable size (30.5 cm high), it became the fifteenth entry in the inventory in order of size, and the volume consequently received the class-mark Or. 15, by which it has been known in scholarly literature ever since. The most important catalogues containing references to the manuscript are De Jong and De Goeje's of 1865 (pp. 246–9), and Voorhoeve's *Handlist*, p. 243.[4]

1. The medical materials are given in a rough alphabetical order by their names, divided into sections in the following order: *alif, bāʾ, jīm, dāl, hāʾ, wāw, zāy, ḥā, ṭāʾ, yāʾ, kāf, lām, mīm, nūn, sīn, ʿayn, fāʾ, qāf, rāʾ, ṣād, tāʾ, thāʾ, khāʾ, dhāl, ghayn, shīn*. This order is neither the Maghribi nor the Mashriqi order of *abjad*. The sequence of the lemmata within each letter (the first six simplicia given are: *amīr bārīs, aqāqiyā, aqḥawān, abhal, anjara, anjarān*; the last ones are *shaḥm al-rubb, shaḥm al-thaʿlab, shaḥm al-ḥimār, shaḥm al-baṭṭ, shaḥm al-dajāj, shuḥūm mukhtalifa*) does not follow this alphabetical order, nor does the order of the letters within each lemma.
2. In fact the Golius collection now comprises 211 inventory numbers, several of which consist of more than one volume, and which together contain many more texts.
3. At the time of writing (February 2006), the highest number was Cod. Or. 26,515.
4. Piet De Jong and Michael Jan De Goeje, *Catalogus Codicum Orientalium Bibliothecae Academiae Lugduno Batavae*, vol. 3, Leiden 1865; Petrus Voorhoeve, *Handlist of Arabic Manuscripts in the Library of the University of Leiden and other Collections in The Netherlands*, 2nd edition, The Hague 1980.

Provenance of the Leiden manuscript

Fig. 28.
Letter from Ahmad b. Qasim al-Andalusi in Marrakesh to Jacobus Golius in Safi, dated 12 Rabīʿ II 1033 A.H. (Friday 2 February 1624 A.D.). Manchester, John Rylands University Library, MS Persian 913, fol. 159

We are more than usually well informed about the Leiden manuscript's earlier provenance and history. While in Morocco Golius corresponded with an old acquaintance of his professor of Arabic in Leiden, Thomas Erpenius (1584–1624). This learned Muslim was Ahmad b. Qasim al-Andalusi (*c.* 1570–after 1640), an experienced traveller *in partibus infidelium.*[5] Jacobus Golius and Ahmad b. Qasim corresponded. Golius was in Safi on the Atlantic coast, acting as an engineer attached to the Dutch diplomatic mission, while his correspondent was in Marrakesh in an influential position in the Moroccan court.[6] Hardly surprisingly, books are indeed among the subject of the correspondence and the *Kitāb al-Mustaʿīnī* is mentioned several times. Two of Ahmad b. Qasim's letters to Golius are particularly relevant to the earlier provenance of the Leiden manuscript of the *Kitāb al-Mustaʿīnī* and deserve to be quoted in full.[7] On 12 Rabīʿ II 1033 (Friday 2 February 1624) Ahmad b. Qasim wrote from Marrakech to Jacobus Golius [Fig. 28]:[8]

5. See Gerard Wiegers, *A Learned Muslim Acquaintance of Erpenius and Golius: Aḥmad b. Ḳasim al-Andalusī and Arabic Studies in the Netherlands*, Leiden 1988; Ahmad ibn Qasim al-Hajari, *Kitāb Nāṣir al-dīn ʿalā ʾl-qawm al-kāfirīn* (*The supporter of Religion against the Infidels*), historical study, critical edition and annotated translation by P.S. van Koningsveld, Q. al-Samarrai and G.A. Wiegers. Madrid 1997 (Fuentes Arábico-Hispanas, 21).
6. Ahmad b. Qasim's letters are now kept in Leiden Cod. Or. 1228, nos. 32, 33, 34, 101, 114. Not so long ago, the former companion volume of Leiden Cod. Or. 1228 was discovered by Jan Schmidt in the John Rylands Library, Manchester, MS Persian no. 913. A film of that manuscript is in Leiden (A 2092). See Jan Schmidt, 'An Ostrich Egg for Golius; The Heyman Papers Preserved in the Leiden and Manchester University Libraries and Early-Modern Contacts between the Netherlands and the Middle East', in his *The Joys of Philology: Studies in Ottoman Literature, History and Orientalism (1500–1923)*, vol. 2: *Orientalists, Travelers and Merchants in the Ottoman Empire, Political Relations between Europe and the Porte*, Istanbul 2002, pp. 9–74, esp. pp. 19–20. The Manchester manuscript also contains other materials in the hand of Ahmad b. Qasim. Ahmad b. Qasim left other traces during his peregrinations. In their historical study on Ahmad b. Qasim's memoirs, van Koningsveld, al-Samarrai and Wiegers (p. 31, n. 83) mention several manuscripts in the Bibliothèque Nationale de France in Paris which contain notes in Ahmad's hand (MSS ar. 1181, 4119, 4213 and 4348). Ahmad b. Qasim's somewhat nostalgic note in MS ar. 1181, fol. 99b, deserves to be quoted here in full, if only to enable us to dismiss the fantasies of the three Dutch scholars about Ahmad b. Qasim's way of writing his own name:

كنت فى مدينة برّش ورايت هذا الكتاب وعرفت انه كتب فى بلادنا وهى بالمغرب اعادنا الله اليها بأمانه والسلام احمد بن قاسم فقير
الاندلسى عفا الله عنه

'I was in the town of Barrish [Paris] and I saw this book and I knew that it had been written in our land, which is in the Maghrib, may God return us to it safe and sound, *wa-l-Salām*. Ahmad b. Qasim, poor [servant of God], the Andalusian, may God forgive him.'

The writer of these lines was in France between 1610 and 1613. MS Paris ar. 1181 (containing al-Jazuli's *Dalāʾil al-Khayrāt*, dated 1 Ramaḍān 1007/1599 and copied by a certain Ahmad b. Ibrahim) was then in the possession of Etienne Hubert (a mutual friend of Ahmad b. Qasim and Thomas Erpenius), as becomes clear from Hubert's owner's note on the second flyleaf at the end of the volume: 'De la Bibliothecque de E. Hubert Lecteur du Roy en langue Arabicque sil se perd il vous supplie luy rendre.' Hubert apparently acquired the manuscript, still almost brand-new, when he himself was in Morocco, a few years earlier.
7. Golius' part of the correspondence is not known to have been preserved.
8. John Rylands Library, Manchester, MS Persian no. 913, fol. 169 (no. 57).

الحمد لله والصلاة والسلام على رسله الاكرمين وعلى من تبعهم الى يوم الدين

الكتاب الى صاحبنا المكرم النبيه الكاتب الفقيه النصراني الفلمنك
يعقوب جول وبعد فان كتابك العربي بلغنا وفرحنا به غاية
وفهمنا خطابكم وما تضمنه اما ما ذكرت عن النسخة التي انسخناها
من الكتاب المسمى بالمستعيني فاني ابذلت جهدي في اتقانها كما سيظهر لك
من تراجمها اذ ثم جملة اكثر اسماء مفردات فيها بالاعجمية ليسهل عليك فهمها
و تستنسخ نسخة اخرى زايدة على نسخة صاحبنا الطبيب ومنهما تصحح ما
نسخته وحملني على ذلك مسئلتان الاولى قول نبينا عليه السلام رحم الله من
عمل صنعة فاتقنها والثانية ظننت انكم تدخلونها في القالب ولا ينبغي ان
يصنع فيه الا ما هو صحيح واما ما ذكرت عن معرفة بلاد المولف اظنها بلاد الاندلس
ولا نحققه في اي زمان كان وربما يظهر ذلك من كتاب مروج الذهب لانه
ذكر في اول كتاب الطب انه هداه لفلان بن فلان وفي تلك التاريخ يظهر في
اي زمان كان المهدى له وفي غير هذا اليوم نكتب لك الجواب الى شيخك العالم
المدرس ارتبينيوس ان شا الله نسئله ان يزيدك نعمة ويردك سالما الى بلادك
وكتبنا في مراكش حرسها الله في الثالث عشر من ربيع الثاني عام ثلث وثلاثين
والف سنة ومن الحساب العجمي في الثاني من شهر فبراير اربع وعشرين وستمائة
والف سنة وكتب مملوك المقام العلي واسير ذنبه

احمد بنقاسم
[illegible]

Alseñor jacob gul[9]

الحمد لله والصلاة والسلام على رسله الاكرمين وعلى من تبعهم الى يوم الدين

الكتاب الى صاحبنا المكرم النبيه الكايس الفقيه النصرانى الافلمنك يعقوب چول وبعد فان كتابك العزيز
بلغنا وفرحنا به غاية وفهمنا خطابكم وما تضمنه اما ما ذكرت عن النسخة التي انسخناها من الكتاب
المسمى بالمستعين فانى ابذلت جهدى فى اتقانها كما سيظهر لك من تراجمها اذ ترجمت اكثر اسمآء
مفرداتها بالاعجمية ليسهل عليك فهمها وفتشت نسخة اخرى زآئدة على نسخة صاحبنا الطبيب ومنهما
صححنا نسختك وحملنى على ذلك مسئلتان الاولى قول نبئنا عليه السلام رحم الله من عمل صنعة بأتقانها
والثانية ظننت انكم تدخّلونها فى الغالب ولا ينبغى ان يصنع فيه الا ما هو صحيح واما ما ذكرت عن معرفة
بلاد المؤلف اظنها بلاد الاندلس ولا تحققت فى اي زمان كان وربما يظهر ذلك من كتاب مروج الذهب لانه
ذكر فى اول كتاب الطيب انه هداه لفلان بن فلان وفى تلك التاريخ يظهر في اى زمان كان المهدى له وفى
غير هذا اليوم نكتب لك الجواب الى شيخك العالم المدرس اربنيوش ان شا الله نسئله ان يزيدك نعمة ويردك
سالما الى بلادك وكتبنا فى مراكش حرسها الله فى الثان عشر من ربيع الثانى عام ثلاث وثلاثين والف سنة
ومن الحساب العجمى فى الثانى من شهر فبراير اربع وعشرين وست مائة والف سنة وكتب مملوك المقام
العلى واسير ذنبه

احمد بن قاسم
لطف الله به

To Mr Jacob Gool

Praise be to God, and blessing and peace be upon His most noble messengers and on those who follow them till the Day of Judgement.

This letter is to our honoured, intelligent, courteous, learned, Christian, Dutch friend, Jacob Gool.

Your kind letter has reached us and we rejoiced at it very much, and we have understood what you wrote and what was contained in the letter. In connection with what you said about the manuscript that we had copied of the book entitled al-Mustaʿīnī, *I did my best to do this in a perfect way, as will be clear to you from the translations in it, as I have translated most of the names of the simple medicines into Spanish bi-l-aʿjamiyya* [sic], *which should facilitate your comprehension of it, and I have collated it with another copy, an additional one to the copy of our friend, the doctor. From these two we corrected your copy. I was induced to do this by two matters. The first is the word of our Prophet, peace be upon him: 'God has mercy on whoever performs his craft to perfection.'*[10] *The second is that I assumed that you wanted, mostly, to have these included, and that it is only appropriate to include something in it which is correct. As to what you said about information concerning the land of origin of the author, I think this is Andalusia, but I was unable to ascertain from*

9. This line in Spanish, on the reverse side of the paper.

10. Quotation not found in the canonical collections.

11. This particular manuscript of al-Masʿudi's *Murūj al-Dhahab* cannot be identified. Golius had apparently wanted to acquire it, but the copy was stolen, as is clear from Ahmad b. Qasim's letter to Golius of 29 February 1624. Therefore the identification by Wiegers (*A Learned Muslim Acquaintance*, p. 65, n. 155) of the stolen copy of the *Murūj al-Dhahab* as mentioned in Ahmad b. Qasim's letter of 29 February 1624, with Leiden Cod. Or. 127 seems impossible. His claim is silently corrected by van Koningsveld, al-Samarrai and Wiegers (n. 6 above), p. 43, n. 111. Leiden Cod. Or. 127, a medieval manuscript which does indeed contain part (namely the second book) of the *Murūj al-Dhahab*, is in so far remarkable that it has, among several other similar notes, a

which period. This may become clear from the book 'The Golden Meadows', since it was said at the beginning of the Kitāb al-Ṭīb *that he presented it to so-and-so, and from that date it is clear in which period the person to whom it was presented lived.*[11] *On another day I will write for you the answer to your Sheikh, the learned professor Erpenius, God willing, and from Him we ask to enlarge your blessings and to bring you back safely to your country. Thus written in Marrakesh, may God protect it, on twelve Rabīʿ II of the year one thousand and thirty-three, and in the Christian era on the second of February of the year one thousand six hundred and twenty-four. Thus written by the servant of the High Authority and the prisoner of his sins, Aḥmad b. Qāsim, may God treat him with kindness.*

Preliminary remarks on the basis of this letter:

~ *allatī ansakhnā* 'that we had copied', and which was therefore a manuscript which was apparently not copied by Ahmad b. Qasim himself. The owner of the first original was the medical doctor, whose name is not mentioned in either letter.
~ 'translations into Spanish'. These were apparently made by Ahmad b. Qasim.
~ 'I have collated it with another copy, an additional one to the copy of our friend, the doctor.' This means that there was another, presumably unrelated, manuscript copy of the *Kitāb al-Mustaʿīnī* around and available.
~ 'From these two we corrected your copy.' From this sentence, in which the grammatical dual is clearly visible, we may conclude that at least three copies of the *Kitāb al-Mustaʿīnī* are involved: the copy belonging to the doctor, the other copy, and finally 'your copy' (= Golius' copy).
~ 'may become clear from the book "The Golden Meadows"'. But the copy of that manuscript, which may have contained valuable information on the provenance of MS Leiden Or. 15, was stolen (as we read in Ahmad b. Qasim's letter to Golius of 29 February 1624, quoted below), and that information must now be regarded as lost.
~ 'the beginning of the *Kitāb al-Ṭīb*'. The meaning of this passage is unclear, unless al-Ṭīb is to be understood as al-Ṭibb, and then refers to the *Kitāb al-Mustaʿīnī*.

On 10 Jumādā I 1033 (Thursday 29 February 1624) Ahmad b. Qasim wrote again from Marrakesh to Jacob Golius in Safi [Fig. 29]:[12]

Alseñor jacob gul flamenco en safi

الحمد لله والصلاة والسلام على رسله

اما بعد حمد الله الواحد الاحد الفرد الصمد الذى لم يلد ولم يولد ولم يكن له كفوا احد فانى قبلت كتابك
وفرحت بما رايت من ضبط خطك ففهمت معناه ومرماه اما ما ذكرت من كتاب مرج الذهب انه لم يبلغ اليك

birth note on its title page (added later) for a boy ʿAbd al-Malik born on a Tuesday 12 June or 17 or 15 Rajab (year not clear, but after 988/1580, the date mentioned in a previously written birth note). May we conclude from the double calendar notation that this manuscript was once in the possession of Moriscos such as Ahmad b. Qasim, or were Christian dates used more often than one would think? In his first letter to Golius Ahmad b. Qasim also refers to both calendars.

12. Leiden Cod. Or. 1228, no. 32.

Fig. 29.
Letter from Ahmad b. Qasim in Marrakesh to Jacobus Golius in Safi, dated 10 Jumādā I 1033 A.H. (Thursday 29 February 1624 A.D.). Leiden, University Library, Cod. Or. 1228, no. 32

وانه نهبه العرب من ايدى حامله فذلك عادتهم فى هذه البلاد وفى هذا الزمان الصعب وفرحت اذ جاء
على غرضك الكتاب المستعينى فى صناعة الطب ما زلت نكتب لك فى شانه شيئ الان في غالب ظنى ان
النسخة التى بيد صاحبنا الطبيب ظهر لى انّ لها مكتوبة نحو الاربع مائة سنة وهو هذاك الكتاب المذكور
عجيب مقبول عند المسلمين وكنت ذكرت لى ان عندك حروفا محفوظة لميل الشمس لو امكان ان تردها
عربية او فى لسان الاشبانيول وتبعث لى نفرح بذلك والسلام وكتب فى مراكش المحروسة فى العاشر من
شهر جمادى الاوّل من عام ثلاث وثلاثين والف سنة

خديم المقام العلى

احمد بن قاسم
لطف الله به

To Mr Jacob Gool, Dutchman in Safi[13]

Praise be to God. Blessing and peace be to His messengers.
After thanking God, the One, the Unique, the Eternal, Who is not born, and to Whom no one is born, and to Whom there is no equal.[14] *I have received your letter and I was glad to see how well you can write, and I have understood its content and meaning. What you wrote about the 'Book of the Golden Meadows', namely that it had not arrived with you and that the Arabs had taken it from its bearer, well this is their habit in this land and in this difficult time.*[15] *It gives me pleasure to receive the news that it is your purpose to acquire* Kitāb al-Mustaʿīnī *on the Art of Medicine. I am writing to you once more about this because I think strongly that the copy, which is with its owner, the doctor, was written about four hundred years ago. It is a marvellous book and it is very much appreciated by the Muslims. You mentioned that you had with you a text*[16] *on astronomy [literally: 'the declination of the Sun']. If it would be possible to translate this into Arabic or Spanish, and then send it to me, that would give us pleasure. Greetings.*
Thus done in Marrākush, may God preserve it, on ten Jumādā I of the year one-thousand and thirty-three.
The Servant of the High Authority,
Aḥmad b. Qasīm, may God be kind to him.[17]

13. This line in Spanish is written on the reverse side.
14. *Qur'ān* 112.
15. It is probable that another (incomplete) copy, of the second volume only, of the *Murūj al-Dhahab* in Maghribi script later came into Golius' possession anyhow. It is now in Leiden, Cod. Or. 127. As I have already said, it is hardly possible that this volume was the same as the copy of the *Murūj al-Dhahab* which was stolen in Morocco while being brought to Golius.
16. Wiegers, *A Learned Muslim Acquaintance*, p. 65, translates *ḥurūfan maḥfūẓatan* as 'mnemonic words', a translation which he connects with work by Ahmad b. Qasim on *al-Risāla al-Zakūṭiyya* (p. 66). Van Koningsveld, al-Samarrai and Wiegers further elaborate on this in their historical study of 1997 (pp. 44–5).
17. The letter has been fully translated by Wiegers, *A Learned Muslim Acquaintance*, p. 65. Wieger's references to Ahmad b. Qasim's letters in manuscript Leiden Cod. Or. 1228 are confused, but his captions on pp. 80, 83–4 are correct. This letter was previously edited by Reinhardt Dozy in *Catalogus Codicum Orientalium Bibliothecae Academiae Lugduno Batavae*, vol. 1, Leiden 1851, pp. 161–2, and later once more edited and translated (into Dutch) by Martijn Theodor Houtsma, *Uit de Oostersche correspondentie van Th. Erpenius, Jac. Golius en Lev. Warner. Eene bijdrage tot de geschiedenis van de beoefening der Oostersche letteren in Nederland* (Verhandelingen der Koninklijke Akademie van Wetenschappen, Afdeeling Letterkunde, vol. 17, pt. 3), Amsterdam 1887, no. 5.

الحمد لله والصلاة والسلام على رسله

اما بعد حمد الله الواحد الاحد الفرد الصمد الذي لم يلد ولم يولد ولم يكن
له كفوا احد جاءني قبلت كتابك وفرحت بما رايت من ضبط
خطك وفهمت معناه ومرماه اما ما ذكرت من كتاب مروج
الذهب انه لم يبلغ اليك وانه نهبه العرب من ايدي حامله فذلك
عادتهم في هذه البلاد وفي هذا الزمان الصعب وفرحت اذ جاء
على غير ذلك الكتاب المستعينين في صناعة الطب مازلت نكتب لك
في شانه شيئا الا في غالب ظني ان النسخة التي بيد صاحبنا
الطبيب ظهر لي ان لها مكتوبة نحو لاربع مائة سنة وهو
هذاك الكتاب المذكور عجيب مقبول عند المسلمين وكنت
ذكرت لي ان عندك حروفا محفوظة لميل الشمس لو امكن
ان تردها عربية او في لسان الاشبانيول وتبعثها لي نعمل بذلك
والسلام وكتب في مراكش الحمراء وسه في العاشر من شهر جمادى
الاول من عام ثلاث وثلاثين والف سنة

خديم المقام العلي

احمد بن قاسم
الحجري لطف الله به

Preliminary remarks on the basis of this letter:

~ The present owner of *Kitāb al-Musta'īnī* is, again, said to be a medical doctor.
~ The book is said to be held in high esteem.
~ The doctor's manuscript is said to be four hundred years old.
~ Nothing is said about an incomplete or damaged manuscript.

The first two details can be taken at face value, but not so Ahmad b. Qasim's note on the antiquity of the manuscript. If this applies to Leiden Cod. Or. 15 (which is by no means sure) it can only apply to the old part of the manuscript, which is certainly medieval.

From the two letters of Ahmad b. Qasim we can gather that Golius' appetite for *Kitāb al-Musta'īnī* was whetted by the first letter. To this he may have answered that he wished to acquire a copy of the work, and we can assume that his interest was further aroused by the four-hundred-year-old manuscript mentioned in the second letter.

Physical description of the Leiden manuscript

When leafing through the Leiden manuscript the reader is immediately struck by the fact that the physical constitution of the volume is diverse. At first glance it is evident that a medieval manuscript of the *Kitāb al-Musta'īnī* had become very incomplete in the course of time, and that this incomplete copy (still containing 101 folios of old paper) had been supplemented by 34 newly written paper leaves. Old and new leaves together more or less make up the entire work, although only a full review of all existing witnesses of the text can confirm this. A clue for the dating of the repaired part of the text is the watermark in the new paper: an ornamented and crowned pot, with a crescent on top.

Although Briquet and Heawood give many pots in watermarks dating from the latter part of the sixteenth and the early seventeenth centuries,[18] none of these is similar to the watermark in Leiden Cod. Or. 15, nor is the identification of the watermark as given by Wiegers correct.[19] In Heawood,[20] as in Briquet, several of the pots have peculiarities very similar to those in the watermark in Leiden Cod. Or. 15, but none is positively identifiable with it. It shows, once more, that the reference works on watermarks can only be used as rough guides, not as precision instruments. The world of papermaking is infinitely more complex than can be described in such books. Personally I only use them for the purpose of corroboration, or refutation, and always in order to have an additional argument.

18. Charles M. Briquet, *Les filigranes: dictionnaire historique des marques du papier dès leur apparition vers 1282 jusqu'en 1600. A Facsimile of the 1907 Edition with Supplementary Material Contributed by a Number of Scholars*, ed. Alan Stevenson, Amsterdam, 1968.
19. Wiegers, *A Learned Muslim Acquaintance*, p. 66, n. 159, where there is a reference to Heawood No. 3563. Heawood's No. 3563, however, is not dated 1620, but 1600. The letters PR in Heawood 3563 are also at variance with what the watermark actually has: HL, as can been seen clearly in fol. 135.
20. Edward Heawood, *Watermarks Mainly of the 17th and 18th Centuries*, Hilversum 1950.

Wiegers was the first scholar to point out that the supplemented leaves in the Leiden manuscript of the *Kitāb al-Mustaʿīnī* are in fact written by Ahmad b. Qasim himself. For this he convincingly adduces palaeographical evidence, by a simple juxtaposition of Ahmad b. Qasim's letter in Or. 1228, no. 32, to a random supplemented page in Or. 15.[21] If we compare this with the words by Ahmad b. Qasim in his letter of 2 February 1624 (*ansakhnāhā*, 'we had it copied') it is clear that this cannot apply to MS Leiden Cod. Or. 15, which Ahmad b. Qasim did copy, but to another manuscript of the *Kitāb al-Mustaʿīnī*, which must have been copied by someone else. In the time immediately preceding Golius' acquisition of his copy of the *Kitāb al-Mustaʿīnī* there must have been at least three manuscripts of the text around.

It may also be assumed from this that the *Kitāb al-Mustaʿīnī* was not a very rare work. When Ahmad b. Qasim writes to Golius on 29 February 1624 that the *Kitāb al-Mustaʿīnī* 'is a marvellous book and ... very much appreciated by the Muslims', this implies a certain popularity and availability of the text. If Ahmad b. Qasim, in that same letter to Golius, mentions four centuries as the age of the manuscript, and if he is writing about the manuscript which is now Leiden Cod. Or. 15, this can only apply to the part of the text on old paper. Ahmad b. Qasim's estimate is not meant as an accurate dating, but even if the four centuries are an exact indication of the manuscript's age in 1624, the old part of the manuscript would date from around 1224.[22] I do not wish to exclude this as a possible estimate for the age of the old, original parts of the Leiden manuscript.

The division between the old part and the supplement on new paper is as follows:

New paper	Old paper
folios 1–13	folios 14–15
16	17
18	19
20–23	24–29
30	31–43
44	45–47
48	49–82
83	84–96

21. Wiegers, *A Learned Muslim Acquaintance*, p. 66. Wiegers' remark on Golius completing the manuscript is wrong. A rather puzzling remark about Or. 15 was already made by Dozy, *Catalogus*, vol. 1, p. 162, n. 1. It would imply that Or. 15 also contained copies of other books. This is not the case at present, nor, in all probability, was it the case in Dozy's time, since the previous printed catalogue of the Leiden Library (*Catalogus Librorum tam Impressorum quam Manuscriptorum Bibliothecae Publicae Universitatis Lugduno Batavae*, Leiden 1716, p. 443, no. 809) mentions the text as the only one in the binding. In the description of Or. 15 (De Jong and De Goeje, *Catalogus*, vol. 3, no. 1339), p. 249, n. 1, we find the further specification that the supplemented leaves were probably made *Golii jussu*, at Golius' request. Dozy, De Jong and De Goeje did not realize that Ahmad b. Qasim was in fact the copyist himself, but they all knew Golius' handwriting too well to commit the error which Wiegers ascribes to them.

22. This 'four hundred years' may be based on knowledge of part of Leiden Cod. Or. 15, which is now lost. This may be a colophon or some owner's note. We do not know. It is also possible that such information was somehow preserved in the (stolen) copy of the *Murūj al-Dhahab*.

97	98–100
101	102–115
116	117–125
126	127
128–135	
Total: 34 folios	Total: 101 folios

The manuscript as a whole now consists of 135 leaves, which were numbered in the 1970s by a Leiden librarian, in pencil, as 1–135 in the upper margin of each recto page. All references to the Leiden manuscript in this article follow this foliation. Roughly three-quarters have been preserved on old paper and one quarter was supplemented by Ahmad b. Qasim on new paper. The structure of the old paper occasionally shows a pair of parallel chain lines (e.g. fol. 95) and is evidently of much older date than the newly added leaves, the early thirteenth century having been mentioned already as a possibility. The old paper is of a somewhat smaller size (26.7 x 19.2 cm and sometimes less because of wear and tear) than the new paper (29 x 19.5 cm). The volume is now bound in a European-style full parchment binding, which may mean that the pages were only bound when Golius brought them back to Leiden. He did the same with other piles of paper which he collected, such as the Leiden Cod. Or. 14.

All the old leaves, and a number of the new ones, have been fixed on guards of paper, with the result that no bifolium of the old part of the manuscript has been preserved. If there were still bifolia intact when Golius acquired the manuscript, these must have been cut into single folia for the purpose of the restoration scheme which was applied to the entire manuscript. These guards of paper of about 1 cm width have been made in such a way that they constitute quires and give the book as a whole a quired structure. A conspectus of the quires of Leiden Cod. Or. 15 is a follows: I (1–8), II (9–14), III (15–23), IV (24–31), V (32–9), VI (40–7), VII (48–55), VIII (56–63), IX (64–71), X (72–9), XI (80–7), XII (88–95), XIII (96–103), XIV (104–11), XV (112–19), XVI (120–7), XVII (128–35). There is an evident preference of Ahmad b. Qasim, who did the restoration work, to make quires of eight leaves. Bifolia of the newly supplied paper were kept intact as far as possible: quires I and XVII consist entirely of the new paper and these therefore consist of bifolia. The fact that these quires had to be fully replaced shows, again, that the most vulnerable parts of a book block are the beginning and the end.[23] All the other quires are of mixed composition and only rarely do we see bifolia in the new paper in such mixed quires (fols. 10–13, 11–12 and 21–2 only).

23. One might even wonder whether the traditional Islamic horizontal storage of books may have been more likely to aggravate this type of damage, which would be less likely to occur in, or would be less detrimental to, books which are stored vertically.

Maintaining the order of the leaves

That several owners of the manuscript have tried to maintain the correct order of the leaves becomes clear by their numbering of the leaves or pages. Apart from the modern foliation, the Leiden manuscript shows five older systems of foliation or pagination, only one of which was made on both the old and the new paper. This full foliation was probably made by Ahmad b. Qasim. He did not number the folios of the introductory part, since the correct order of the leaves there is secured by a system of catchwords. The double-page openings with the *jadāwil*, the first being fols. 12b–13a, are numbered by Ahmad b. Qasim from the first one onwards. These numbers (1–122) are written, almost without a break, in the upper right-hand corner of each verso (i.e. right-hand) page, from fol. 12b onwards. Sometimes one can see corrections in mistakenly written numbers. The purpose of this numbering was to count the double openings of the text. Where a double opening has text which may be disregarded, this page has been crossed out and the opening is not numbered [fols. 13b–14a: Fig. 30]. This system of numbering is therefore related to the restoration work on the Leiden manuscript.

The other numbering systems are older, since they can only be seen on the leaves of old paper. Their relative age could not be established, but there may be a relationship between some of them:

~ A foliation with roman numerals on fols. 14a, 15a, 17a, 19a, at the bottom of each recto page, sometimes somewhat centred. It shows the numbers 3, 4, 6 and 8, respectively. Note that numbers 1, 2, 5 and 7 are missing, but for these the old paper was replaced by the new, meaning that the foliation was added when the old paper part of the manuscript was (more) complete.

~ A pagination with roman numerals (2–11) at the bottom of the page in the section consisting of fols. 25a–29b. There is no numeral visible on fol. 24a. Fols. 24 and 25 are apparently the leaves that were on top of the pile and have suffered most from wear and tear. The pagination had been added when these leaves were on top of the bundle of paper.

~ A system of foliation in large *ghubārī* numerals, written with a thick pen in the upper margin of a recto page. The first of these that can be observed is on fol. 28a, followed by a fragment of a numeral which is on fol. 29a; neither can be identified with certainty. The tens seem to be written in reverse order: '03' for '30' (fol. 43a), '04' for '40' (fol. 52a), '05' for '50' (fol. 60a). To this series of *ghubārī* numerals belong the numbers within the section consisting of fols. 42a–65a [Fig. 31]. After fol. 65a this thick numbering suddenly stops. Not all of these *ghubārī* numerals are very legible, but remnants of most numerals can still be seen. Several lacunae in the numbering can be observed as well (if '40' is on fol. 52a and '50' on fol. 60a, either two leaves are missing or the scribe has skipped two numbers by mistake). To find out whether these lacunae in the numbering coincide with lacunae in the text is the editor's task.

~ Another system of foliation in large *ghubārī* numerals, now written with a thinner pen in the upper margin of each recto page. Between fols. 59a and 63a there is an overlap of the two *ghubārī* foliation systems. The thinner one there is possibly meant to be a correction to the thicker one. The entire system of these thin *ghubārī* numerals

OVERLEAF
Fig. 30.
The first leaf of old (original) paper of the Leiden MS of the *Kitāb al-Musta'īnī*. The text on this recto page of the old part, being only half of a double page with information (?), could not be used by Ahmad b. Qasim al-Andalusi in his restoration programme, and was therefore crossed out. Later, he supplied the text in his own hand on fol. 22a. Leiden, University Library, Cod. Or. 15, fol. 14a

FOLLOWING OVERLEAF
Fig. 31.
The long passage in Spanish, probably written by Ahmad b. Qasim al-Andalusi. The passage reads: 'que virtud pueden criar las ymagines pues llevan a quien las haze y a quien las adora al ynfierno y si fueren de oro o plata no se pueden servir dellas antes deven echarlas en el fuego'. On the basis of this passage, Dozy (in a note loosely inserted in the MS) assumed that the author of this note is of the Jewish faith, apparently because of the abhorrence of idols. Over the text the numeral '39' has been written in the older *ghubārī* foliation. Leiden, University Library, Cod. Or. 15, fol. 49a

مسيح اللاذخر يثقل الراس ... ابر الجن ... احود ... ... الحي

... ... واذا استعط بعصارته ... المخالفة للصرع او حبه
... ... اشد من البارد وفي صبغه قبض وقوة تنضج وتحلل مجرب لفم الافعي

منافعها وخواصها ووجوه استعمالها

قوتها الاولى قوة تسخن قليلا وتجفف بغير لذع والثانية قوة تجلو جلاء بليغا وتجذب والثالثة قوة تخرج السلى من بطن الحمل وعصارتها تنفع مما في الدماغ وتخرجه من المنخرين وتدمل الجراحات وتمسك انتشار القروح الخبيثة في البدن واذا تغرغر بعصارته نقا الراس من البلغم وقد يستعط بذلك واذا شرب بشراب نفع من نهش الافاعي ومن وجع الكبد والكلى

حسن اكليل الملك قابض ملين للاورام الحارة ولا سيما الاورام العارضة في العين والرحم والمقعدة والانثيين واذا طبخ بالميبختج وتضمد به وربما خلط مع صفرة بيضة او دقيق الحلبة او دقيق بزر الكتان اذا استعمل وحده شفى القروح الشهدية واستعمل بالعفص والشراب واذا شرب بالشراب سكن وجع المعدة

ح يصلح لاوجاع الرحم اذا طبخت وجلس في مائها وهي نافعة اذا وقعت في اخلاط الدهن والادهان التي تحلل الاعياء وقد تقع في اخلاط دهن البان وسائر الادهان واذا انقعت في شراب انام ذلك الشراب نوما عرقا ونفعت المعدة وطيبتها واذا مضغت نفع البخر والقيء

هو محلل نفاخ منق للرطوبات الزايدة في المعدة مفتح لسدد الكبد ويحلل غشاء الطحال وغلظه مدر للبول والطمث واقوى شيء الدواء الحاطله وبعده الثمر والحب ثم الورق والزهر واذا شرب بقصب ... نفع وجع النقرس من الاورام ... وقد يضمد به الطحال ... الشعير للورم العارض فيه وقد يحلل ... والاورام الصلبة

في الحزير تقوية القلب وتصبية لدمه وهو جيد للخفقان اذا استعمل في دواء المسك ... ليسهل سحقه ويزيد للطبيعة وبعضهم لا يرى ذلك لئلا تذهب قوته ويغرضه قرطا رقيقا ويسحق مع اللولو والكهربا والبسد حتى ينسحق وبعضهم يستخرج قوة الكثير منه في ماء بالطبخ ويسقى ذلك الماء الادوية

طه قوته بالجملة مسخنة ميبسة وهي تعين على ... الرياح عن البدن وتسكن الوجع محللة مدرة للبول والعرق مذيبة للفضول وتوافق ذوات السموم من الهوام ويقطع سيلان الرطوبات التي لونها ابيض من الرحم وتدر البول واللبن وتنهض شهوة الجماع وقيل انه حار يابس في الدرجة الثالثة

والحواقة ... اكثر والقعومة ... واخفى ويذكر ... معلا للاورام الحاسية الباطنة والظاهرة
باعتدال الطبع جيد للقلب مقو لجرمه ح اجود الابنسبوز ما كان منه ... كبير الحب قوي الرائحة

بالادكرك المعروف بلبين الزهبار من غير ان يكون معه اللبن لا كن جمتد كما تجتمد الصمغ كى قيل ان الورس لا يكون الا باليمن
[illegible] اجبد اداكه تهتت خوايكه بينتعض منها الورس البارد و هو
يخرج صبغها صبغ خالص الصفرة و البارد في صبغها حمرة وبغ شل لسورس بسورس العو عر

منافعها وخواصها و وجوه استعمالها

ملطف منق للجراح تنبعنه يسيرة ويجرب جزبا مستريا وجوهره لطيف جدا ويهيج العطاش دا **اسحق** من فعله انه يسخن اسخانا قويا و يجزب من العمق ويخرج السل من باطن اللحم واذا انجور به نفع من السعال واذا لطخ على الفوابد ابرا ها **اسحق** طبيعته طبيعة الثوم

قابض ينفع وينفع الكلف وله قوة صباغة وينفع اذا شرب من البهق الابيض د **لبعض الاطباء** اذا لطخ على البهق والبثور الكاينة في سطح الجسم والحكة نفعهما **ابو حنيفة** اجود الورس الحديثة ويسمى البادرة وهي الخضراء تعتق شجرتها والعتيقة منه ما نقام شجره. اجوده حديثه

مسيح ذو قوة ملينة حارة قليل التحليل نافع من الاورام الجاسية التي تعرض في العصب ويحلل حب الجمال ويحلل الخنا زير **جم** يحلل الصلابة الثالولية الحادثة في المفاصل واذا شرب اسهل البطن ويجذب الحيض واذا شرب منه مقدار درهمين يحلل وزم الجمال وقد يعرض [illegible] المفاصل وعروق النساء اذا العق بعسل وخلط بما الشعير وينفع من الورم الرخو وعض النعيس والشوكة [illegible] اليم الى مستقلال

يحلل ويسخن اللحم ويوافق الشقاق الذي في المقعدة والبواسير اذا لطخ عليها ويلين تعقد الامعاء

نافع للاورام الحادثة في التدبير وذلك انه يطفي لهيبها ويمنع ما ينصب و يحلل ما قد انصب لانه مركب من عنبار [illegible] وينفع من العفن العارضة في الرحم اذا وضع عليها وينفع عرق النسا اذا وضع عليه ويحلل الخراجات العسرة التحلل ويوافق السحوج والقروح العارضة للمشيوخ

نافع محلل ملين **لبعض الاطبا** يحلل الخراجات غير النضجة **وقال** اما وسخ التماثيل بانه يكتسب حرة من التماثيل النحاس..

que birtud pueden criar cal y mas si nes pues lleuan a quien las haze y a quien la labra al yn fierno y si fueren de oro o plata no se pueden seruir dellas antes deuen echarlas en el fuego

بالزعفران المعروف **ابن عمران** الورس صنفان حبشي و [illegible] فالمغربي يقال له [illegible] و هو يقتل حب القرع ويبري الكلف والحول والبول ويخرج الحصوات من البدن **ابن ماسويه** خاصته النفع من النقرس ووجع
منفعة [illegible] انفعا عه في المطبوخ ويقو [illegible] مفردا او مركبا مع غيره

can be observed on the old paper, from fols. 59a to 127a. On fol. 59a the thin *ghubārī* numbering has '48', whereas the thick *ghubārī* numbering has '49'. The thinly written large *ghubārī* numerals continue until the last leaf of old paper ('117'; Fig. 33). This series too has lacunae. Its '50' is on fol. 61a, whereas its '60' is on fol. 70a. This means that somewhere one old leaf is missing (or otherwise that this is an instance of ancient miscounting). Later on, the leaf that should have carried '90' is missing. It should have been between fols. 99a and 100a, but these are numbered '89' and '91' respectively. At the end of the section written on old paper, which is far more heavily damaged than the part in the middle of the book block, several leaves would be missing if the defective numbering were a decisive argument.

Ahmad b. Qasim's restoration of the Leiden manuscript

The tabular structure of the *Kitāb al-Mustaʿīnī* makes it possible for the copyist to copy the work double-page by double-page. Both the Leiden and the Arcadian manuscripts have a layout of seven rows per page, the upper row being used in both manuscripts for the titles of the columns, the six remaining rows for the explanatory text. By maintaining the tabular layout of their copy according to the one in the exemplar copyists made their task easier. In this case, this may be somewhat misleading, however, since this open structure of the *Kitāb al-Mustaʿīnī* also allows for all sorts of additions by owners and readers, which may affect the integrity of the text. That this has happened is clear from the numerous variants which can be observed between the Leiden and the Arcadian manuscript, but I leave remarks about variant readings in the manuscripts to the editors of the critical edition of the *Kitāb al-Mustaʿīnī*. Another aspect of the vulnerable integrity of the text in tabular books such as the present one is that, when one leaf is lost, the right and left sides of the opening are no longer a conceptual unit.

Notes and additions by a great number[24] of readers can be observed on many of the pages on the old paper, some very faded. They are often introduced with the word *quf*, the equivalent of *nota* in Latin manuscripts. It is tempting to identify the thickly written note on *dawā al-khanāzir* (fol. 57a) with the hand which also wrote the thick *ghubārī* numerals.

On fol. 97a of the Leiden manuscript (a leaf of modern paper) we can observe that an extra or explanatory text was struck out at the bottom of the page. The text contains an old medical judgement against the use of copper eating and drinking vessels (*ad* نحاس). Ahmad b. Qasim, the copyist, may have struck it out because he believed it was not part of the text. The Arcadian manuscript (pp. 196–7) has a similar addition at the bottom of the page at the same lemma, but of two lines only, with the mention of Aristotle (as in the penultimate line of the Leiden manuscript). It shows, again, the enormous variety of readings. The philological significance, however, of these variants, notes and additions falls outside the scope of the present study.

A few more isolated details in the Leiden manuscript of *Kitāb al-Mustaʿīnī* may be observed here:

24. I have desisted from specifying and counting them.

~ The title in the Leiden manuscript (over the beginning of the text, on fol. 1b [Fig. 32]) is given in a somewhat confused way, certainly as compared to the Arcadian manuscript, which has a regular title page. Title and author are mentioned in a marginal addition written over the beginning of the introduction:

كتاب المستعينى فى الادوية المفردة مما عني بجمعه وتاليفه يونس بن اسحاق بن بكلارش الاسرآئيلى

للمستعين بالله تعلى ابى جعفر احمد بن المؤتمن بالله

Kitāb al-Mustaʿīnī *on simple medicines from what was collected and composed by Yūnus b. Isḥāq b. B·k·lār·sh al-Isrāʾīlī for al-Mustaʿīn bi-llāh (the Exalted) Abu Jaʿfar Aḥmad b. al-Muʾtamin bi-llah*

Over the beginning is also written in bold script:

كتاب المستعينى فى المفردات الطبيه

Kitāb al-Mustaʿīnī *on medical simples*

This may be due to a damaged exemplar. Textually speaking, the addition in the Leiden manuscript does not greatly differ from the title in the Arcadian manuscript.
~ There are a few conjectures of Ahmad b. Qasim in the margin, which are not confirmed by the Arcadian manuscript. For example, on fol. 1b: اظنه يحق the Arcadian manuscript has *ḥaqīq*, the reading in the body of the Leiden manuscript. The same goes for the conjecture in the last line of fol. 1b of the Leiden manuscript, where the text in the body of the page is not so clear, whereas the copyist in the margin conjectures: اظنه مهيها. The copyist has also written under the last line: سببها, —a reading supported by the Arcadian manuscript, p. 5, line 6. There is a marginal correction for الرجلج in the body of fol. 10a of the Leiden manuscript :قال فى نسخة اخرى الزاج which refers to a manuscript other than the exemplar. This remark may be understood in connection with the other manuscript mentioned by Ahmad b. Qasim in his letter to Golius of 2 February 1624. The marginal conjecture *al-zāj* seems to be correct. The originally written *al-rajlaj* does not seem to make sense, nor does *al-zajāj* in the Arcadian manuscript, p. 24, line 4 from the bottom.
~ The first double page of the tabular text in the Leiden manuscript *Kitāb al-Mustaʿīnī* (fols. 12b–13a) is in fact the beginning of the text, with the six lemmata *amīr bārīs*, *aqāqiyā*, *aqḥawān*, *abhal*, *anjara*, *anjarān*. The Arcadian manuscript opens its tabular text (pp. 32–33) with the same six lemmas in the same order. This continues for a while, but then the two manuscripts first diverge and later reconverge again:

~ Arcadian, pp. 34–5	=	Leiden Or. 15, fols. 20b–21a
~ Arcadian, pp. 36–7	=	Leiden Or. 15, fols. 21b–22a
~ Arcadian, pp. 38–9	=	Leiden Or. 15, fols. 14b–15a
~ Arcadian, pp. 40–1	=	Leiden Or. 15, fols. 15b–16a
~ Arcadian, pp. 42–3	=	Leiden Or. 15, fols. 16b–17a
~ Arcadian, pp. 44–5	=	Leiden Or. 15, fols. 17b–18a

Fig. 32.
Opening page of the Leiden MS of the *Kitāb al-Musta'īnī*, showing the beginning of the author's introduction, copied by Ahmad b. Qasim al-Andalusi. Leiden, University Library, Cod. Or. 15, fols. 1b

NEXT OPENING
Fig. 33.
The last available leaf of old paper of the Leiden MS of the *Kitāb al-Musta'īnī*. This page was damaged with loss of text. Ahmad b. Qasim hastily restored it with modern paper and supplied the missing text. See also the numeral '117' in *ghubārī* numerals written in the upper outer margin. The number was written when this leaf was already considerably damaged. Leiden, University Library, Cod. Or. 15, fol. 127a

Fig. 34.
Marginal addition in the modern part of the Leiden MS of the *Kitāb al-Musta'īnī*. The marginal addition supplies text which initially had been overlooked by Ahmad b. Qasim al-Andalusi. Leiden, University Library, Cod. Or. 15, fol. 10b

~ Arcadian, pp. 46–7 = Leiden Or. 15, fols. 18b–19a
~ Arcadian, pp. 48–9 = Leiden Or. 15, fols. 19b–20a
~ Arcadian, pp. 50–1 = Leiden Or. 15, fols. 23b–24a
~ Arcadian, pp. 52–3 = Leiden Or. 15, fols. 24b–25a
~ Arcadian, pp. 54–5 = Leiden Or. 15, fols. 25b–26a, and so on.

It is evident that the copyist of the modern part of Leiden Or. 15, Ahmad b. Qasim, had become confused, probably because the beginning of the old part of the manuscript, the text of which he intended to complete, was still quite defective. He therefore skipped fol. 14a, which contains the old version of the text (now struck out), and replaced it by a new text on fol. 22a (see the corresponding text in the Arcadian manuscript, pp. 36–7). The newly made text on fol. 23a was skipped as well, since it was already available on fol. 15a on old paper.
~ All lemmata have been provided with Spanish translations in the margins. These may be identified with the translations mentioned by Ahmad b. Qasim in his letter to Golius of 2 February 1624.
~ Not only did Ahmad b. Qasim number the openings, which was essential for maintaining order in what was then just a pile of loose leaves, and not only did he translate the lemmata in order to help his young friend Golius about whose proficiency in Arabic he apparently had his doubts, but he also improved the legibility of some of the illegible and faded text by writing over it, and he added text inside the rows and in the margins of many pages [Fig. 34].
~ On fols. 108, 109, 127, Ahmad b. Qasim has partially repaired the old paper by sticking some modern paper on the upper side of the original, and substituted the lost text on these strips in his own handwriting [Fig. 33]. This restoration lacks the neatness with which he usually worked, and we may, perhaps, assume that he was in haste, and lacked time now that he had come near the end of his restoration work.

The difference is striking. In the beginning of his reconstruction work on the text he replaced entire pages when this was not necessary (compare fols. 14a, 22a), but now he may have had a deadline to keep. From fol. 117 onwards the Leiden manuscript shows, mostly at the top of the pages, considerable damage with the consequent loss of entire lines of text. Apparently this lost text could not be supplemented. Ahmad b. Qasim's two other manuscripts may not have given him the text he needed to complete the copy for Golius. But, again, lack of time may also have been the actual reason why his ambitious restoration programme of the manuscript was not entirely completed. Another consequence of lack of time may be seen in the last quire, which is entirely in the hand of Ahmad b. Qasim. His haste to finish the copying was apparently such that he forgot to use one top row (fol. 132a) for the title of the page, a mistake he could only correct by leaving the bottom row empty. On fol. 131a he even forgot to make this correction and filled in seven rows of text, but then struck out the text in the bottom row. These are not essential mistakes, but Ahmad b. Qasim, who by now had almost completed what must have been an extensive editing job, made them, one assumes, because he was in a hurry and had no time to replace the faulty leaves neatly.

كتاب المستعيني في الادوية المفردة مما عني بجمعه وتاليفه يونس بن اسحاق بن بكلارش
للمستعين بالله تعالى ابي جعفر احمد بن المؤتمن بالله قال الحمد لله الذي تفرد بالكمال ولم يبرح احدا من النقصان خير العزة [illegible]
والجلال والقوة والسلطان خالق الانس ومعلمه البيان جاعله مبرزا على جميع الحيوان بما خصه به من نور العقل وابانه من المزية والفضل
حمدا يقضي حق الائه ويوجب المزيد من نعمائه

كتاب المستعيني في المفردات الطبية

قال المؤلف ان كان المتقدمون قد الفوا ودونوا وصنفوا فاحسنوا فليس
ذلك بمباح لهم دون من تاخر زمانه لكنه حقا يلزم من يوثق علمه واحسانه فهو واجب
على من علم ان يدون ويضع ويحفظ من جاء بحكمة ان ينفع ويسمع فمن اوتي علما لزمه
بيانه ولم يحل له كتمانه لكن عليه ان يخص به اهله ولا يودعه غير مستاهل له وان يشح عليه
كشح ضنين ولا يذيعه لذي جاهل باضاعته كظنين حتى يضعه في مكانه ويجريه في ميدانه
فقد تلحق افة التقصير من طرح الدر بين ارجل الخنازير واني لما رايت المستعين بالله ابا جعفر
احمد ابن المؤتمن بالله بن هود ادام الله امره واعز نصره اوحد يا في زمانه احوذيا
في علمه وبيانه قد حاز الفضل برمته وفاقه بازمته يخلص بالمجد خلوص الابريز وبرز
في السودد غاية التبريز خلد الله دولته وادام على الايام بهجته ولا زال الزهر مشوقا بدوام
سلطانه ومتمكن سعده وعلو شانه جعلت وسيلة اليه احسن ما لدي وافضل ما
عرضه الاختيار علي ولم ار فضل لجوهرته الرفيعة وروحانيته البديعة التي فضل الله
تعالى بها اهل عصرنا وشرف بشرافها ابناء دهرنا مرار اخصه ادام الله تاييده ووصل
نصره وتمهيده بكتاب جمعت فيه ما افترق من جواهر الحكما ونظمت فيه ما انتثر
من جواهر العلما الملتقطة في عرصات الدواوين المستخرجة من سيرهم المكنون في الادوية
المفردة التي هي العمدة في علاج الابدان على تقلب الايام وتغيير الازمان وطرزته باسمه العالي
اعلى الله كلمته وايده ووصل اقباله وسعده فسميته المستعيني ليتشرف به وتتشوف
بسببه واستشعرت فيما اوردته واصدرته وجمعته وحصرته الادعان لجسمه الرايع
والاستسلام بين يدي علمه البارع علما باني كمن جلب التمر الى هجر واهدى الى جهينة الخبر
وسلكت فيه طريقة المتقدمين وسقته على عادة المتفلسفين وذلك انهم ذكروا
ان التاليف لا يتم حتى يتضمن احدى ثلاث خصال احدها جمع مفترق والثانية اختصار
بطول والثالثة ايضاح مشكل وكتابي هذا قد جمع ذلك الثلاث خصال وذلك اني لم ار
قط كتابا لمن تقدمني من كتب الادوية المفردة جمع ما جمعته في هذا الكتاب لاني
جمعت الدواء وطبعه وفي اي درجة هو من الحرارة والبرودة والرطوبة واليبوسة ثم
جعلت ما له من الاسماء الشاذة وغير الشاذة على حساب الالسنة منها سريانية ومنها فارسية
ومنها يونانية ومنها عربية ومنها رومية ومنها عجمية عامية وجعلت على كل دواء من
هذه الاسما بقدر ما وجدت منها مفرقا في كتب جمة لاني رايت الضرورة داعية الى
مثل ذلك لتحير الناس فيها وضلالهم بسببها مني وقعت في نسخة من النسخ مبهمة باسم ما

من هذه

على انه ممار لمن ضعفت حرارته الغريزية وكان الغالب على مزاجه فلبه حرارة عرضية مثل اصحاب حمى الرف
ان يتحد رجسد الدماغ وربما هلك الانسان في اقرب مدة فيجب ان يتحفظ من استعماله من كان على هذا السبيل
واما قشور الخشخاش فانه اذا طبخ وحمل على الراس منه مقدار معتدل جلب نوما معتدلا واذا اكثر منه جلب سباتا

منافعها وخواصها ووجوه استعمالها

وشي الفضة
escoria
deplata

117 مسبع يختم الجراحات ويجذب الرطوبات [illegible] نافع من قروح العين والقروح الخبيثة في سائر البدن وتمنع الجراحات وينقي وسخها وينقص اللحم الزائد ويستعمل كثيرا في الاكحال ومنه انواع منها ذهبية ومنها نحاسية ومنها مغربية

مبرد يحبس نزف الدم من العضا ويمنع الحبل ويحلل الاورام الحارة والانتفاخ وينفع من الظفرة سود الاجفان وينفع من النقرس وداء الثعلب [illegible] اذا سحق وعلي بخل وصمغ وقطر ذلك في الاذن جفف رطوبتها [illegible] اذا انقع في الخل وشرب منه قوى المعدة

252 البرم — الخل مسبع مبرد في الدرجة الثالثة مقبض صالح للمعدة حابس لكل سيلان رداع نافع من القروح الدموية والاورام ويبرد المعدة الحارة وينفع من استرخاء اللثة والاكلة والنملة والبرص والنواصير والطعوة

اذا دق وخلط بها وضمد به الجبهة والصدغان نفع من الصداع ومن برق بزر الخشخاش الاسود دقا ناعما ويشرب بشراب لاسهال البطن وسيلان الرطوبة المزمنة من الرحم وخارج الجسد وللعلة من الغايلة اذا استعمل

ينفع اصحاب البلغم والرطوبة المتولدة في المعدة ويهضم الطعام ويسخن المعدة ويحلله واذا البلغم وينفع من القولنج ويسخن الكليتين ويحل البلة ويهيجه واذا اخذ منه في الم عود وامسك قليلا بانه ينفع الغلظ شربا

بدر البقل نافع من حرارة المعدة مسكن للدع العقارب وفيها من حرة المرة الصفرا ويسكن العطش ويطفي حرة الدم والتهابه ويجلب النوم ولذلك اذا استعمل على نغاذ المعدة ولا يستعمل في اثر شيء حتى ينهضم واذا اعمل منه ضماد وحمل على الجبين نفع من الصداع الصفراوي والدموي والاكثار منه يولد ظلمة في البصر ويطفي نور القوة المضرة وينفع بزره من الاحتلام ويقطع شهوة الجماع

ومن الناس من يسميه الخشخاش البحري والصنف الثاني يعرف بالزبريبو من كل قوم انه الماميثا وليس عصيها والمعجونات النافعة من ارواح البواسير ونجار الحديد قابض اذا تحملته المراة في [illegible] عنها نزف فان لم يتدارك بان يسقى وزن نصف مثقال من المغنطس مع كلاء حتى يخرجه من البطن والا قتل

جواهرها ولو كانت الادوية انما تفعل بطبايعها دون خواصها التي تخفى على العقل ولا توجد في الوهم لكان كل دواء حار في الدرجة الاولى فيبدل عن دواء ثان في تلك الدرجة من الحرارة وساير الكيفيات على هذه الجهة فلما ثبت في الادوية هذه الدلايل اعني فعلها بخواص في جواهرها لا بطبيعتها فقط تلطف الاوايل في استخراج الابدال وذلك انهم جعلوا الكثير من الادوية عوضا من دواء واحد او زادوا في الاوزان او نقصوا منها كيما يقوم مقامه ويؤدي الخاصية التي في ذلك العقير الواحد كما فعل بديفورس بالفاونيا التي خاصتها النفع من الصرع العارض للصبيان اذا علق عليهم فجعل بدلا منه ليؤدي عن خاصته قشور الرمان الشمور وعظام سوق الغزلان فان هذه الثلاثة اذا اجتمعت فعلها ما يفعل بالفاونيا ادت عن خاصتها وكذلك البلادر فان من خاصته اذهاب النسيان وتصفية الذهن فان جعل بدله اذا عدم وزنه خمس مرات بنكرفا و وزنه دهن بلسان وسدس وزنه نفطا ابيضا قامت مقامه فعلى هذا المثال فعل المتقدمون الابدال للادوية فان وجدوا بدلا للدواء الذي يرومون بدله من دواء واحد بمثل وزنه بالسواء من دواء اخر كان ذلك بلوغ المطلوب ونهاية المرغوب على ما نجد ذلك في السقمونيا التي من خاصتها اسهال المرة الصفرا وهي رديئة للمعدة ويجعل البدل منها اذا عدمت وزنها لبن الشبرم لانه يسهل الماء الاصفر والمرة الصفرا بقوة وهو ردي للمعدة ايضا وكذلك قثا الحمار يفعل قريبا من فعل السقمونيا ولكنه ليس يبلغ مبلغها الا ان يجعل بدل درهم سقمونيا وزن درهمين من عصارة قثا الحمار اقل ذلك واوسط بدل الدرهم ثلاثة امثاله وما كان من الادوية تفعل بطبايعها فقط جعل بدلها بالسواء ما كان في تلك الطبيعة نفسها وفي تلك الدرجة بعينها من الحرارة او البرودة او الرطوبة او اليبوسة واكثر ما يصحب ذلك في ردع مادة او تصليب عضو او تغيير مزاج الى احد الكيفيات او جذب او تحليل او نحوها ومنها

ادوية لنقص زيادة اللحم مثل اصل الحنظل واصل اللقاح

الرطب ودهن قثاء الحمار ورماد الحلزون وقشر النحاس والتنكار والزنجار ونحوها ومنها ادوية تدمل وتختم الجراحات مثل النحاس المحروق المغسول والعفص وقشور الرمان اليابسة وخبث الرصاص والمرداسنج والرصاص المحرق والاثمد المحرق واسفيداج الرصاص والتنكار والقلقطار المحرق وقشور النحاس وقشور الحديد والزنجار والنورة المحرقة فهذه كلها تدمل وتختم لكنها تختلف في افعالها لان منها ما يفعل بلذع ومنها ما يفعل بلا لذع فيجب للطبيب ايضا ان يتحرى هذا الموضع متى اراد البدل لان الدواء الذي يلذع يحتاج الا يستعمل في بدن حساس البتة والدواء الذي لا لذع معه يقصد به البدن الحساس ومنها ادوية مقرحة لظاهر البدن مثل اصل السلق والثوم وحب الماء والخردل والزرنيخ وزبيب الجبل وزهر النحاس وعاقر قرحا والكلس ولحاء اصل الكبر والشونيز والثافسيا ومنها

Concluding remarks

In addition to the numerous new details that can be gathered from a close inspection of the Leiden manuscript, the following conclusions may be drawn. The earlier view that Leiden Cod. Or. 15 was a copy of the *Kitāb al-Mustaʿīnī* made by Ahmad b. Qasim at the request of Jacobus Golius, on the basis of a single manuscript, is no longer tenable. A newly discovered letter by Ahmad b. Qasim in the Manchester library shows that at least two *exemplaria* were involved, one to be copied from and the other for advanced collation work. Traces of both can be discerned in the Leiden manuscript.

Notwithstanding the new information, Ahmad b. Qasim's involvement in procuring a copy for Golius has not become any clearer. It has, if anything, become harder to understand. His was an exhausting editorial task, for which time almost failed him. An analysis of the traces of several pagination systems in the Leiden manuscript shows that the old part, apart from being incomplete at the beginning and at the end, seems to have had lacunae in the text.

Finally, the description of the Leiden manuscript of the *Kitāb al-Mustaʿīnī*, here undertaken for the first time since Dozy's remarks in 1851 and the description of 1865 by De Jong and De Goeje, together with newly discovered material in Manchester, shows that the Leiden manuscript is one of several codices that clearly need to play a key role in a critical edition of the *Kitāb al-Mustaʿīnī*. It is to be hoped that such a project will receive an extra impulse now that the important manuscript of the Arcadian Library has come to light.

GEOFFREY KHAN

THE SYRIAC WORDS IN THE *KITĀB AL-MUSTAʿĪNĪ* IN THE ARCADIAN LIBRARY MANUSCRIPT

In the third column in the synoptic tables of *Kitāb al-Mustaʿīnī* Ibn Baklarish presents synonyms of the Arabic names of the simple medicines in a variety of languages, including Persian, Greek, Latin, Berber, 'Roman vernacular' (*ʿajamiyya rūmiyya* [Byzantine Greek]), 'common vernacular' (*ʿajamiyya ʿāmmiyya*) and Syriac (*suryāniyya*). He says in his introduction to the work: 'I mentioned all that I could gather from different books about each drug whenever I found it necessary to enlighten people about it in case they come across unknown names in prescriptions.'[1] The presentation of synonyms, therefore, would seem to have had a practical purpose of facilitating the identification of drugs.

Little is known about the life of Ibn Baklarish. He was associated with the court of Ahmad al-Mustaʿin, the Hudid ruler of Saragossa from 1085 to 1109. The work is dedicated to his patron al-Mustaʿin. Ibn Baklarish does not speak about journeys or first-hand observations. It appears that the material that he presents in his work is based largely on books that were at his disposal in Spain. Some of the synonyms in different languages may have been gathered orally from informants, though this could have been done within the Iberian peninsula. This was, of course, the case with the 'common vernacular' (*ʿajamiyya ʿāmmiyya*), which referred to the local Romance vernacular. On some occasions he referred specially to the vernacular of Saragossa (*ʿajamiyyat Saraquṣṭa*).[2] The Berber words also could have been collected within Spain, where there were numerous Berber-speaking immigrants at that period.[3]

The large number of references to the medical works of his predecessors does not necessarily imply that he consulted all their works first-hand. It is likely that a large proportion of them are secondary references that he culled from other compilations.[4] This may apply also to the citation of many of the synonyms. One of his sources was the *Kitāb al-Taṣrīf* of the physician al-Zahrawi (died early eleventh century) from Madinat al-Zahraʾ near Córdoba. The 29th treatise of this work gives synonyms in Persian, Syriac, Greek and Romance.[5] Another source may have been a work known as *Kitāb al-Talkhīṣ* by Yonah Ibn Janah (died *c.* 1050) from Saragossa. This is now lost, but we know it contained an inventory of simples with synonyms in Persian, Syriac, Greek, Berber and Romance.[6]

The fact that Ibn Baklarish cites synonyms in numerous languages does not imply that he was familiar with these languages. He is likely to have spoken the Romance

1. Martin Levey, 'The Pharmacological Table of IbIbn Biklārish', *Journal of the History of Medicine and Allied Sciences*, 26, 1971, pp. 413–21 (see p. 414); Martin Levey and Safwat S. Souryal, 'The Introduction to the *Kitāb al-Mustaʿīnī* of Ibn Biklārish (fl. 1106)', *Janus*, 55, 1969, pp. 134–66 (see p. 136).
2. Henri P. J. Renaud, 'Trois études d'histoire de la médicine arabe en occident', *Hespéris*, 10, 1930, p. 142.
3. Renaud, 'Trois études', p. 146.
4. Ana Labarta, 'La farmacologia de Ibn Buklāriš: sus fuentes' in: *Actas del IV Coloquio Hispano-Tunecino*, Madrid 1983, pp. 163–74, see pp. 164–5. See also the articles by Labarta and Ricordel in this volume.
5. Sami Khalaf Hamarneh and Glenn Sonnedecker, *A Pharmaceutical View of Abulcasis al-Zahrāwī in Moorish Spain*, Leiden 1963, p. 65; Labarta, 'La farmacologia de Ibn Buklāriš', p. 168.
6. Labarta, 'La farmacologia de Ibn Buklāriš', p. 168.

dialect of Saragossa, referred to as *ʿajamiyyat Saraquṣṭa*. Obviously he was well acquainted with Arabic, though it is not clear whether this was anything more than a literary language for him. We know that he was Jewish[7] and may, therefore, have had some knowledge of Hebrew and Talmudic Aramaic. He may not, however, have had first-hand knowledge of the other languages he cites.

After examining the citation of Berber words, Renaud concluded that, because of the frequent confusions in these citations, Ibn Baklarish is unlikely to have been familiar with the Berber language. He also observed that the Berber synonyms did not reflect a uniform linguistic background but rather exhibit considerable dialectal diversity and appear to have been taken from a wide variety of sources.[8]

My own investigations have led to similar conclusions regarding the Syriac synonyms.[9] The Syriac synonyms are not uniform in linguistic background and it is unlikely that Ibn Baklarish was familiar with all the different varieties of the language that they reflect. They must have been collected from a wide range of sources. Such is the diversity of the background of these synonyms that, although they are designated as *suryāniyya*, it is not always appropriate to refer to them all as 'Syriac', according to the normal usage of this term by modern scholars.

The term 'Syriac' is generally used to designate a literary variety of the Aramaic language that was used by eastern Christians in their writings. In Ibn Baklarish's time it was used by Christians in Syria, south-eastern Turkey, Iraq and western Iran, and also by some Christian communities further afield, mainly to the east where the missionaries of the Nestorian church brought their language together with their faith. This literary form of Aramaic remained essentially uniform in structure wherever it was used throughout this wide geographical area. Considerable differences did exist, however, in the way it was pronounced when read aloud. Two main reading traditions developed, which came to be characteristic of the two main denominations of eastern Christianity, namely the Jacobite and Nestorian churches. The Jacobite communities were located mainly in Syria whereas the Nestorians resided for the most part in the Mesopotamian area and further east. The two reading traditions, therefore, are sometimes designated as the western tradition (Jacobite) and the eastern tradition (Nestorian) of Syriac.

Many of the Christian communities who used Syriac as a written language would have spoken Aramaic as a vernacular language. Indeed Aramaic has survived down to modern times as the vernacular of several Christian communities in Syria, south-eastern Turkey, northern Iraq and north-west Iran. The vernacular form of Aramaic that exists today ('Neo-Aramaic') is by no means uniform but exihibits considerable dialectal diversity. The Christian dialects are usually classified into three main groups: (1) the western group spoken in Maʿlula and various other villages in the region of Damascus, (2) the Turoyo group, spoken in Tur ʿAbdin in south-eastern Turkey, and (3) the north-eastern Neo-Aramaic group, which survived into modern times across a wide area encompassing northern Iraq, north-west Iran and

7. In some sources he has the *nisba* epithet *al-Isrāʾīlī* (cf. Labarta, 'La farmacologia de Ibn Buklāriš', p. 163).
8. Renaud, 'Trois études', p. 146.
9. These investigations were carried out on the Arcadian Library manuscript, in which 31 Syriac synonyms have been identified. Labarta ('La farmacologia de Ibn Buklāriš', p. 169) has counted 29 Syriac synonyms in the Madrid manuscript (Biblioteca Nacional, MS ar. 5009).

south-eastern Turkey east of the Tigris. These Neo-Aramaic dialects are not direct descendants of literary Syriac. They have existed as vernaculars for centuries side-by-side with Syriac.

The words designated as *suryāniyya* by Ibn Baklarish include both those that can be identified as literary Syriac and those that can be identified as vernacular Neo-Aramaic. This distinction is reflected by different types of phonetic structure, which can be discerned since the words are presented in Arabic transcription, as is the case with the synonyms in other languages. Within the words from literary Syriac, moreover, the transcription reflects one particular reading system, namely the eastern Nestorian tradition. The crucial distinctive feature is the realization of an original long *ā* vowel. In the eastern reading tradition this retains its quality as a low unrounded vowel, which would be represented in Arabic transcription by the vowel letter *alif*. In the western reading tradition, on the other hand, an original long *ā* shifted to the rounded vowel *ō* which would be represented in Arabic script by the vowel letter *wāw*. Some transcriptions of Syriac that are found in other medieval Arabic texts reflect this western type of pronunciation, with *wāw* representing original long *ā*, e.g. the citations from the Syriac Gospels by the Ismaʿili scholar al-Kirmani (386–411 A.H./996–1020 A.D.), *Kitāb al-Masābīḥ*:[10]

Gospel of Saint John (15:26):

موذوثى فارقليطو هو ذينو مشادرنو لخون روحو شرورو

ܡܐ ܕܐܬܐ ܦܪܩܠܝܛܐ ܗܘ ܕܐܢܐ ܡܫܕܪܢܐ ܠܟܘܢ ܪܘܚܐ (ܕ)ܫܪܪܐ

When the Counsellor (παράκλητος) comes, whom I shall send to you ..., the Spirit of truth ...

In all the transcriptions of literary Syriac words cited by Ibn Baklarish an original long *ā* is represented by the vowel letter *alif*. This is shown by the transcription of the final vowel in the following: جوزا ('nut' = Syriac: ܓܘܙܐ *gawzā*, p. 76), دَبا ('bear' = Syriac: ܕܒܐ *debbā*, p. 90), كركما ('saffron crocus' = Syriac: ܟܘܪܟܡܐ *kurkmā*, p. 108), كبريتا ('sulphur' = Syriac: ܟܒܪܝܬܐ *kebrīthā*, p. 164), بسْرا ('flesh' =Syriac: ܒܣܪܐ *besrā*, p. 172).

In a number of words an original final long *ā* is represented in the transcription by *tā marbūṭa*, which reflects the shortening of the vowel. The shortening of final vowels is a feature of the Neo-Aramaic vernaculars. It is conditioned by the incidence of stress on the penultimate rather than on the final syllable. The source of this set of words, therefore, can be identified as vernacular Neo-Aramaic rather than the literary Syriac language. Other features in this set of words allow us to establish that they come specifically from the north-eastern Neo-Aramaic (NENA) group of dialects. Thus *tā marbūṭa* clearly reflects final short *-a*, which is characteristic of the NENA group, rather than short *-o*, a characteristic of the Turoyo dialect, e.g. سُستة ('mare' =Syriac: ܣܘܣܬܐ *sūstā*, NENA *susta*, p. 170).

The transcription, furthermore, reflects the retention of the original stop realization of initial *bgdkpt* consonants, as is the case in the NENA group, and not

10. Paul Kraus, 'Hebräische und syrische Zitate in Ismaʿīlitischen Schriften', *Der Islam* 19, 1931, pp. 243–63.

their fricativization, as in the Maʿlula group. Examples: قِلدة (= Syriac: ܓܠܕܐ *geldā*, NENA *gilda*, p. 78), قملة (= Syriac: ܓܡܠܐ *gamlā*, NENA *gumla*, p. 88).

Note also the shortening of the original long medial *ā* vowel in a closed syllable that is reflected in the transcription حَمُرتَة (=Syriac: ܚܡܪܬܐ *ḥmārtā*, p. 170). This also is a feature of NENA dialects, in which the word has the form *khmarta*. The *ḍamma* vowel after the *mīm* in the transcription may reflect the further raising and attenuation of this vowel that is attested in several dialects (*khmərta* < *khmarta*).

The word بختة, which is given as the synonym of النسا 'women' in the phrase لبن النسا 'women's milk' (p. 180) can be identified with NENA *baxta* 'woman'. The lexical item *baxta* is found exclusively in the NENA dialects, where it has replaced the original Syriac word *ʾattā*. The etymology of *baxta* is uncertain, the one favoured in recent scholarship being Syriac *bākheθtā* 'weaveress'.[11]

The sound *g* is transcribed by the Arabic letters *jīm, qāf* or *ghayn*, the one unique occurrence of the latter being given as an alternative to a transcription with *qāf*: جوزا ('nut' = Syriac: ܓܘܙܐ *gawzā*, p. 76), قِلدة (= Syriac: ܓܠܕܐ *geldā*, NENA *gilda*, p. 78), غملة وقيل قملة (= Syriac: ܓܡܠܐ *gamlā*, NENA *gumla*, p. 88). These can be regarded as attempts to represent the voiced stop *g*. It is likely that none of the letters were pronounced exactly as *g* in the Arabic of the person who created the transcription, but only approximated to it. All three letters were used in medieval Arabic texts to arabicize the letter *g* sound in Persian loan words.[12]

Two of the words designated by Ibn Baklarish as *suryāniyya* are, in fact, not Aramaic at all, but rather Hebrew. The first is the synonym given for مخيْطة 'sebesten plum', which is said to be 'known as اكساس in *suryāniyya*' (p. 178). This can be identified with Hebrew אַגָּס *aggās* 'pear'. The form اكساس would be a copyist's error for اكاس, an easy mistake given the fact that the letter *sīn* is often written without 'teeth' in cursive Arabic script. The second case is the synonym of Arabic فُجل 'radish', which is said to be سِينون in *suryāniyya* (p. 218). This can be identified with Hebrew צְנוֹן *ṣenōn* 'radish'. Note that both words lack the Aramaic definite article suffix *-ā*. They belong to the lexicon of Rabbinic Hebrew. They are not attested in Biblical Hebrew. Rabbinic texts were typically written in a mixture of Hebrew and Aramaic. This is the case, for example, with the Babylonian Talmud, one of the central Rabbinic texts. It is possible that Ibn Baklarish, or his source, did not distinguish the two linguistic layers, but designated the Rabbinic language in general as *suryāniyya*. This would clearly not correspond to the modern usage of the term 'Syriac', which is used to refer to the literary Aramaic of the eastern Christians. In the transcription of سِينون (צְנוֹן) the *shewa* under the first letter is represented by *yāʾ*. This no doubt reflects the pronunciation of the *shewa* as an *e* vowel, which was characteristic of the Sephardi pronunciation of Hebrew. This would have been used among the Jews of Spain at the time of Ibn Baklarish. The initial *ṣade* of the Hebrew word is represented by Arabic *sīn*, which indicates that it

11. Cf. Georg Krotkoff, 'Studies in Neo-Aramaic Lexicography' in: Ann Kort and Scott Morschauser (eds.), *Biblical and Related Studies Presented to Samuel Iwry*, Winona Lake 1985, pp. 131–2; Hezy Mutzafi, *The Jewish Neo-Aramaic Dialect of Koy Sanjaq*, Wiesbaden 2004, p. 218. According to this etymology the singular form *baxta* would, in fact, be derived, by back formation, from the plural *bakhtāthā*. An alternative etymology that has been proposed is Kurdish *baxt* 'luck, good fortune', this being a euphemistic substitution (cf. Krotkoff, 'Studies in Neo-Aramaic Lexicography', p. 131).

12. Cf. Asya Asbaghi, *Persische Lehnwörter im Arabischen*, Wiesbaden 1988, p. xviii.

was not pronounced as emphatic ṣ. In the pronunciation traditions of Hebrew that have come down to modern times the letter *ṣade* is pronounced as emphatic ṣ in Arabic-speaking communities. In communities where Arabic is not the vernacular, on the other hand, the letter is mostly pronounced without emphasis. The Persian-speaking communities, for example, pronounce it as non-emphatic *s* and in the Ladino (Judaeo-Spanish)-speaking communities it is pronounced as an affricate *ts*.[13] This suggests that the transcription سِينون has its origin in a non-Arabic-speaking community. It is possible that this was the Romance-speaking local community of Ibn Baklarish himself.

In conclusion, the synonyms designated by Ibn Baklarish as *suryāniyya* have a variety of different backgrounds. These can be divided into the following categories (1) literary Syriac with an eastern pronunciation, (2) a form of vernacular Aramaic belonging to the north-eastern Neo-Aramaic dialect group and (3) the language of Jewish Rabbinic texts. There is no evidence that Ibn Baklarish travelled in the East, so it is likely that he drew the first two categories of transcriptions from written sources that were eastern in origin. The sources for words of category (1) must have been written in areas where the eastern pronunciation of Syriac was current, most likely Iraq. The transcriptions of category (2) are likely to have been records of fieldwork conducted orally among speakers of north-eastern Neo-Aramaic dialects in Iraq or adjacent regions east of the Tigris. The source for the words in category (3) may have been nearer to home, in a non-Arabic-speaking Jewish community in Spain, possibly that of Ibn Baklarish himself. It is possible that Ibn Baklarish did not take the transcriptions in categories (1) and (2) directly from their original sources, but rather indirectly from citations in other compilations. We know that he drew on previous works that included Syriac synonyms, such as *Kitāb al-Taṣrīf* of al-Zahrawi (see above).

Finally, it should be noted that several of the transcriptions have become corrupted by scribal error. This may have arisen from mistakes made by copyists of the text. However, given the indirect transmission of the transcriptions, as well as Ibn Baklarish's apparent ignorance of Syriac and most likely also of any other Aramaic dialect, it is possible that many of these corruptions existed in the original text of the work.

Inventory of transcriptions[14]

1. p. 76

جوز الاكل : جوزا

'Edible nut: جوزا'

Syriac: ܓܘܙܐ *gawzā* 'nut'

13. Shlomo Morag, 'The Pronunciations of Hebrew', *Encyclopaedia Judaica*, XIII, p. 1133.

14. The following abbreviations are used: *DBJA* = Michael Sokoloff, *A Dictionary of Jewish Babylonian Aramaic of the Talmudic and Geonic Periods*, Ramat-Gan and Baltimore 2002. *LS* = Carl Brockelmann, *Lexicon Syriacum. Editio Secunda Aucta et Emendata*, Halle 1928. NENA = north-eastern Neo-Aramaic. The page numbers refer to those of the Arcadian Library manuscript.

2. p. 78
جلد الكبش والتيس : قِـــلدة
'The skin of a ram and male goat : قلدة'
NENA : *gilda* 'skin'

3. p. 88
دماغ القنفذ والجمل : يعرف الجمل .... بالسريانية غَملة وقيل قملة
'The brains of a hedgehog and a camel: camel is known in *suryāniyya* as غملة and one also says [i.e. an alternative form of the word is] قملة'
NENA : *gumla*.

4. p. 90
دم الدب : دَبا والذكر منها دُخرًا
'The blood of a bear : دَبا and the male (is called) دُخرًا'
Syriac: ܕܶܒܐ *debbā* 'bear', ܕܶܟܪܳܐ *dekhrā*.
In Syriac the word ܕܶܒܐ when used generically often has feminine gender. In other dialects of Aramaic this is regularly the case, e.g. Babylonian Jewish Aramaic (דּוּבָּא f.), NENA (*dubba* f.). In order to designate a male bear, therefore, the word has to been accompanied by the term for 'male' ܕܶܟܪܳܐ . The vocalization of the transcription ܕܶܟܪܳܐ indicates that Ibn Baklarish or at least the copyist of the manuscript misunderstood the final *alif* as a marker of *tanwīn*.

5. p. 103
زوف رطب : قلفا
'Grease of hyssop wool : قلفا'
The transcription appears to represent the Aramaic word for 'peel, skin'. In Syriac this is ܩܠܳܦܬܳܐ *qlāphtā* with the feminine ending *-tā* (cf. Jewish Babylonian Aramaic קְלָפְתָא *qlāphthā DJBA* 1022). The masculine form ܩܠܳܦܐ *qlāphā* has the sense of 'leaf of a book' (*LS* 670), which does not seem to be appropriate in this context. The transcription, moreover, does not represent the medial long *ā* vowel of these Syriac words. It is noteworthy that in north-eastern Neo-Aramaic the word *qalpa* is used in the sense of 'peel'. If the transcription is reliable and has not been altered by scribal corruption, one could interpret it as representing *qalpā*, which would be essentially the north-eastern Neo-Aramaic form *qalpa* but with the final long vowel of Syriac retained. Another possibility is that it represents Hebrew קְלִפָּה *qlippā* 'peel'.

6. p. 108
زعفران : كرْكما
'Saffron : كرْكما'
Syriac: ܟܘܪܟܡܐ *kurkmā*.

7. p. 114
زبل خنزير : الخنزير ... بالسريانية حزرا
'Dung of a pig : pig ... in *suryāniyya* is حزرا'
The Syriac for pig is ܚܙܝܪܐ *ḥzīrā*. The transcription is likely to be a corruption of an original حزيرا.

8. p. 114
زبل الذيب : خراوة
'Dung of a wolf: خراوة'
This appears to be a scribal corruption of خردوة, which could be interpreted as NENA *xre d-dewa* 'dung of a wolf', corresponding to ܚܪܝܐ ܕܕܐܒܐ *ḥrayyā d-dēwā* in Syriac. The final short *-a* in the transcription and also the occurrence of *kh* for original *ḥ* are distinctive features of NENA.

9. p. 122
حب الراس هو الميرُبَرْج بالسريانية
'The seed of the head is *myrbrj* in *suryāniyya*'
The form *myrbrj* is an unidentifiable word, which is apparently a scribal corruption. In the Madrid manuscript (fol. 62b) the form is *mnwyrj*. Ibn Baklarish attributes this Syriac synonym to al-Zahrawi.[15]

10. p. 122
حماما هو بالسريانية القشرا ومَاسرمنيس
'*Ḥamāma* in *suryāniyya* is القشرا and مَاسرمنيس'
The interpretation of the Syriac words is unclear.

11. p. 148
يتوع : حلباديا
'Tithymal [Euphorbia]: حلباديا'
Syriac: ܚܠܒ ܕܒܐ *ḥleb debba* (*LS* 232: 'Euphorbia', literally 'milk of the bear'). The transcription must be a scribal corruption of حلبا دبا *ḥalbā d-debbā*.

12. p. 162
كبد الدب : يعرف الدب بالسريانية دبا ويقولون دُبّا دَخْرَا ومعناه دُب ذكر
'Liver of the bear: the bear in *suryāniyya* is known as دبا and they say دُبّا دَخْرَا, which means: male bear'
Syriac: ܕܶܒܳܐ *debbā* 'bear' (common gender), ܕܶܟܪܳܐ *dekhrā* 'male'. See the remarks on دم الدب (no. 4 above). The vocalization of دُبّا with *ḍamma* corresponds to what is found in NENA (*dubba*) and also Babylonian Jewish Aramaic (דּוּבָּא). Another possibility is that the vocalization is influenced by the Arabic form of the word: دُبّ.

13. p. 164
كبريث : كبريتا
'Sulphur: كبريتا'
Syriac: ܟܶܒܪܺܝܬܳܐ *kebrīthā*. In the Arabic word the final *tā'* has the diacritical marks of *thā* rather than of *tā*, which is its normal pronunciation. Conversely the corresponding letter in the transcription of the Syriac has the diacritical marks of *tā*, reflecting the stop *t* rather than the expected fricative *th*.

15. I am grateful to Ana Labarta for informing me of the reading in the Madrid manuscript.

14. p. 166
لاذن : الاذنيا
'Gum ladanum : الاذنيا'
Both the Arabic and Syriac are derived from Greek λάδανον. The attested Syriac forms are ܠܕܢܐ *ladnā*, ܠܐܕܐܢܘܢ *lādānūn* and ܠܐܕܢ *lādēn* (*LS* 359). The transcription does not correspond exactly to any of these. There may have been some scribal corruption. The initial *alif* and *lām* of the transcription are presumably to be identified as the Arabic definite article.

15. p. 168
لك : اللكا
'Lacquer : اللكا'
Syriac : ܠܟܐ *lakā* The transcription is prefixed with the Arabic definite article.

16. p. 168
لبن الكلبة ... بالسريانية لبنا كلبة
'Milk of a bitch ... in *suryāniyya* is لبنا كلبة'
The form كلبة could be interpreted as the NENA form of 'dog' *kalba*, with a short final vowel. The form لبنا does not correspond to anything in Aramaic with the meaning of milk. It appears to be the Arabic word *laban* with a Syriac inflectional ending added to it. In the light of this the whole phrase may simply be a repetition of the Arabic with a Syriac ending added artificially to the first word to give it the flavour of Syriac.

17. p. 170
لبن البقر ... يعرف بالسريانية لـبنى توتا
'Milk of the cow ... is known in *suryāniyya* as لَبنى توتا '
The second word can be interpreted as a corruption of تورتا which would correspond to Syriac ܬܘܪܬܐ *tawrtā* 'cow'. The first word in the phrase appears to be a corrupt transcription of the Arabic word for milk.

18. p. 170
لبن الماعز ... يعرف بالسريانية لبنى عَزيا
'Milk of the goat .... is known in *suryāniyya* as لبنى عَزيا'
The second word appears to be a corruption of Syriac ܥܙܐ *ʿezzā* 'goat'. The first word in the phrase appears to be a corrupt transcription of the Arabic word for milk.

19. p. 180
لبن النسا : ... يعرف النسا ... بالسريانية بختة
'The milk of women : [the word] "women" are known ... in *suryāniyya* as بختة'
NENA : *bakhta*.

20. p. 170
لبن الخيل : بالفارسية معين بالسريانية سُستة
'The milk of horses : in Persian *maʿīn* ['mare'] and in *suryāniyya* سُستة'
NENA : *susta* 'mare'.

21. p. 170
لبن الاتن : انثة الحمار بالسريانية حَمُرتـة
'Milk of a she-ass: the female of an ass in *suryāniyya* is حَمُرتـة'
NENA: *khmarta* or *khmərta*. The occurrence of *ḥā'* rather than *khā'* in the transcription may be due to scribal corruption. It should be noted that in some dialects of NENA that are spoken today (e.g. Hertevin, Derabun) the original pharyngal *ḥ* is retained (*ḥmarta*).

22. p. 172
لحم الحرباء : اللحم ... بالسريالنية بسْرا
'The flesh of a chameleon: flesh ... in *suryāniyya* is بسْرا'
Syriac: ܒܶܣܪܳܐ *besrā*.

23. p. 172
لحم الفار : الفار ... يعرف ... بالسريانية جردًا وهي الجردان
'The flesh of a mouse: mouse ... is known ... in *suryāniyya* as جردًا, which are rats'
Syriac: ܓܱܪܕܳܐ *gardā*. The final *alif* of the transcription is vocalized with *tanwīn* owing to scribal error.

24. p. 178
مخيْطة : ... يعرف اكســاس بالسريانية
'Sebesten plum: ... it is known as اكســاس in *suryāniyya*'
Scribal corruption for اكــاس = Rabbinic Hebrew אַגָּס *aggās* 'pear'.

25. p. 184
مرارة الدب : يعرف الدب بالسريانية دبا ولذكره دَخرَاء
'The gall bladder of a bear: the bear in *suryāniyya* is known as دبا and its male (is known as) دَخرَاء'
See the comment on دم الدب (no. 4 above). Syriac: ܕܶܒܳܐ *debbā* 'bear', ܕܶܟܪܳܐ *dekhrā*. The *hamza* after the final *alif* in the transcription دَخرَاء has been written by scribal error due to the influence of Arabic orthography.

26. p. 192
نر سيان دار : ... وهو عصا الراعى ... يسمى بالسريانية نرعانا ومعناه راعى الغنم لان الغنم بالسريانية عانا
'Nirsiyandar: ... this is "the stick of the shepherd" ... it is called in *suryāniyya* نرعانا, meaning "the shepherd of the sheep", since sheep in *suryāniyya* is عانا'
The form عانا is clearly Syriac ܥܳܢܳܐ 'sheep'. The background of the transcription نر is unclear. Likewise the Arabic rubric نر سيان دار and its gloss as 'the stick of the shepherd' are unclear. Perhaps سيان is a scribal corruption of شبان, which represents Persian *shubān* 'shepherd'.

27. p. 208
سوس : سوُما
'Sus: suma'
The transcription may perhaps be identified with Syriac: ܣܰܡܳܐ 'drug, medicine'.

This word occurs in numerous names of medicinal herbs, e.g. ܦܡ ܒܝܥܬܐ 'gentian'. The medial *wāw* could reflect the shift of original *a* to *u* before the labial consonant *m*, which is not uncommon in Aramaic dialects, though not attested specifically in this word in Syriac.

28. p. 218
فُجل : سِينون
'Radish : سِينون'
Rabbinic Hebrew : צְנוֹן *ṣenōn* 'radish'. The *sīn* of the transcription reflects the non-emphatic pronunciation of the *ṣade*. The *yā'* reflects the pronunciation of the vocalic *shewa* as an *e* vowel.

29. p. 248
تُوتِيَا : الطرطوة
'Tutiya : الطرطوة'
Syriac : ܛܘܪܛܒܐ *turṭwā* 'tribulus' (plant) (*LS* 288) = ܬܘܪܛܒܐ (*LS* 695). The final *tā' marbūṭa* reflects the shortening of the final long *ā*, which is a characteristic of Neo-Aramaic. The transcription of the original *beth* by *wāw* reflects the pronunciation *w*, which is characteristic of the eastern reading tradition of Syriac and also of NENA.

30. p. 266
شَيطرَج : هو بالسريانية لبنذُون ... وهو لببديون
'Lepidium latifolium : in *suryāniyya* it is لبنذُون and لببديون'
The two transcriptions can be traced back to the Greek : λεπίδιον. Presumably they are Arabic transcriptions of original Syriac transcriptions of the Greek word. The Arabic transcriptions have suffered from scribal error. Their original form, no doubt, was لبيديون.

31. p. 270
شحم الدُب : ... يعرف بالسريانية دَبا والشحم بالسريانية شَحْمَة
'The fat of the bear' : [the bear] is known in *suryāniyya* as دَبا and fat in *suryāniyya* is شَحْمَة'
Syriac : ܕܒܐ *debbā* 'bear'. The background of the transcription شَحْمَة is unclear. The Syriac word ܫܚܡܐ *shaḥmā* means 'black' (*LS* 769) ; cf. Babylonian Jewish Aramaic : שַׁחְמָא 'dark colour, black spot' (*DJBA* 1128). There appears to have been a confusion with the Arabic word for 'fat'.

DAVID J. WASSERSTEIN

IBN BIKLARISH – ISRA'ILI

We have now quite a respectable number of copies of Ibn Biklarish's work. I stress this only to draw attention to the fact that it is fairly rare to have more than a single manuscript, or at most a couple, of Arabic texts of the Middle Ages. Of some, it is true, we have lots, but not of very many, and the fact that we have some half a dozen of this one should tell us something of its popularity and even, perhaps, of its importance. That it is by a Jew makes this all the more striking. Ibn Biklarish was a Jew, and he was active in a period of extraordinary variety and productivity among Jews of the medieval Islamic world, and of al-Andalus, Islamic Spain, in particular.[1] However, there is, I think, more (or perhaps rather less) to be said about his activity as a Jew in the time and place of his work.

Let me begin with a glance at his name. He is called 'Yunus b. Ishaq Ibn Biklarish'. The first two names, whether we give them an Arabic, as I have done here, or a Hebrew dress, are clearly recognizable.[2] They present no problems and might easily be those of a Jew (or, for that matter, of a Muslim, even, at a pinch, of a Christian) of the general time and area. But it is worthy of note that *all* our sources uniformly give them an Arabic dress, not a Hebrew one.

'Biklarish' presents more of a puzzle. Thomas Glick vocalizes it 'Buklarish', 'Baklarish' has been adopted in this volume, while I and most others make it 'Biklarish'.[3] I do not think that there is much more than random or vaguely aesthetic reasons for the choice, but you will see that it may also have reason; of course the last syllable could equally be vocalized with an 'u', not necessarily with an 'i'; and the first and last vowels could even in theory both be 'a'. Biklarish/Biklarush/Buklarush/Buklarish is not Hebrew, nor is it Arabic. Nor is it obviously the name of a grandfather: Yunus son of Ishaq *son of Biklarish*. While I do not exclude that genetic possibility entirely, it seems far more likely that it is some sort of by-name, of the type so well known in Islamic society of the Middle Ages. Ibn Rushd is one obvious example; dozens could be cited. They are not usually ancestors in the strict sense of the word. But if it is neither Hebrew nor Arabic, what is it? The obvious answer is that it must be some form of Latin/Romance; the exact definition of the linguistic background is of no significance, the general area is. The ending '-(u/i)sh' in this case looks like a normal Latin ending in '-(u/i)s', such as we find not uncommmonly in Iberian names in Arabic dress.[4]

But if the name is Latin/Romance, then we face a problem—not that fact in itself,

1. See generally Bernard Lewis, *The Jews of Islam*, Princeton 1984; Mark R. Cohen, *Under Crescent and Cross. The Jews in the Middle Ages*, Princeton 1994; Moritz Steinschneider, *Die arabische Literatur der Juden*, Frankfurt-am-Main 1902 (for Ibn Buklarish see pp. 147–8, no. 99).

2. Angel Sáenz-Badillos and Judit Targarona Borras, *Diccionario de autores judíos (Sefarad. Siglos X–XV)*, Córdoba 1988, pp. 176–7, by contrast, give him only a Hebrew form.

3. For the variants see the article by Labarta in this volume, pp. 20–2.

4. Adhfunsh (for Ildefonsus/Alfonso), Farghalush, Furtish (= fortis?), Bibish (= Vives? but *avant la lettre*), Balakayash (Latinate?), Armalyuth (Latinate?) (though we also have *M·w·r·q·'·t*, without an ending - for Mauregato/us? But this presumably reflects a later stage in linguistic development away from Latin and towards Romance). These examples come from my 'Inventing Tradition and Constructing Identity: the Genealogy of 'Umar ibn Hafsun between Christianity and Islam', *Al-Qantara*, 23, 2002, pp. 269–97.

for we have good examples of Iberian Jews, from al-Andalus, from this very period, with such names: the best-known is Samuel ha-Nagid who was Ibn Naghrela, explained very persuasively long ago now by Samuel Stern as 'son of the little/young darkie' (Lat. nigra).[5] The problem is rather the fact that it is difficult to say what lies behind this name. Fortunately, it is not, quite, unique; we also have the sixth-century Gothic historian known as John of Biclar (Biclaro/a, the ending is unclear: masculine or feminine?). He died soon after 621, thus long before the period and cultural mix in question here, but he is our only witness, so far as I know, to this name, so we must see how far and indeed whether he can be of help. In fact I think he can. While this John was born, we are told, in Portugal, he founded a monastery in Biclar (the great Spanish Espasa-Calpe encyclopedia, under this writer, gives us the forms Biclaro and Vallclara,[6] which latter form may be a pointer to something). A search through other reference books and scholarly monographs confirms that all agree that he did this, but only Edward Colbert, in the *New Catholic Encyclopedia*, has the courage to add 'location unknown' to the name. Apparently no one knows where Biclar is or was. However, for our purposes it may be of interest, and even possibly relevance, that this John 'of Biclar' seems to have spent his life, following his return to the peninsula after a stay of many years in Constantinople, in the area of north-eastern Spain. He was in Barcelona, then in Biclar; he attended councils in Saragossa and Barcelona, as well as in Toledo, in the centre of the peninsula, and in Egara (in the region of Barcelona); and he was also bishop of Gerona.[7] May we assume that Biclaro/Biclara (possibly = Vallclara) as the location of the monastery founded by John, who lived and worked in the general area of Saragossa in the sixth–seventh centuries, is the same as the Biklar/Buklar behind the name of Yunus b. Ishaq, who lived and worked in Saragossa in the eleventh? I do not want to push this further than it can reasonably go, but these are, I think, our only occurrences of the name, and, despite the apparent clarity of Vallclara as given to us by Espasa-Calpe, that place-name, if it is one, does not solve anything for us, and we have nothing else to help us here. If the two are the same, then this may well offer us an indication or a confirmation of a local connection, even origin, for our Ibn Biklarish, one tying him not only in a geographical sense but also in a linguistic and a cultural sense to the area of Saragossa, and possibly even to a small and obscure place nearby.[8] This is of value for our understanding of his context as a Jew.

We are not quite finished with the man's name. He is also called 'al-Isra'ili'. Goitein, in his entry on the Banu Isra'il in the *Encyclopaedia of Islam*, describes the expression al-Isra'ili as 'a more polite designation for a Jew than Yahudi', but the only

5. Samuel M. Stern, 'Les vers finaux en espagnol dans les muwaššahs hispano-hébraïques: une contribution à l'histoire du muwaššah et à l'étude du vieux dialecte espagnol "mozarabe"', *Al-Andalus*, 13, 1948, pp. 299–346, at p. 330 (= 'The final Lines of Hebrew Muwashshahs from Spain', in idem, *Hispano-Arabic Strophic Poetry. Studies by Samuel Miklos Stern*, selected and edited by Leonard Patrick Harvey, Oxford 1974, pp. 123–60, at p. 148, with n. 33). See also idem, 'Contributions to the History of Samuel Hanagid', *Zion*, 15, 1950, pp. 135–45, at p. 135, n. 2 (Hebrew).

6. *Enciclopedia universal ilustrada europeo-americana*, 70 vols. in 72, Barcelona 1907–30, vol. 8, p. 763.

7. See Edward P. Colbert 'John of Biclaro' in: *New Catholic Encyclopedia*, New York etc. 1967, VII, p. 1036; 2nd edition, 2003, VII, p. 965, with an enlarged bibliography.

8. That he is also said to have a connection to Almería does not necessarily conflict with this; see also Ana Labarta's essay in this volume (above pp. 22–3).

examples whom he gives of individuals who are thus designated are Isaac al-Isra'ili, the famous ninth-tenth-century Jewish doctor and philosopher from North Africa, and Ibrahim b. Sahl al-Isra'ili, the Jewish poet from Seville who converted to Islam around 1100.[9] 'Al-Isra'ili' as a name can of course have come into existence only in an Islamic context: Jews would not have called one of their own 'the Jew', or 'the Israelite'.[10] It would have been like naming a man from Frankfurt 'the Frankfurter'. It does happen, but not in Frankfurt. There everyone is a Frankfurter. A person could be called that only somewhere else, outside that context. And both the examples cited by Goitein, Isaac al-Isra'ili and Ibrahim b. Sahl al-Isra'ili, were in fact known thus in Muslim contexts, not Jewish, because their principal activity, that for which they are known and remembered, took place largely in a Muslim, not a Jewish, context—Isaac al-Isra'ili as a doctor and scientist in the service of North African rulers, Ibn Sahl al-Isra'ili as a poet writing Arabic verse for Muslim rulers in al-Andalus, and converting to Islam (before drowning in the straits between Spain and North Africa while on a diplomatic mission). It can scarcely have been otherwise with Ibn Biklarish.

The picture of Ibn Biklarish that begins to emerge is of a Jew who is not perhaps all that Jewish. This impression can be confirmed and deepened by our other information, or lack of it. Ibn Biklarish seems not to be known to our Jewish sources for the Jews of al-Andalus, sources which it is worth noting are not very sparse. Furthermore, Saragossa at the time of Ibn Biklarish's activity was home to a Jewish community of some size.[11] We need not accept the estimate of Ashtor for this (some 1,200 or so, in a population estimated by Glick as somewhere between 10,000 and 20,000)—it is more precise than we can believe accurate, and perhaps somewhat larger than is really acceptable—but it is clear that for its day this was not an insignificant community. We know of at least half a dozen intellectuals and otherwise culturally creative Jews who were active there in the eleventh century, including two, Solomon Ibn Gabirol and Bahya Ibn Paquda, of the first rank. Both of these were well acquainted with a wide range of Jewish texts, including the Talmud, and we may assume that these were available in that city to those with an interest in reading them. Was Ibn Biklarish among those with such an interest?

We cannot be certain of the answer to this question, but we can make an informed guess. The linguistic character of Ibn Biklarish's work is of relevance in this connection: I have not checked this thoroughly in the manuscript of the Arcadian Library, but my impression is that, while Ibn Biklarish's work contains examples of words in what is for the medieval Islamic world a very respectably wide range

9. Shlomo D. Goitein, 'Banū Isrā'īl', *Encyclopaedia of Islam*, new edition, I, pp. 1020–4.

10. We can contrast here usefully the Arabic name 'al-Islami', meaning 'the convert to Islam' (distinguished in our source from al-Aslami, which means belonging to a particular tribe, that of Aslam). See my 'Inventing Tradition', p. 272.

11. See, e.g., Eliyahu Ashtor, *The Jews of Moslem Spain*, 3 vols, Philadelphia 1973–84, II, pp. 253–63 and index. See also idem, 'The Number of the Jews in Muslim Spain', *Zion*, 28, 1963, pp. 34–56 (Hebrew), for the size of the Jewish population of Saragossa. Thomas F. Glick, *Islamic and Christian Spain in the Early Middle Ages. Comparative Perspectives on Social and Cultural Formation*, Princeton 1979, pp. 113–14, suggests that between the tenth and the eleventh century Saragossa increased in size from 12,000 to 17,000. Such precision seems implausible.

of languages, it contains no Hebrew at all. What is described by the cataloguers for Sotheby's as a single Hebrew word on the margin of fol. 119b (p. 236) of this manuscript is actually several words, not only in the margin, and not in Hebrew, though they are in Hebrew script.[12] His range of languages is of great interest, both for its own sake and as it tells us something of the limits of the material available to Ibn Biklarish in his work, available both in the sense of what he could find and in the sense of what he could read: the languages which Ibn Biklarish refers to, alongside Arabic, are Greek, Persian, Syriac, Latin, Romance, and Berber. At first sight impressive, particularly in a society where foreign languages were generally little or unknown, this list nonetheless raises more than one important problem. Here is one of them: it is a commonplace of writing about the Middle Ages that Jews knew lots of languages. But linguistic skills, far less knowledge, are not a genetic trait, and among the Jews no less than among their neighbours both general and specific claims to wide and varied linguistic knowledge need to be weighed very carefully. Here, where the subject is botanico-pharmacological onomastics and lexicography, we should hesitate to ascribe too much linguistic knowledge to him and consider the possibility that in this case, as in so many others, both botanico-pharmacological and apparent linguistic skill is actually the ability to use other people's dictionaries.[13] *Al-Kitāb al-Mustaʿīnī* is a sort of dictionary and certainly uses other people's work—we can see this by opening it almost anywhere and looking for the citations which are sometimes helpfully identified for us in this manuscript by the slightly larger writing for their authors' names. Did Ibn Biklarish really know all these languages? Very probably not. Certainly the ability to give translations or equivalents of words which, in their specific context, are fairly well known does not of itself show that he did. Did he have access to such earlier works? Certainly, as he refers to them so often—though this need not mean always direct access. But we can say more than this: as he makes no reference to earlier Jewish material on the subject of this work, it seems certain also that either he had no access to it or he did not know how to use the access to it that was available to him in Saragossa. Thus the Talmud, for example, contains much material of relevance to a work like this.[14] We can be sure that the Talmud was available in Saragossa in his time. We know that the Talmud, or parts of it, had been available in Spain in the tenth century.[15] And from the presence in Saragossa in the eleventh century itself of Bahya Ibn Paquda, who was certainly acquainted with the Talmud, we can be confident that it and texts like it were available there at that time. If, working in this sort of context, Ibn Biklarish did not use them, and if he gives no

12. The 'Hebrew' says *bārid yābis fī b* ('cool and dry in the second "degree"'); this is written once inside the column listing the character of the item in this lemma and repeated in the right-hand margin. While it is written in Hebrew characters it is actually Arabic; it is apparently a correction of what is written here in Arabic in Arabic characters: *ḥārr yābis fī b* ('hot and dry in the second "degree"').

13. A comparison between Reinhardt Dozy, *Supplément aux dictionnaires arabes*, Leiden 1881, and Federico Corriente, *Dictionary of Andalusi Arabic*, Leiden 1997, suggests somewhat similar conclusions.

14. See, e.g., Immanuel Loew, *Die Flora der Juden*, 4 vols., Vienna–Leipzig 1924–34, repr. 1967; Julius Preuss, *Biblisch-talmudische Medizin. Beiträge zur Geschichte der Heilkunde und der Kultur überhaupt*, Berlin 1911; trans. Fred Rosner, *Biblical and Talmudic Medicine*, New York 1978; see also Samuel Krauss, *Griechische und lateinische Lehnwörter im Talmud, Midrasch und Targum*, Berlin 1898–9.

15. See my 'An Arabic version of Abot 1:3 from Umayyad Spain', *Arabica*, 34, 1987, pp. 370–4; and 'Encore une fois Abot 1:3 dans l'Espagne omeyyade', *Arabica*, 38, 1991, pp. 275–7.

indication whatever of having any knowledge of anything Hebrew, then it is a fair assumption that he knew nothing of that language or of texts written in it.

This is very different from a case like that of Moses Maimonides, not only because of the towering figure that he was but also because he too wrote in such fields and displays much varied linguistic knowledge and experience.[16]

Let me return now to the question with which I began: what sort of Jew was Ibn Biklarish? To answer that question, now that we are a little better informed about him, means trying to locate him on a multi-dimensional spectrum. Jews in al-Andalus, as in the medieval Arabo-Islamic world in general, were part of a complex linguistic and cultural set-up, with complicated relationships to the social nexus of their environments. They usually spoke the language of their environment.[17] This generally meant a form of Arabic, but in al-Andalus—especially, we may assume, in the north-east, an isolated and far-off corner of the Islamic world—at the end of the eleventh century, this was probably accompanied by what we have come to call Romance, a derivative of late Latin, creating a very unusual linguistic situation in the medieval world of Arab Islam, with in effect two parallel languages of speech. Ibn Biklarish could write literary Arabic; that much we know. And we can presume that he spoke spoken Arabic and Romance. Can we move beyond that?

For reading and writing, among those Jews who possessed these skills, a form of Arabic and different forms of Hebrew and Aramaic were available—but only to those who knew these languages and had learned how to read and write them. Being Jewish did not of itself confer such knowledge. In general, the Arabic written (and read) by such Jews was written, like those other languages, in Hebrew characters. The employment of a single script for all languages in use within a particular religious community occurs elsewhere in the Islamic world. It has some clear advantages—as it also exacts a price. Advantages and price can be described as one of the barriers between different communities.[18] On the one hand, it can offer protection of various sorts, especially to a culture facing different kinds of threats and temptations, while on the other it can cut one community off from its neighbours. And it is rare, though far from impossible, to find people who are skilled and productive both in the internal script of the community and in that of the broader environment.[19] A consequence of this is that texts written in Arabic by members of the Jewish community were generally written in Hebrew characters, often on topics

16. See, e.g., Moses Maimonides, *Sharḥ asmāʾ al-ʿuqqār (L'explication des noms de drogues): un glossaire de matière médicale*, ed. Max Meyerhof, Cairo 1940. See also the article by Emilie Savage-Smith in this volume, where it is suggested that Maimonides too did not necessarily know all the languages of his pharmacological sources, but relied on indirect sources, including Ibn Biklarish himself. She wonders whether Maimonides might have known Ibn Biklarish's work because they were both Jewish scholars. We have, however, nothing but the note in Hebrew characters in the Arcadian manuscript to suggest a Jewish link for any Ibn Biklarish manuscript, and nothing else to support such a link of any significance for Ibn Biklarish himself.

17. For what follows see David J. Wasserstein, 'The Language Situation in al-Andalus', in *Studies on the Muwaššah and the Kharja*, ed. Alan Jones and Richard Hitchcock, Reading 1991, pp. 1–15 (repr. in Maribel Fierro and Julio Samsó (eds.), *The Formation of al-Andalus*, Part 2: *Language, Religion, Culture and the Sciences*, The Formation of the Classical Islamic World, 47, Aldershot 1998, pp. 3–17).

18. See e.g., David J. Wasserstein, 'Langues et frontières entre juifs et musulmans en al-Andalus' in: *Judíos y musulmanes en al-Andalus y el Magreb. Contactos intelectuales*, ed. Maribel Fierro, Madrid 2002, pp. 1–11.

19. For examples, see Shlomo D. Goitein, *A Mediterranean Society. The Jewish Communities of the Arab World as Portrayed in the Documents of the Cairo Geniza*, Berkeley etc., 6 vols., 1967–93, passim.

of interest mainly or exclusively to members of the community. They would thus generally not become known or even be of interest to outsiders. Outsiders who might wish to read such texts, as they did occasionally, would generally need to have them transcribed into Arabic characters, as may have happened, for example, with one text of Maimonides (and this process might also involve a change in the register or the type of the language itself, from one type of written Arabic to another).[20] At the other extreme, this means that Jews who wrote in *Arabic* characters were more or less consciously and deliberately choosing to write for a particular audience, in this case a Muslim one, and equally consciously not for another—the more natural?—the Jewish one.[21]

We can confirm this very easily, both positively and negatively. On the positive side, we have the woman poet Qasmuna. Material on her survives at all probably just because she was a woman and because woman poets are so rare. We have a tiny handful of Arabic verses by her preserved in entries in an Arabic biographical dictionary of poets and *littérateurs*. It is only in the last couple of decades or so that her identity has been clarified: she turns out to have been the daughter of Samuel ha-Nagid, the great Hebrew poet and vizier of Zirid Granada in the eleventh century, to whom I referred earlier.[22] In her writing she offers a stark contrast to her father: he wrote his poetry in Hebrew, for a very self-consciously Jewish audience. She wrote in Arabic, clearly for an Arabic-reading audience, and it is in Arabic, among Muslims alone, that a few of her verses have survived.[23] There is no trace of her or of her activity as a poet in the Jewish tradition.

On the negative side, if we look at the two major figures of eleventh-century Saragossan Jewish intellectual life, Bahya b. Paquda and Solomon ibn Gabirol, we get a dramatically different result: Bahya b. Paquda is known principally for a single work, the *Farā'iḍ al-Qulūb*, *Hovot ha-Levavot*, *Duties of the Heart*, written in Judaeo-Arabic, Arabic in Hebrew characters. Composed around 1080, this was translated into Hebrew by Judah Ibn Tibbon, that prince of translators, in 1161—but for a Hebrew-reading audience in Christian Europe, one that knew no Arabic of any sort.

20. Mubahat Türker, *Mūsā b. Maymūn'un Makala fī Sinā'at al Mantik'i*, *Review of the Institute of Islamic Studies*, Publications of the Faculty of Letters, Istanbul University, III, Parts 1-2, 1959–60; idem, 'Mūsā ibn-i Meymūn'un *Al-Makāla fi Sinā'at al-Mantik*' in: Arpaca Asli, *Türk Tarih Kurumu Basimevi*, Ankara 1961; Israel Efros, 'Maimonides' Arabic Treatise on Logic. Introduction', *Proceedings of the American Academy for Jewish Research*, 34, 1966, pp. 155–60 (English section) and Judaeo-Arabic text, pp. 9–42 (Hebrew section). Herbert A. Davidson, *Moses Maimonides. The Man and his Works*, Oxford 2005, pp. 313–22, argues persuasively that this work is not by Maimonides, that it is by a Muslim, and that it was composed originally in Arabic, and only subsequently transliterated into Hebrew characters. At ibid, pp. 425–6 he also discusses the possibility, or probability, of transliterations of parts of Maimonides' *Guide for the Perplexed* into Arabic characters. His discussion demonstrates both the existence of such transcriptions and how rare they were.

21. For extensive discussion of this and related phenomena see, e.g., Geoffrey Khan, 'The Medieval Karaite Transcriptions of Hebrew into Arabic Script', *Israel Oriental Studies*, 12, 1992, pp. 157–76; idem, 'On the Question of Script in Medieval Karaite Manuscripts: New Evidence from the Genizah', *Bulletin of the John Rylands Library*, 75, 3, 1993, pp. 132–41; idem, 'The Orthography of Karaite Hebrew Bible Manuscripts in Arabic Transcription', *Journal of Semitic Studies*, 38, 1, 1993, pp. 49–70.

22. J. M. Nichols, 'The Arabic Verses of Qasmuna bint Isma'il ibn Baghdala', *International Journal of Middle East Studies*, 13/2, May 1981, pp. 155–8; corrected and extended by James A. Bellamy, 'Qasmuna the Poetess. Who was she?', *Journal of the American Oriental Society*, 103, 1983, pp. 423–4.

23. See David J. Wasserstein, 'Samuel Ibn Nagrila ha-Nagid and Islamic Historiography in al-Andalus', *Al-Qantara*, 14, 1993, pp. 109–25.

Among Jews in Islamic lands, it continued to be read in the original Arabic—but in Hebrew characters. As a result, despite its language, and despite the fact that it draws heavily on Islamic sources, it was not read by Muslims and acquired no reputation outside Jewish circles there.

Ibn Gabirol was more productive than Bahya: in Hebrew he wrote a great deal of poetry, much of which has survived, under his name. In Arabic, he composed a philosophical work. It was translated into Latin in the Middle Ages, as *Fons Vitae*, and nothing was known of its author, Latinized as Avicebron. Parts of it were also translated into Hebrew in Christian Spain in the thirteenth century, and on the basis of these fragments Solomon Munk was able in the nineteenth century to establish its authorship. In its original Arabic, however, the work was totally lost—which means also wholly ignored, by an audience which probably had no access to it because of the script in which it was written and copied. Very few works written in Judaeo-Arabic, Arabic in Hebrew characters, attracted attention in Islamic circles, and they could do so only because—or if—they were transliterated or transcribed into Arabic characters.

Script, as much as, perhaps even more than, language, acted as a major barrier between people of different, related cultures and religions in the medieval Islamic world. One result, or perhaps just reflection—and I stress just reflection—of this that we can see fairly easily is indifference on the majority, dominant, Islamic side to what the members of the small Jewish minority did. We happen to possess a brief account of Jewish intellectual life in eleventh-century al-Andalus by a contemporary Muslim, Saʿid al-Andalusi of Toledo. He shows himself totally unaware of the achievements or the significance of this vastly important period.[24]

We should also consider the field in which Ibn Biklarish was active and productive. Medieval poetry, as Samuel Stern argued, needed both poets and patrons. Muslim patrons would not be interested in supporting Jewish poets writing in Arabic. The result was Jewish patrons who supported Jewish poets writing in Hebrew. Philosophical texts tended, like theological ones, to have a religious flavour, and thus they too were not likely to excite interest among Muslims. So while these texts were written in Arabic, it was actually Judaeo-Arabic, hidden behind the barrier of the Hebrew script.[25] Scientific texts, medical texts, texts of botanical or pharmacological onomastic lexicography, these were all culturally much more neutral, and hence those working in such areas could straddle cultural and social boundaries much more easily.[26] But this did not mean that they sought or brought linguistic or cultural stuff across those barriers.

I return to Ibn Biklarish: he shows no knowledge of Hebrew; he does not use and seems to be unacquainted with Jewish material of relevance for his work; he does not appear to be part of the thriving Jewish culture of his city, Saragossa; he is known

24. See David J. Wasserstein, 'The Muslims and the Golden Age of the Jews in al-Andalus' in: *Israel Oriental Studies*, 17: *Dhimmis and Others. Jews and Christians and the World of Classical Islam*, ed. Uri Rubin and David J. Wasserstein, 1997, pp. 179–96.

25. Cf. Chaim Rabin, 'Hebrew and Arabic in Medieval Jewish Philosophy', in *Studies in Jewish Religious and Intellectual History Presented to Alexander Altmann on the Occasion of his Seventieth Birthday*, ed. Siegfried Stein and Raphael Loewe, Birmingham, Alabama, and London, 1979, pp. 235–45.

26. See, e.g., David J. Wasserstein, *The Rise and Fall of the Party-Kings. Politics and Society in Islamic Spain, 1002–1086*, Princeton 1985, pp. 220–1, with references.

only in the Muslim tradition; what he writes is preserved, as it was almost certainly produced, in a form directed exclusively at a Muslim audience, in Arabic language and in Arabic characters. In a world where cultural identity, cultural belonging, was marked not just by religion and by language but also by script, here we have a case very close to one end of that multi-dimensional spectrum that I mentioned earlier. On one hand this points to the real possibilities that existed for full cultural integration of Jews in the surrounding Islamic society, through education, for example. On the other it tells us something of the price that this integration exacted. Very like Qasmuna and only a little bit like Ibn Gabirol, at least in his *Fons Vitae*, but unlike Maimonides and quite unlike Bahya Ibn Paquda, Ibn Biklarish was fully absorbed linguistically and culturally into his Islamic environment and shows no signs of the cultural mixing so characteristic of the Jewish–Islamic encounter in the Middle Ages.[27] If he were not called al-Isra'ili, what should we think he was?[28]

27. Glick, *Islamic and Christian Spain*, p. 258, discusses the role of Jews in the overall translation process in medieval Iberia, drawing attention to the importance of their contribution. At p. 353, n. 14 (to this passage), he adds that 'Jews had played a similar polycultural role in al-Andalus, as when ibn Buklārish of Zaragoza composed tables of synonyms, including Romance variants, of different simples.' As my argument here suggests, this may not be quite accurate. For the importance of Jews in the translation process, see the articles of Pieter Sjoerd van Koningsveld, 'Andalusian-Arabic Manuscripts from Christian Spain: a Comparative Intercultural Approach', *Israel Oriental Studies*, 12, 1992, pp. 75–110; 'Christian-Arabic manuscripts from the Iberian Peninsula and North Africa: a Historical Interpretation', *Al-Qantara*, 15, 1994, pp. 423–51; 'Christian Arabic Literature from Medieval Spain: an Attempt at Periodization' in: *Christian Arabic Apologetics during the Abbasid Period (750–1258)*, ed. Samir Khalil Samir and Jorgen S. Nielsen, Leiden 1994, pp. 203–24.
28. See now also Z. Ammar and Y. Seri, 'Ibn Biklarish, One of the Greatest Sefarad Physicians', *Korot* 15, 2001, pp. 79–91 (in Hebrew).

EMILIE SAVAGE-SMITH

IBN BAKLARISH IN THE ARABIC TRADITION OF SYNONYMATIC TEXTS AND TABULAR PRESENTATIONS

The most immediately distinctive feature of the treatise on medicinal substances written in the city of Almería by Ibn Baklarish al-Isra'ili at the turn of the eleventh to twelfth century is its tabular format. In the course of 121 synoptic tables, Ibn Baklarish discussed the properties and uses, as well as alternative names, for 704 medicinal substances. An example of one of the tables can be seen in Figure 35, an opening from the copy recently acquired by the Arcadian Library that was, according to the colophon, completed on 'Saturday in the middle ten days of the month of Ṣafar of the year 524' [= 18 January 1130 A.D.].[1] The purpose of this paper is to explore where Ibn Baklarish fits into the didactic tradition of presenting medical material in synoptic tables and the concern for establishing synonyms for a medicinal substance.

NEXT OPENING
Fig. 35.
The Arcadian Library manuscript, pp. 42–3

The origin of synoptic tables is unknown, though their occurrence in an Arabic *jawāmiʿ*, or summary, of the treatise by Galen (d. *c.* 216 A.D.) on simple drugs, *Peri kraseōs kai dunameōs tōn haplōn pharmakōn*, known in Latin as *De simplicium medicamentorum temperamentis et facultatibus libri XI*, suggests they may have been devised in Alexandria. The so-called 'Alexandrian Summaries' (*Jawāmiʿ al-Iskandaraniyyīn*) of Galenic treatises were originally written in Greek, though they survive only in Arabic, Hebrew, and Latin translations, and they (or at least their Arabic versions) employed various popular didactic devices such as branch-diagrams and synoptic tables.

Figure 36 shows one of the synoptic tables in an early thirteenth-century copy of the *jawāmiʿ* of Galen's treatise on simple drugs.[2] It consists of fourteen leaves of synoptic tables, each with seven columns, whose headings are, reading right to left: (1) the name of the drug (*asmāʾ al-adwiya*), such as feverfew (or camomile, *uqḥuwān*); (2) the nature of the drug (*ṭabāʾiʿ al-adwiya*), cold, dry, etc.; (3) the uses of the drug (*manāfiʿ al-adwiya*), for example, easing phlegm; (4) the dangers of the drug (*aḍrār al-adwiya*), as in causing inflammation of the spleen (*al-ṭuḥāl*); (5) an antidote for the drug (*iṣlāḥ al-adwiya*), usually another medicament; (6) the preferred form of the drug (*al-mukhtāt min al-adwiya*), such as fresh or green; and (7) the recommended quantity of the drug (*awzān al-adwiya*) usually given in *dirhams*.

Immediately before the start of the synoptic tables in this manuscript there is a note that apparently occurred in the exemplar used by the unnamed copyist. In it the compiler of the epitome stated, 'I found seven chapters of the book, and so I

1. The colophon occurs on p. 273 of the manuscript.

2. Oxford, Bodleian Library, Oriental Collections, MS Hunt. 600, fol. 20a (undated, twelfth–thirteenth century). The *Kitāb Jawāmiʿ iḥdā ʿashrat maqāla min kitāb Jālīnūs fī al-adwiya al-mufrada* occupies folios 15a–35a of the volume. See Emilie Savage-Smith, 'Galen's Lost Ophthalmology and the *Summaria Alexandrinorum*' in: Vivian Nutton (ed.), *The Unknown Galen* (Bulletin of the Institute of Classical Studies, Suppl. 77), London 2002, pp. 121–38, esp. pp. 122–5. For further details concerning this manuscript, see Emilie Savage-Smith, *A New Catalogue of Arabic Manuscripts in the Bodleian Library, Oxford*, vol. 1: *Arabic Manuscripts on Medicine and Related Topics*, Oxford forthcoming.

٢٣

والرشيش وعرجه اجراجا لقوة مع شي من المرة الصفرا ويسهل الادويه اخراج
بشرب معردا ان نلث برمعز اللوز الحلو ويكون الرمعز معزار وزنه عشره مرات والشربه
والصبر والمقل والاشق وبزر الكرفس والنانخاه وتجود لها ان غابلته كثيرة ونحاله

منافعها وخواصها ووجوه استعمالها

د له قوه ملزقه للجراحات ويقطع الرطوبه السايله من العين وينفع في اخلاط المراهم
ابو جريج باكل اللحم العفن من الجراحات وله في الزمر قوه بالغه وخاصته اخراج العزا
من العين اسيما ان خلط بالنشا والسكر وحجر التوتي ويلحم القروح. ابن ماسويه
خاصيته اسهال البلغم اللزج واذا سحق بنا في البيض او باللبن جيد ثم سعود رونا نفع
من الرمد

ف وله قوه حاره تحلله والحجاره له تو جرد الا تصفي للعروق فونها فويحب
ويفتت الحصاه المتولده في المثانه والك... رذلك عرفها الطبيب واذا وضع وهو
جاف في القروح الرطبه العتيقه التي لها محاريد في الاعضاء جففها واذا استعمل بالخل
قطع النزف وقد يحرق ويصلح للرمد والجلا وللغشي

هو ملزق للجراحات مدمل للقروح وقوته قوة تجيب والورق اليابس اكثر من الرطب
وقوة النابته قوة جاليه مانعه اذا وضع في خارج البدن وقوته بالجمله ملاصه ولها
طبخ نافع من سيلان الرطوبات من الرحم اذا اغتسل وعصارة تشد اللثه وتحلو البهر
وتقطر في الاذن له تسيل منها القيح وتقطع الرعاب مع الخل ويقطع نفث الدم والاسهال
ويدر البول ويسكن اللذع الحادث في المثانه وينفع من نهش الرتيلات ولسع العقرب من عبد لام

ق واما تخلعه في القبض والتحليل عن ميسح الزهراوي هو بزر تجيب الخردل وهو حاره
يابسه مقطعه للشرد العارضه في الراس مقويه للدماغ ومعها شي من قبض وافضلها
اكبرها واشدها حراره وارزانها ويدخل في اعمال الطيب ولا تدخل في اعمال النار

يلين الطبيعه وينفع من اوجاع الحلق والربو العارضه من الدم وينفع من الاوجاع
الحادثه من ... المرة الصفرا ۞

ميسح ... معها شي من قبض مع لطافه وينفع من المعده والكبد والارحام بطبعها
بولس
ومال الذي يسمها اكثر من جرمها تنبه المراه التي بها اختناق الرحم واحتباس القرع
وان شربت تحل حركة البطن ۞

الى اكلتسيها منه محموطه لانه اذا طالت به المده ذهبت عنه ولم يحب ان يستعمل
برمها واذا بل بالما ... والخل قطع انبجاس الدم العارض عن القطع والبط بعض الاطبا
تريحها ... في ... الجنه شي يسير من راحه الجنة باشر

ابن ماسويه خاصة الانزروت اسهال البلغم الغليظ الذي يجتمع في المفاصل والوركين
الادوا عن الابدان وربما نفع العصب والامعا وجردها ويجمعها نحوه فلذلك يجب ان
منه مفردا من درهمين الى ثلاثة دراهم وقد يصلح بالشحم والمليح والتربد

	الاسماء	الطبايع والدرج	تفسير معاني الاسما واللغات	الابدال منها
Sarcocolle	انزروت	حار يابس في الثانية	موضع شجرة تنبت ببلاد فارس ويعرف بجل فارس ومنه العنزروت ويقال له ايضا اسر فيلش ومن غير الام اضراره بالمعا اصلاحه بالصمغ العربي وقيل ان اصلاحه ان ينقع في ماء الشراب والخلتيت اصلاحه برمن اللوز وذلك ان ينقع في المطبوخ حتى ينحل ويخلط بالصمغ العربي	[illegible]
Spogni	اسفنج البحر	حار يابس في الاولى	هو القيم ومنه الغمام ومنه رغوة الحجامين وتسمى بالعجمية اشبنجة	انزروت
Iarhi:	آس	بارد يابس في الثانية	هو الريحان ومنه المردسان ومنه المورد بانج ومنه المرتة بالرومية ومنه المارتة وقيل ان هذه الاسماء كلها واقعة على حب الريحان دون الورق والاغصان . من غير الام اصلاحه بالكثيرا .	ثمر الريحان [illegible]
	[illegible]	حار يابس في الثانية	قيل انها حشيشة تنفع في الغالية ومنها ملتحة وحبه مثل حب الريحان او الخردل والاكبر منها غبيراني صغار مثل العصفر والاكبر منها اجودها ومنه الريت جالراي ومنه رجل الجراد	[illegible]
Spanachi	اسفاناخ	بارد رطب في الاولى	ويقال الاسباناخ بالبا واسفاناخ والعامة تعرفه اسبانخ	[illegible]
Vngulas my repsicas	اظفار الطيب	حار يابس في الثانية	ابن وافد هو عطر صنف من ذوات الاصداف ومنه شبيه بصدف العرقير ويقال له مارح عن الزهراوي وابن جناح	[illegible]

خطرة جـ . افضل اسفنج البحر ما كان قريب العهد بالبحر وكانت فيه القوة ~~وقوة الاول~~ وقوة الاول
قوة تجفف والثالثة قوة ترمل والثالثة قوة تلزق الجراحات الطرية .
رائحة اظفار الطيب عطرة لان الحيوان الذي هو منه يرعى الناردين فلذا

اسما الادويه	سوان	بعولل	[illegible]	اوسان	[illegible]	[illegible]	[illegible]	[illegible]	[illegible]
طبايع الادويه	حار يابس	حار يابس	حار يابس	حار يابس	حار يابس	حار يابس	حار يابس	حار رطب	حار يابس
منافع الادويه	مسهل الصفرا	مسهل الراس والمعده	اسهال البلغم والسودا	اسهال الصفرا	اسهال الدود وجع الفرج	اسهال الدود وجع الفرج	من الحكه والجرب	من عرق النسا	من الصداع الفالج
اضرار الادويه	بالطحال	بالامعا	بالامعا	بالامعا	بالمقعده	بالقلب	بالامعا	بالكلى	بالمعده
اصلاح الادويه	بالانيسون	بزر الرازيانج	بالكثيرا	بالمصطكي	بالشيح الارمني	بالشل الارمني	بالاهليلج الاصفر	بالزوفا	بزر الكرفس
المختار من الادويه	الاصفر الخفيف	الاحمر سقطري	الابيض الاسود الخفيف	الاخضر	الخفيف الاسمر	الحديث	الكبار منه	الاسود الصمغي	الزاهي
اوزان الادويه	وزنه نصف درهم	وزن درهمين	وزن درهم	وزنه نصف درهم	وزن ثلثه دراهم	وزن نصف درهم	وزنه نصف درهم	وزن درهمين	وزن ثلثه دراهم

decided to arrange them in branch-diagrams (*tashjīr*) and tables (*jadāwil*) so that the book would be a better abridgement, more worthy of being taken seriously, more attractive to see, easier to read, and not so boring.'[3]

The table format lent itself particularly well to the presentation of rules for food and drug use, but it was also used for listing diseases and aligning them with appropriate therapies. Such charts are found, for example, in the therapeutic handbook *The Almanac of Bodily Parts for the Treatment of People* by Ibn Jazla (d. 1100), a Christian convert to Islam who practised as a physician in his native Baghdad, and also in *The Ultimate Book on the Treatment of Diseases and the Knowledge of Afflictions and Affections* by his Baghdad contemporary Saʿid ibn Hibat Allah (d. 1101).[4] In the following century synoptic tables are found in *The Quintessence of Medicine,* a medical manual on the causes and symptoms of disease composed in the province of Khwarazm in Persia by Ismaʿil ibn al-Husayn al-Jurjani (d. *c.* 1136), and in *What is Sufficient for the Medical Art* by ʿAdnan ibn Nasr al-ʿAynzarbi (d. 1153), a court physician in Fatimid Egypt.[5]

For the purposes of this paper, comparison of Ibn Baklarish's treatise with other synoptic tables will be limited to Arabic treatises concerned with medicinal substances, in which the entries are by the name of the medicament. I will begin with the most influential of all treatises employing this format: *The Almanac of Health (Kitāb Taqwīm al-ṣiḥḥa)* by Ibn Butlan (d. 1066), a Christian physician of Baghdad.[6] In the course of 40 tables, he presented 210 plants and animals and 70 other items and procedures useful for maintaining good health, including the use of music, regulation of sleep and exercise, bathing, fumigations, and alteration of air quality. He accompanied all 280 topics by recommendations from various authorities whose names were represented by abbreviations. This imaginatively structured manual enjoyed wide currency not only in the Arabic-speaking world but also in medieval and Renaissance Europe where elaborate illustrations were introduced to enhance the visual structure.

While the *Almanac of Health* is concerned with more than simply *materia medica*, it nonetheless includes as main entries several medicinal substances. I have chosen to look at the entry for myrtle, a low-growing evergreen shrub (*Myrtus communis* L.) notable for its fragrant leaves, because it is a substance that is an entry in all the tabular treatises that were available for comparison.

Figure 37 shows a table from Ibn Butlan's treatise in which myrtle is the first of the seven entries.[7] Above and below the table, there are registers containing 40 canons

Fig. 36.
Oxford, Bodleian Library, MS Hunt. 600, fol. 20a

NEXT OPENING
Fig. 37.
Oxford, Bodleian Library, MS Bodl. Or. 266, fols. 30b–31a

3. Oxford, Bodleian Library, Oriental Collections, MS Hunt. 600, fol. 19b.

4. For *Kitāb Taqwīm al-abdān fī tadbīr al-insān* of Ibn Jazlah, and *al-Kitāb al-Mughnī fī tadbīr al-amrāḍ wa-maʿrifat al-ʿilāl wa-l-aʿrāḍ* by Saʿid ibn Hibat Allah, see Manfred Ullmann, *Die Medizin im Islam*, Leiden 1970, p. 160. Both treatises were dedicated to the ʿAbbasid caliph al-Muqtadi bi-amr Allah (ruled 1075–94).

5. For *Kitāb Zubdat al-ṭibb* by al-Jurjani, better known for his important Persian-language medical compendium, see Ullmann, *Medizin im Islam*, p. 161. For al-ʿAynzarbi and his al-*Kitāb al-Kafī fī ṣināʿat al-ṭibb*, see also Ullmann, *Medizin im Islam*, p. 161. For samples of synoptic tables from both these treatises, see under 'Encyclopedias' in the online catalogue by Emilie Savage-Smith, *Islamic Medical Manuscripts at the National Library of Medicine* (www.nlm.nih.gov/hmd/arabic).

6. For Ibn Butlan, who died 8 Shawwāl 458/2 September 1066, see Ullmann, *Medizin im Islam*, pp. 157–8; and Hosam Elkhadem, *Le 'Taqwīm al-ṣiḥḥa' (Tacuini sanitatis) d'Ibn Buṭlān: un traité medical du XIe siècle. Histoire du texte, édition critique, traduction, commentaire*, Louvain 1990.

7. Oxford, Bodleian Library, MS Bodl. Or. 266, fols. 30b–31a (undated, thirteenth–fourteenth century); for

البارد منها

… النافعة لها ولا لتلذذ حاسة الشم ولتكمل منها لذات الحواس الخمس وتنقسم بحسب الازمنة الى ما يوجد
… الشتاء كالنارنج والمنثور والى ما يوجد في كانون الاول من كتاب الفواكه وفي كانون الثاني … تار
… وفي نيسان كالياسمين والتفاح وفي ايار البطيخ والعوسج والنسرين والى ما يوجد في حزيران

الاختيارات

… لقبضه بارد يابس ولمرارته صار فيه ادنى حرارة مع لطافة **الياسمين** قوي الحرارة وا…
… يابس نافع لاصحاب اللقوة والفالج والصداع من برد **النسرين** قريب من قوة الياسمين الا انه
… ونه والدهن منه **النرجس** معتدل في الحرارة واليبس ملطف محلل للرطوبات والبرى
قوي واحد من السنبل والمحرق اذا شق بصله صليبيا وغرس صار مضاعفا

الورد عدة انواع منه الجوري ومنه الاحمر الناصع ومنه الابيض ومنه الاصفر ومنه ما
… الهز وقه اسود وظاهره اصفر فاما طباعه نقية قوى مختلفة الا انه الى البرد ما هو
… ولذلك صار يبرد الدماغ ويجمعه ويسكن حرارته ويحرك للباردي الادمغة زكاما
… ما يسيرا فاما **الخيري** فالاصفر فيه حرارة ما والاسود معتدل **لو** قول حار يابس في الثانية

الشاهسفرم فيه حرارة بها يحلل فضلات الدماغ في رفق واذا القي عليه الماء برد ورطب **النمام**
حار يابس في الثالثة قوي التحليل لرطوبات الدماغ وعصارته نافعة للقوا فع …لا **المرزجوش**
حار يابس في الثالثة لطيف يحلل الرياح من الدماغ ويفتح سدده ويلطف رطوبته ودهنه ينفع
… وجاع الاذن من ريح غليظة واذا اعتصر ماؤه في محجمة على القفا بعد الحجامة اذهب اثار الشرط

… للدماغ لتبريده وفي السهر لسرعة تنويمه اذا اشتم واذا وضع على الراس وهو طري
… يجعل البول مثل رائحته على مثال ما ينصبغ بول المختضب بالحنا احمر بلونه فاما **اللينوفر**
… شبيه بالبنفسج في قوته ومنفعته الا انه ابرد ولذلك صار يسكن الصداع الكاين من حرارة
… هو نوعان اصفر بري وازرق بستاني والازرق ارطب **والمرماحوز** حار يابس وادا نبع

السوسن عدة انواع كلها منسوبة الى الحرارة محللة لارياح الدماغ **الخيري** اما الاصفر فحار
… لطف يحلل باعتدال وبقية انواعه معتدلة في الحر والبرد **الافرنجمشك** قريب
… المرزجوش في افعاله **البهرامج** معتدل المزاج طيب الريح عند النفس ينفع الرياح الحقيقة
… التي في الدماغ **البرم** يجري مجرى البهرامج المحبب قوتها كقوة البرم

… يسفوريلس يقول كثيرا اما باكله الحوامل عند ما يحدث عليهن الشهوات الرديه
… وهو مقاوم للسموم القاتلة **ح** قشره حار يابس حريف وحماضه بارد يابس
… الثالثة وشحمه بينهما وحرارته وعطريته تقوي المعدة وتعين على الاستمرا وحرارته قريبة
… من الاعتدال وحماضه يقطع ويلطف ولحمه متوسط من قشره وحماضه **كسوع** في

التفاح يبرد الدماغ ويرطبه ويخدره **النارنج** يحلل الرياح الباردة منه وهو الطف من الترنج
الليمون شبيه بالترنج في رائحته وفعله في الدماغ **التفاح والسفرجل** رائحتهما مبردة
مقوية للدماغ والنفس ورائحة السفرجل تقطع الغثيان والقيء

… الحارة وتتاخر في البلاد الباردة و… ربا الفواكه نفعا ما هي مشمومة لا ما هي ماكولة والعلة
… ها دون بعض مشابهة الفق في امزجتها والشبيه ينتفع بشبيهه ولهذا صار المعتدل المزاج
المضاده من بعاد عن الصحة قليلا كما ان اهل البلاد الحرورون ياكلون اشيا الباردة ومن دماغه بخار غليظ
… والاحر … ه عنها ومثل ذلك نوجد اثنين في الطعوم واحدا يشتهي طعما واحرا يلتذ به ولا يشتهيه

رحان

ع النيلنفر السكر … في البيت كحرة اللامونيه ان اكله … بالبيت كحرث الحول

الرياحين والمشموم في المجلس لاصلاح الهوا ولتقوية الدماغ حتى لا تفعل بخارات الخمر المفسدة له ور...
في ايلول كالاترج والدستنبويا والليمون والجلسد... وفي تشرين الاول كالتفاح والنرجس والمرزجوش
كالتبق وفي شباط منثور الورد والشاهسفرم وورد السيحر والخيري ما يوجد في اذار كالمنهاد ...

الرياحين والازهار

الرياحين

	الاسم	الطبع	الدرج	جيده	منفعته	مضرته	دفع مضرته	[illegible]	الامزجه	الاسنان	الاوقات
قصو	الاس	بارد يابس ... [illegible]	[illegible]	الخضر الى العفص	للسلح الحار ضماد	السهر	بالبنفسج الطري	٤	الحار الرطب	الشباب	الصيف
قح	الورد	[illegible]	[illegible]	الفارسي الطري	للدماغ الحار	يحدث ... زكام	بالكافور	٤	الحار	الشباب	[illegible]
قصط	الشاهسفرم	[illegible]	[illegible]	السعتري ...	يحلل فضلات الدماغ	يصدع الدماغ البارد	بالنيلوفر	٤	[illegible]	الكهول	[illegible]
ذ	البنفسج	بارد رطب ... [illegible]	[illegible]	اللازوردي المضاعف	شمه نافع في البرسام وشربه يسهل الصفرا	[illegible]	بالخيري والنرجس	٤	الملتهب	الشباب	[illegible]
ذا	السوسن	[illegible]	[illegible]	الاسمانجوني	يحلل العفونة في الدماغ ... [illegible]	الصداع	بالكافور	٤	البارد	الشيوخ	الشتا
ذب	الاترج	[illegible]	[illegible]	السوسي الكبار	[illegible]	بالدماغ الحار ... [illegible]	بالبنفسج الطري ... [illegible]	٤	البارد	الشيوخ	الشتا
ذج	اللفاح	[illegible]	[illegible]	الكبار الرحي	نافع للصداع والطلق ... [illegible]	[illegible]	[illegible]	٤	البارد	الشباب	الصيف

منفعته بقياس

كالتفاح والبطيخ الشامي وفي تموز السفرجل وفي آب ... الترنج الاخضر وجميع الفواكه ...
في اختلاف الوانها وارايحها احتلاف مترجعها في الحار والبارد والرطب واليابس والدليل ...
يلتذون بالالوان الخضر لا عند الهوا واصحاب الماليخوليا يوثرون السود في المواضع المظلمة ...
الروايح الحارة كالمسك والعنبر ولا بعجب من هذا الاختلاف فمثل ذلك يوجد في علم الموسيقي واخ...

(*qānūn*), expounding the principles of dietetics and regimen. Within the frame of the table itself, the titles of the columns are given in large script, and below the titles the entries for each of the seven substances extend across the two facing pages. The first column, reading from the right, gives a number for the entry, in this instance 197 (out of 280). Columns 2–8 are grouped under the larger heading 'aromatic plants and blossoms' (*al-rayāḥīn wa-l-azhār*). The second column contains the Arabic name —in this case *ās*, meaning myrtle. For the third column, labelled 'nature' (*al-ṭibāʿ*), the entry for myrtle reads: 'ʿIsa and Hunayn [say] cold, dry'. Two authorities are cited: Hunayn ibn Ishaq (d. *c.* 873 or 877) and ʿIsa ibn Massah al-Basri (d. *c.* 888), both Baghdadi physicians.[8] The fourth column gives the 'degree' (*daraj*): cold in the 2nd degree and dry in the 3rd degree, in keeping with the system established by Galen in which each substance was assigned a pair of primary qualities (dry or moist, warm or cool) and an intensity on a scale from one (weakest) to four (strongest).

In the fifth column, labelled 'its best form' (*jayyiduhu*), it is said that the preferable type of myrtle is 'fresh *al-khusrawānī*', an unidentified species whose name apparently means 'regal', from Khusraw, the name of a sixth-century Persian king.[9] Its use (*manāfiʿ*), given in column six, is for an inflamed liver, used as a dressing (*ḍimādan*). Its dangers (*maḍarra*), entered in column seven, consist of insomnia (*sahar*), while the antidote for countering or avoiding the danger (*dafʿ maḍarratihi*) is given in column eight as fresh violet (*banafsaj al-ṭariyy*).

The ninth column has a vertical title reading 'that which is produced from it', and for myrtle the entry is zero. For other substances you get such products as a moderate or large amount of blood. Columns 10–13 are grouped together under the heading 'its use by analogy' (*manāfiʿuhu bi-qiyās*), referring to the types of patients or conditions for which the drug is suitable. Under this umbrella, column 10 states that myrtle is useful for those whose temperaments are hot and moist; column 11 for those in the age category of youth; column 12 for use when the season is hot; and column 13 for those living in hot countries.

Columns 14 and 15 occupy the entire left page of the opening. The narrow fourteenth column, with its vertical title, provides (using abbreviations) the names of three authorities: ʿIsa ibn Massah, Hunayn ibn Ishaq, and Yuhanna ibn Masawayh. The latter was also a ninth-century Baghdadi physician and teacher of Hunayn ibn Ishaq. The final cell provides further details regarding the medicinal substance, according to the authorities cited in column 14. In the case of the entry for myrtle, this last cell reads:

Myrtle because of its astringency is cold and dry, but [thanks to] its bitterness there is fragrance and heat in it. Jasmine [al-yāsmīn] *is very warm and very dry. It is not* [?] *useful*

---

further details concerning this manuscript, see Savage-Smith, *A New Catalogue of Arabic Manuscripts in the Bodleian Library*. See also Elkhadem, *Le 'Taqwīm al-ṣiḥḥa' (Tacuini sanitatis)*, table no. 20, item 197.

8. ʿIsa ibn Massah was a contemporary of the more famous translator and physician Hunayn, and he wrote on dietetics amongst other topics; see Ullmann, *Medizin im Islam*, pp. 122–3.

9. The term designates something regal, and is derived from Khusraw, the name of a Persian king who ruled from 531 to 579; it also can refer to a type of wine and a type of cloth (see Francis Steingass, *Persian–English Dictionary*, London 1892, p. 460). The recent editor of Ibn Butlan's *Taqwīm* is of no help regarding this curious term; see Eklhadem, *Le 'Taqwīm al-ṣiḥḥa'*, table no. 20.

for those suffering from one-sided facial paralysis [al-laqwa] *and partial paralysis* [al-fālij, *hemiplegia*] *and headache* [ṣudāʿ] *arising from cold. Jonquil* [al-nisrīn] *has almost the same strength as jasmine except that it is weaker and is more fragrant. Narcissus* [al-narjis] *is moderately warm and dry; it is an emollient and reduces moistures; the wild form has more force and more sharpness than the narcissus of the garden. If the bulb of the garden narcissus is split in a cross before being planted, the florescence is increased.*

Something seems to have gone amiss with the text of Ibn Butlan at this point, for the subject inexplicably shifts from myrtle to jasmine and spring bulbs. The recent edition of Ibn Butlan's treatise presents an identical text, but the editor does not note the unexplained change of subject.

Forty years later, and in Muslim Spain, Ibn Baklarish composed his treatise encompassing 704 medicinal substances. Figure 35 illustrates the table that contains his entry on myrtle.[10] The running header and footer on the folios both concern sarcocol (*anzarūt*), a gum resin of a shrub resembling frankincense, which is also the topic of the first entry in the table itself. The third entry in the table concerns myrtle, and at the right-hand margin has the Latin annotation 'iaris'. The first column gives its Arabic name (*ās*), followed in the next column by its 'nature and degrees' (*al-ṭibāʿ wa-l-daraj*), given as 'cold in the 1st and dry in the 2nd'. The third column, and largest on the right-hand side of the table, is titled 'its explanation in different languages' (*tafsīruhā bi-khtilāf al-lughāt*), and reads as follows:

It is al-rayḥān*, and it is* al-mardiyān, *and it is* al-mardiyānaj, *and it is* al-martah *in Byzantine Greek* [bi-l-rūmiyya]. *And it is* al-mārnah. *It is said that all of these names apply to the seed of* al-rayḥān,[11] *but not to the leaf nor to the branches. In another source its antidote* [iṣlaḥ] *is gum tragacanth* [kathīrā'].[12]

Column 4 of the Ibn Baklarish table provides substitutes, and for myrtle this is specified as rind of pomegranate (*al-rumān*) or gall-nut (*ʿafṣ*). The left-hand side of the table has only one column, labelled 'Usefulness, Properties (*khawāṣṣ*), and Modes (*wujūh*) of Employment'. For myrtle it reads:

It is a sticking-plaster for wounds and cures ulcers. Its strength is the drying power. Its secondary strength is its powerful seizing [jābis] *force when it is placed externally on the body. Its strength in general is its astringent* [qābiḍ] *force. The extract* [*lit.*, *boiled juice*] *is useful for the excessive flow of moisture from the uterus,* [*used*] *when washing. Powdered, it dries up the gums,* ***and it stops breathlessness*** [? al-buhr]. ***Dropping it into an ear from which purulent matter*** [qayḥ] ***is flowing*** [***stops it***]. ***And it stops nosebleeds*** [al-ruʿāf] [***when***

10. The Arcadian Library manuscript, pp. 42–3.

11. *al-rayḥān* is a comprehensive term meaning *any* aromatic or sweet-smelling plant, though it can also apply specifically to sweet basil.

12. The Leiden copy of Ibn Baklarish used by Martin Levey differs, for the last sentence is omitted, and replaced by a sentence giving three additional names: *hīrbān*, *simsin*, and in Persian *mūrtush*. Furthermore, the names *mardiyānaj* and *mardiyān* are specified as Persian names in the Leiden copy, and the Greek name *al-mursīn* is also provided. See Martin Levey, 'The Pharmacological Table of ibn Biklārish', *Journal of the History of Medicine*, 26, 1971, pp. 413–21, esp. p. 418.

applied] mixed with wine, and stops expectoration [nafth] ***of blood and diarrhoea, but it hastens urination. It soothes prickling that occurs around the navel*** [al-maʾana], ***and it is useful for the bite of the tarantula*** [al-rutaylāt], ***the bite of a scorpion, and other complaints.***[13]

When comparing Ibn Baklarish with Ibn Butlan it is evident that a common source (presently unknown) provided a guide to the general layout, with both employing continuous running headers and footers though Ibn Butlan has fifteen columns under six headings while Ibn Baklarish only five columns. The source of the content, however, differed for each author. Ibn Butlan cites authorities within his tabular presentation while Ibn Baklarish generally does not. When it comes to the nature and degree of the substance, they differ with regard to both attributes. As for the use of myrtle, the only one given by Ibn Butlan (for an inflamed liver) is not even mentioned by Ibn Baklarish. The latter gives the antidote as gum tragacanth while the former says it is fresh violet. Ibn Baklarish has no category for 'preferred form' of the substance, and therefore we cannot know if he knew of the mysterious *al-khusrawānī*, while Ibn Butlan does not exhibit a particular interest in synonyms.

Let us now compare Ibn Baklarish with later twelfth-century tabular presentations of medicinal substances. Ibrahim ibn Abi Saʿid ibn Ibrahim al-ʿAlaʾi al-Maghribi composed such a treatise for a member of the Danishmendid dynasty in Anatolia who was active at the middle of the twelfth century.[14] Al-ʿAlaʾi's popular synoptic tables of 550 drugs circulated under several titles, most commonly the *Almanac of Simple Drugs (Kitāb Taqwīm al-adwiya al-mufrada)* or *Success in Medicine and in Therapy among the Categories of Diseases and Complaints* (*Kitāb al-Munjiḥ fī al-ṭibb wa-l-tadāwī min ṣunūf al-amrāḍ wa-l-shakāwā*).[15] Figure 38 illustrates the opening table from a copy completed on 17 Rabīʿ II 896 (= 27 February 1491) by an unnamed scribe and now in the collections of the Bodleian Library. This particular copy was owned by an important Ottoman theologian and legalist who was *qāḍī* of Edirne from 1491 to 1501; his Turkish annotations are evident in the margins.[16]

Note that in al-ʿAlaʾi's treatise there are no running headers or footers, and the numeral assigned each medicinal substance runs down the left-most column of the left-hand page, in contrast to the right-hand column in Ibn Butlan's table. The myrtle plant is second in the sequence given by al-ʿAlaʾi—that is, the second row on this table, under the row of column headings. On the right-hand page of al-ʿAlaʾi's treatise, the table has on the right six narrow columns presenting (1) the name, in this case *ās*, myrtle; (2) the nature *(al-māhiyya)*, said in this instance to be 'leaves of a

13. The portion of the translated text in bold type is missing from the Leiden copy used by Martin Levey (Levey, 'The Pharmacological Table', p. 419).

14. The treatise was apparently composed for Dhu al-Qarnayn ibn Ismaʿil Danishmendid, who governed from the city of Malatya from 1152 to 1162 (547–57 A.H.). See Henri P. J. Renaud, 'Un problème de bibliographie arabe: le *Taqwīm al-Adwiya* d'al-ʿAlaʾaī,' *Hespéris*, 16, 1933, pp. 60–98, esp. pp. 79–81; and Irène Mélikoff, 'Dānishmendids', *Encyclopedia of Islam*, new edition, II, pp. 110–11.

15. See Ullmann, *Medizin im Islam*, pp. 275–6.

16. ʿAbd al-Rahman ibn ʿAli Muʾayyad-zade Čelebi, who was the first Ottoman to form a private library, of over 7,000 volumes (see Theodor Menzel, 'Muʾayyad-zāde', *Encyclopedia of Islam*, new edition, VII, p. 272), For further details concerning Oxford, Bodleian Library, MS Hyde 35, see Savage-Smith, *A New Catalogue of Arabic Manuscripts in the Bodleian Library*.

shrub, sweet-smelling, known for [use in] washing'; (3) the type (*al-nawʿ*), 'garden and mountainous'; (4) the preferred form (*al-ikhtiyār*), 'fresh, young, savoury, fragrant'; (5) the temperament (*al-mizāj*), 'cold in 1st degree, dry in 2nd'; and (6) the potency (*al-quwwa*), 'very strong astringent'.

NEXT OPENING
Fig. 38.
Oxford, Bodleian Library, MS Hyde 35, fols. 19b–20a

The next two columns (the seventh and the eighth) on the right-hand side are each much larger. The seventh is titled 'Its Usefulness for Parts of the Head' and for myrtle reads:

It strengthens the eye and stops it watering [damʿa] *and prevents water descending to it* [*i.e., a cataract*]. *It quiets ophthalmia and protrusion* [*of the eyeball,* juḥūẓ]. *It prevents dandruff* [ḥazāz], *and strengthens the hair, making it thick and preventing it from falling out. Placing it* [*mixed*] *with wine on the head stops nosebleeds* [al-ruʿāf], *and its ashes* [ramād] [*are useful*] *for pterygium.*

The eighth column is titled 'Its Usefulness for the Chest and Organs of Respiration', and reads:

Fruit of the mature plant is useful against cough [suʿāl], *and it stops expectoration* [al-nafth] *of blood. A syrup of it* [rubb] *is useful for the chest and the lungs* [al-riʾa]. *When it is used as a perfume, it is salutary for the pneuma, strengthens the heart, and is useful against palpitations of the heart* [khafaqān].

Moving to the left-hand side of the table, the ninth column titled 'Uses for the Organs of Digestion and Evacuation' reads:

Its seed calms the stomach and stops loss of blood. It is useful against dribbling of urine and a loosening [istirkhāʾ = irtikhāʾ] *of the bladder* [mathāna] *and its ulcers; it is also suitable for burning urine. When it is cooked in water and one sits in the cooked juice, it is useful against protrusion* [burūz] *of the rectum* [*lit., lower part*] *and against prolapse of the uterus. And it is useful against swelling of an inflamed liver.*

The tenth, and last, of the large columns is titled 'Uses Throughout the Entire Body', and for myrtle the following are given:

When used as a warm compress [*or bath,* nuṭūl], *it obstructs/blocks the vessels and restores the bones. It settles* [?] *the parts that have stopped functioning* [*or become slack*] *and sweetens the odours of the body. It is useful against inflamed swellings and whitlow* [dāḥis, felon], *burning* [?] *and pain of toenails and the dryness in them. And it is useful against fresh scabs.*

The table is then symmetrically balanced by six narrow columns on the left side. They are as follows: (col. 11) Directions for Use: make an oil (*duhn*) from its leaves, and from its seeds a drink (*sharāb*) and a syrup (*rubb*); (12) The Amount to Use: 2 *mithqāl*s of seeds; (13) Its Dangers: sniffing it causes insomnia (*sahar*); (14) Its Antidote: violets (*banafsaj*) and white water lily (*nīlūfar*); (15) Its Substitute: flower of the henna plant (*al-ḥinnā*); and (16) The Number of the Drug: 2.

20

منفعته في آلات اعضاء الغذاء والات النفض	منفعته في جميع البدن	كيفية استعماله	مقدار ما يستعمل منه	مضرته	اصلاحه	بدله	عدد الادوية
حماضه يقطع القي ويوافق المحمومين ويقطع الاسهال المري ويشهي الطعام وربه يدبغ المعدة وورقه يذهب نفخ البطن وقشره يسحج المعدة ودهنه ينفع من البواسير وحبه يلين البطن ويقتل الدود	رايحته يصلح فساد الهوا وهو من المسمنات ويحرق ويطلى به البرص وقشره ينفع من لدغ الافاعي ضمادا وشربا وحبه ينفع من السموم ولدغ العقارب ودهنه للنافض والمفاصل الباردة	يتخذ من قشره شرابا ودهنا ومن حماضه شرابا ومن لحمه مربى	نصف مثقال من حبه	حماضه يضر بالصدر والعصب	الخشخاش شراب	النيمو	كا
حبه يمسك البطن ويقطع نزف الدم وينفع من تقطير البول واستر خاء المثانة وقروحها وهو صالح لحرقة البول واذا طبخ في الماء وجلس في طبيخه نفع من بروز السفل وشق الرحم وينفع من ورم الكبد الحار	يحبس العرق ويجبر العظام نطولا ويقوي الاعضا المسترخية ويطيب رايحة البدن وينفع من الاورام الحارة والداحس وحرق النار ووجع الاظفار واليابس منه ينفع من الجرب الرطب	يتخذ من ورقه دهنا ومن حبه شرابا ورُبا	مثقال من حبه	شمه يحدث سهرا	والنيلوفر البنفسج	زهرة الحنا	كب
قشر اصله يشرب للصفار واليرقان ويضمد به الطحال وينفع من وجع الكبد وورمها وحبه ينقي معد الصبيان من رطوبات اللبن ويقوي المعدة ويدبغها وينفع من بروز المقعدة ويجفف بلة الرحم	يتدخن به فينفع من فساد الهوا ووبايه ودخانه يجفف الجدري ويشفه ويسحق بالخل ويطلى به الثاليل مرارا فتذهبها واذا طبخ ونطل بمائه الاعضاء المشتنجة شددها	يستعمل مشروبا من داخل وموضوعا من خارج	مثقال	بالصدر الخشن	والسكر الطبرزد	عفص او حلبنار	كج
يذهب رياح المعدة ويزيل نفخها ونفختها ويحبس القي ويفتح السدد ويدر الحيض وينفع من الحصاة واذا اشربت بالخل حركت البطن اي نوع كان فيه ودخانها ينفع من اختناق الرحم	اذا دقت وذرت على الاربيتين والابط قوتها ومنعت رايحة الصنان ويقوي الاعضا ضمادا بالخل ويحلل صلابة المفاصل وينفع من الاورام الجاسية	يستعمل شربا ونطولا وذرورا	درهم نصف	بالامعاء	انيسون	وزنها اذخر وربع وزنها سنبل	كد
يذيب الفضول اذا شرب بسكنجبين وينفع من ورم الكبد والمعدة ويحلل ورم الحجبة ويستنقع في مائه فينفع من صلابة الرحم والورم فيه ويعين على الحبل حمولا	يلين الاورام الصلبة في المفاصل وينفع من بحرها مع صفرة البيض والميبختج وينفع من القلموني	اكثر ما يستعمل نطولا وضمادا من خارج	درهمين شربا	بالاعضاء المسترخية	بماء الآس المنبطل	الحلبة	كه

دهن الشونيز بوليو

الادوية	اترج	آس	اثل	اشنه	اكليل الملك
الماهية	معروف	ورق شجر طيب الرايحة يعرف بالغسلة	هو الطرفا البستاني لحب في قدر الحمص شديد القبض يميل عذب	قشور رقيقة لطيفة يلتف على شجر البلوط والجوز والصنوبر فيها عطرية	زهر نبات هلالي الشكل
النوع	حلو وحامض	بستاني وجبلي	البستاني اثل والبري طرفا	واحد	ابيض واصفر
الاختيار	الكبار الاصفر	الغض الطري الذكي الرايحة	الحديث	البيضاء الزكية الرايحة	الحديث الاصفر الصلب
المزاج	قشره حار يابس في ب لحمه ب رب حماضه ب ب في ج ج ح رب	بارد في الاولى يابس في الثانية	باردة في الثانية يابس في الثالثة	معتدل في الحر والبرد	معتدل من الحر والبرد
القوة	قشره ملطف	قابض مقوي	قابض	فيها قبض يسير	محلل ملين
منفعته في اعضاء الرأس	حماضه يجلو الكلف واللون طلاء ويكحل به لبياض العين والظفرة واليرقان ودهنه ينفع من الرعشة وقشره لامراض العصب الباردة وحبه الحل يسقط العلق ويشد اللثة والارنج يطيب النكهة	يقوي العين ويقطع دمعتها ويمنع ما ينحدر اليها ويسكن الرمد والجحوظ وينفع من الحزاز ويثور الراس ويقوي الشعر ويكثفه ويمنع تناثره ويجعل الخل على الراس يقطع الرعاف ورماده للظفرة	ثمرته يقوي الاسنان وينفع من اكلها ويشد اللثة المسترخيه وينفع من بثور الفم والقلاع ويغسل الراس بمائه فيقتل القمل والصيبان ودخان خشبه ينفع من اللقوة	اذا انقعت في الشراب وشرب نومت نوما عميقا واذا وقعت في الاكحال قوت العين ونفعت من رطوبتها ونشفت دمعتها	يعجن الورد اليابس مسحوقا بطبيخه ويضمد به العين فينفع من الرمد ويطلى الراس بمايه فينفع من الصداع وهو ينفع من الكلف واورام الاذنين وفي وجهها ضمادا
منفعته في الصدر وآلات النفس	ربه ينفع من الخفقان الحار وورقه ... المفرحات للقلب وكذلك زهره ... الطف من ورقه وقشره ايضا من المفرح...	ثمرته البالغة ينفع من السعال ويقطع ... الدم وربه ينفع الصدر والرئة والا... لعطريته ملايم للروح مقو للقلب ... الخفقان	اذا استعمل حب الاثل مع غيره من الادو... نفع من قروح الرئة والصدر وحصف... وقطع نفث الدم	فيها تفريح للقلب ونفع من الخفقان	يطبخ مع دقيق الباقلي ودهن الورد ويضمد به الثدي فيحل صلابته و... من ورمه وتعقد اللبن فيه

In his table al-ʿAlaʾi provides no information about synonyms for myrtle, for he devoted the final section of his treatise to a 'Discourse on Drugs Having Multiple Names'. In this concluding chapter, which does not employ synoptic tables, al-ʿAlaʾi does not give any synonyms for *ās*, myrtle.

A second comparative example is taken from the *Almanac of Simple Drugs and Foodstuffs (Kitāb Taqwīm al-adwiya al-mufrada wa-l-aghdhiya)* by Hubaysh ibn Ibrahim al-Tiflisi. Little is known of his life except that he worked at the end of twelfth century and was a prolific medical author.[17] His *Almanac* consists of two books, the first covering 730 commonly used medicaments and foodstuffs discussed in tables of 13 columns with each chart extending over a full opening. The second book lists in simple two-column tables, in alphabetical order, 880 medicaments and foodstuffs more difficult to find and scarcely used, with suggestions for substituting drugs discussed in the first book.

Figure 41 presents the table from Book I of al-Tiflisi's *Almanac* that includes his discussion of myrtle, occupying the bottom row of the table. This example is from a copy completed by an unnamed copyist in Baghdad in middle of the month of Rabīʿ II 876 [September/October 1471] and in the collections of the Bodleian Library (MS Pococke 389). There is a small running header presenting general principles, but no footer; 11 authorities are cited, including Ibn Butlan.

The first five narrow columns are grouped together under the rubric 'Names of the Drug', with the five columns providing (1) the Arabic name, in this instance *ās*; (2) the Persian name *(bi-l-fārisiyya)*: *mūrid*; (3) the Syriac name *(bi-l-suryāniyya)*: *āsā*; (4) the Byzantine Greek name *(bi-l-rūmiyya)*: *mīrsīn*; and (5) the classical Greek name *(bi-l-yūnāniyya)*: *Aṭīqūnus*.

The next six columns (nos. 6–11) on the right-hand page provide brief accounts of the attributes of myrtle: (6) Its Nature *(māhiyya)*: a well-known tree, and in it is a bitterness *(marāra)* along with astringency *(ʿufūṣa)*; (7) Its Preferred Part *(mukhtār)*: rounded *al-khusrawānī*, fresh leaves; (8) Its Natures *(ṭabāʾiʿ)*: [according to] ʿIsa, cold in the 1st degree, dry in the 2nd; (9) Its Uses *(manāfiʿ)*: strengthens the heart and the stomach and destroys palpitation of the heart *(khafaqān)*; (10) Its Dangers *(maḍarra)*: it obstructs the natural disposition *(al-ṭabʿ)* and produces insomnia *(sahar)*; and (11) Its Antidote *(iṣlāḥ)*: by means of 'military' violet *(bi-l-banafsaj al-ʿaskarī)*.

On the left-hand side of the table there is a narrow column (no. 12 counting from the right) that gives the Size of the Dosage *(miqdār al-sharba)*, which for myrtle is specified as two and one-half *dirhams*. The thirteenth and largest column presents the opinions of different physicians regarding the medicaments. For myrtle, al-Tiflisi says:

Dioscorides [*said it*] *blackens hair; when drunk, it curbs jaundice; cleanses the stomach and restrains its nature* [al-ṭabīʿa]*; drys up purulent moistures in the stomach.* ***Galen*** *said it cleanses the thick humours from the body and is useful against loss of hair and baldness*[18] *when it is plastered on them externally, but it is necessary that you scarify the area before embrocating it and then it is smeared on it.* ***Rufus*** [*stated it was useful for*] *severe colic* [maghṣ] *and cleanses the stomach of phlegmatic and putrid humours.*

17. For some of his medical writings, see Ullmann, *Medizin im Islam*, 169–70.
18. al-Tiflisi gives both *dāʾ al-thaʿlab* and *dāʾ al-ḥayya*, alopecia and ophiasis, whose names derive from loss of

As with Ibn Baklarish, it is evident that al-ʿAla'i and al-Tiflisi were working within an established tradition of tabular presentation as exemplified by Ibn Butlan. Moreover, al-Tiflisi cites ʿIsa ibn Massah al-Basri (d. *c.* 888), who was also one of the authorities cited by Ibn Butlan in his discussion of myrtle. The following table [Fig. 39] allows us to compare more easily the four authors we have discussed.

From this (admittedly limited) comparison, it is evident that Ibn Baklarish was not directly influenced by Ibn Butlan, nor does Ibn Baklarish appear to have influenced the other writers we have discussed. With regard to the synonyms given for myrtle, it is seems that the only common point between Ibn Baklarish and al-Tiflisi is the term *mīrsīn* or *mursīn*, which reflects the classical Greek of Dioscorides μυρσίνη; al-Tiflisi, however, calls this term *rūmiyya*, usually applied to the Byzantine Greek of Anatolia, rather than *yūnāniyya*, which is the standard term for classical Greek. For the latter, al-Tiflisi gives the curious synonym of *aṭīqūnus*, for which no parallel is obvious.[19]

While there appears to be no evidence of influence by Ibn Baklarish upon al-ʿAla'i or al-Tiflisi, a comparison of the synonyms with those given by Maimonides (d. 1204) is quite revealing. Maimonides' *Commentary on the Names of Drugs* (*Sharḥ Asmā' al-ʿuqqār*) is preserved in a unique manuscript transcribed in the handwriting of Ibn al-Baytar (d. 1248), who was originally from Malaga in the kingdom of Granada and the author of the most influential of all Arabic treatises on basic medicinal substances.[20] This exercise in pharmacological philology by Maimonides displays considerable similarity to the synonymatic material given Ibn Baklarish. Maimonides' entry for myrtle reads: 'Myrtle (*al-ās*): Its name is well known amongst the people of the Maghrib as *al-rayḥān* (or *al-rīḥān*), but amongst the peoples of Egypt is it *al-mursīn*.'[21] Both of these synonyms are given by Ibn Baklarish.

The similarity is even more striking when we compare entries for the plant called *uqḥuwān* or *aqḥuwān*, whose identity is uncertain but which may be feverfew, an aromatic bushy plant with feathery leaves and daisy-like flowers traditionally used to reduce fever.[22] A comparison of Ibn Baklarish's synonyms for *uqḥuwān* with those

---

hair in foxes and the shedding of skin by snakes respectively; on these terms, see Peter E. Pormann, 'Yūḥannā ibn Sarābiyūn: Further Studies into the Transmission of his Works', *Arabic Sciences and Philosophy*, 14, 2004, pp. 233–62, esp. 246–7.

19. The Persian variants *mūrid*, *mardiyān*, and *mardiyānaj* are all ultimately derived from Greek, μύρτος being a variant of μυρσίνη. The Arabic *ās* comes through the Syriac *āsā* from the Akkadian. The modern Arabic synonyms used in Egypt are *mirsīn* and *riḥān*; see M. A. H. Ducros, *Essai sur le droguier populaire arabe de l'inspectorat des pharmacies du Caire* (Mémoires présentés à l'Institut d'Égypte, 15), Cairo 1930, p. 15.

20. Istanbul, Aya Sofya MS 3711, edited with a French translation by Max Meyerhof, *Sharḥ asmā' al-ʿuqqār (L'explication des noms de drogues), un glossaire de matière médicale composé par Maïmonide.* Texte publié pour la première fois d'après le manuscript unique, Cairo 1940; English trans. Fred Rosner, *Moses Maimonides' Glossary of Drug Names, Translated from Max Meyerhof's French Edition* (Memoirs of the American Philosophical Society, 135), Philadelphia 1979. The attribution to Ibn al-Baytar is made on the basis of an owner's note on the title page; a second note suggests it was copied by Ibn Tarhan al-Suwaydi (d. 1291), but Meyerhof argues convincingly that it was transcribed by Ibn al-Baytar.

21. Meyerhof, *Sharḥ asmā' al-ʿUqqār*, p. 5, no. 10.

22. *Tenacetum parthenium* L. or related species. It has also been identified with camomile. On the difficulty of precisely identifying this plant, see Martin Levey and Noury al-Khaledy, *The Medical Formulary of al-Samarqandī and the Relations of Early Arabic Simples to those Found in the Indigenous Medicine of the Near East and India*, Philadelphia 1967, p. 230; Henri P. J. Renaud and Georges S. Colin (eds.), *Tuḥfat al-aḥbāb. Glossaire*

Fig. 39.
A comparison of Ibn Butlan, Ibn Baklarish, al-ʿAlʾi and al-Tiflisi

	Ibn Butlan	Ibn Baklarish	al-ʿAlʾi	al-Tiflisi
Authorities	ʿIsa Hunayn Ibn Masawayh			ʿIsa Dioscorides Galen Rufus
Preferred Form	*al-khusrawānī*		fresh, savory	*al-khusrawānī*
Dangers	insomnia		insomnia	insomnia
Antidotes	violets	gum tragacanth	violets; lily	'military' violet
Substitutes		pomegranate rind gall-nut	flower of henna plant	
Uses	inflamed liver	wounds, ulcers; discharges from uterus, ear, nose; diarrhoea; aids urination; itching; tarantula, scorpion bites	many uses, incl.: hair; heart/palpitations; inflamed liver [NO bites]	stomach hair heart/palpitations; jaundice [NO bites]
Synonyms		*al-rayḥān* *al-mārna* *al-mardiyān,* *al-mardiyānaj* [*bi-l-fārisiyya,* Leiden MS] *al-martah* (*bi-l-rūmiyya*) [*al-mursīn* (*bi-l-yūnāniyya*); *simsin, hīrbān* Leiden MS]		*āsā* (*bi-l-suryāniyya*) *mūrid* (*bi-l-fārisiyya*) *mīrsīn* (*bi-l-rūmiyya*) *aṭīqūnus* (*bi-l-yūnāniyya*)

Fig. 40.
A comparison of Ibn Baklarish, Maimonides and al-Tiflisi

	Ibn Baklarish	Maimonides	al-Tiflisi
Feverfew (*uqḥuwān*)	*ghashūnish* *bablanīra*, in Saragossa white type: *amārīqūn* yellow type: *amārīṭūn*	*ghashūnish* *bablanīra* in al-Andalus white type: *amārīqūn,* (*bi-l-yūnāniyya*) yellow type: *amārīṭūn* *al-qirāṣ* (*bi-l-ʿarabiyya*)	*kāwajshim* (*bi-l-fārisiyya*) *ʾīnātūrāʾ* (*bi-l-suryāniyya*) *barafthāwamin* (*bi-l-rūmiyya*) *buyalfūn,* (*bi-l-yūnāniyya*)

given by Maimonides is also revealing [Fig. 40].[23]

NEXT OPENING
Fig. 41.
Oxford, Bodleian Library, MS Pococke 389, fols. 6b–7a

Interestingly, neither Ibn Baklarish nor Maimonides include Hebrew terms amongst the synonyms, though both were noted Jewish scholars. For an individual entry, Maimonides often adds one or two additional terms over those included in Ibn Baklarish. Maimonides does not, however, include animal or mineral products in his commentary on drug names, thus limiting it only to medicinal plants, whereas Ibn Baklarish was far more inclusive in his definition of medicinal substances. Moreover, Maimonides sorted or arranged his entries in a different order from that of Ibn Baklarish, sometimes placing an entry under a lead name that was for Ibn Baklarish an alternative synonym.

The close relationship between the synonymatic lists of Ibn Baklarish and Maimonides is even more apparent when the entries for feverfew are compared in Figure 40 with that presented by al-Tiflisi.[24]

The synonyms given by al-Tiflisi for *uqḥuwān* bear virtually no resemblance to those presented by either Maimonides or Ibn Baklarish. On the basis of this small sampling, it suggests that either Maimonides employed the treatise of Ibn Baklarish when composing his commentary or that they shared a common source which varied enormously from any of the sources employed by the other two twelfth-century writers discussed here, al-ʿAla'i and al-Tiflisi.

It is also suggested by the comparisons presented here that Ibn Baklarish employed an already well-established didactic device when he chose to present his material in a tabular format. Moreoever, it appears that Ibn Baklarish's treatise may not have had a great deal of influence amongst later writers who resided in more eastern regions. Could the fact that Ibn Baklarish was a Jewish scholar have any bearing on the dissemination of his treatise? Far more remains to be done before such a question can be answered. A larger number of treatises need to be compared, and a larger sampling of individual entries within each treatise must be undertaken. Nevertheless, since Ibn Baklarish's synonymatic lists appear to resemble closely those of Maimonides, while almost no characteristics are shared in common with the other synoptic drug presentations surveyed here, does this suggest the possibility that certain texts tended to circulate only amongst certain groups of scholars? Could Ibn Baklarish's treatise have circulated primarily amongst the community of Jewish physicians and scholars of the twelfth century and not have been widely read outside that community?

de la matière médicale marocaine, Paris 1934, p. 15, no. 25; and Martin Levey, *Early Arabic Pharmacology. An Introduction Based on Ancient and Medieval Sources*, Leiden 1973, p. 157, note 4.

23. The entry for *uqḥuwān* given by Ibn Baklarish occurs on pp. 32–3 of the Arcadian Library manuscript, and it has been translated into English (from the Leiden MS) by Martin Levey (Levey, *Early Arabic Pharmacology*, pp. 156–7). Maimonides' entry for *uqḥuwān* can be found in Meyerhof, *Sharḥ asmā' al-ʿuqqār*, p. 6, no. 20.

24. Oxford, Bodleian Library, MS Pococke 389, fols. 9b–10a.

فيه جزءا بعد جزء ويداومه يغنى ما بقى منه بقوة حرارته مثل الجندبادستر وما اشبهه فى الطبع من الادوية

اختيارات آراء الاطبا فى خاصيتها

قال بقراط اذا شرب منه مع المطبوخ او المثلث نفع من الادوية القتالة ومن لدغ الهوام قال ديسقوريدس ان المراة الحامل اذا تحملت منه اسقطت الجنين وان تحملت منه مراة لم تحبل اسرعت الحبل قال ابن ماسه ينفع من دا الثعلب ودا الحية مسحوقا بخل الخمر ورماده بالخل ينفع من عرق النسا قال اسحق انه ينفع من السموم كلها وخصوصا من اللدوغ ومن لسع العقارب منفعة بينة

قال الرازى انه يطيب النكهة وضماده ينفع من الاورام الحارة ويحلل الرياح قال اربياسيوس يقوى الدماغ ويشد العمور ويوافق امراض الفم والبثور الحادثة فيه ويقوى اللثة ويمنع انتشار القروح ويدملها بغير لدغ واكلها ينفع من الرمد ويعقل الطبيعة قال بولس ينفع من رمد العين ويقوى القلب والاحشا ويحبس البطن قال ديسقوريدس ينفع من القروح ويدملها ضمادا وكذلك ينفع من الجرب جدا

قال جالينوس انه يعقل الحد والمطبوخ باللبن يزيد فى المنى ولا يعقل قال ارجيجانس الفارسى منه ينفع من قيام الدم ومن بيول الدم وعلل الكلى والمثانة واختناق الرحم قال روفس الفارسى ينفع من الزحير ويسكن ما يعرض من البلغم المالح الذى يحدث منه البواسير والثوثة فى المقعدة ومن اوجاع العارضة فى اسفل البدن والحقنة بما الاحمر المطبوخ مع بعض الادوية القابضة ينفع من سحج الامعا

قال بقراط دمه ينقى الكلف ورماد راسه ينفع من دا الثعلب وخصوصا البحرى قال مسيح دماغه مشويا ينفع من الرعشة الحادثة عقيب المرض واذا اضمد بدماغه عمور الصبيان اسرع نبات الاسنان قال اسحق انفحته اذا احلت بسمن او زبد او عسل وشربت بخل نفعت من الصرع واذا شربت بالخل بعد الطهر ثلثة ايام منعت الحبل ودمه يذهب بالبهق والكلف اذا طلى به عليهما واذا اشوى نفع من قرحة الامعا

قال ابن سينا هى شجرة كبيرة من كبار الشجر يسمونه بطبرستان طاحات فقاحه مفتح للسدد وما ورقه يقتل القمل ويطيل الشعر وخاصة عروقه اذا استعملت مع الخمر قال ماسرجويه عصارته نافعة من السم اذا شربت مع عسل وينفع من القولنج ويفتح سدد الدماغ لاسيما فقاحه قال الرازى طبيخ لحابه مع الشاهترج والهليلج مروقا ينفع من الحميات البلغمية وثمرته ضارة للصدر جدا قاتلة

قال جالينوس انه يقوى الدماغ وينفع من السودا والبلغم قال ديسقوريدس ينفع من الوسواس السوداوى والبلغم اللزج ويقوى الدماغ ويسهل الاخلاط المجتمعة فيه قال قولس ينفع من المغص الشديد ويسهل الاخلاط الردية وهو يقوم مقام احد ادوية الايارج
قال اربياسيوس ينفع من وجع الامعاء وينقى الدماغ والمعدة والاحشا من الاخلاط الباردة الردية وينفع من الصرع وامراض العصب من برد

قال بقراط انه يسهل البلغم اللزج المجتمع فى المعدة والراس ويزيد فى الباه ويطيب النكهة قال اربياسيوس انه يزيد فى الجماع ويذكى الذهن ويصفى اللون ويسمن البدن ويقوى الاعضاء الرخوة وينفض ما فيهما من البلغم اللزج قال مغنس ينفع من نزول الما فى العين ومن السبل وداء الثعلب والحية قال روفس يفتح السدد وينقى المعدة ويحد اللسان وينفع من النسيان وامراض الدماغ وعرق النسا ووجع الوركين

قال الرازى ينفع من الصرع والماليخوليا ويحد البصر وينفع من الربو والسعال العتيق وخشونة الصوت قال جالينوس ينفع من صلابة الطحال ويقوى المعدة وكذلك خله وينفع من الاستسقا والبرقان ويدر البول قال مسيح المسلوق منه مع عسل يلين الطبيعة وينفع من وجع المقعدة والرحم قال اسحق ينفع من المغص وخله ينفع من الحميات المزمنة وطلاوه يقلع الثواليل ومع العسل ينفع من الثعلب والحية

قال جالينوس ينفع من القروح والسعفة والبثور وداء الثعلب وداء الحية اذا طلى عليها مع دهن الورد قال ديسقوريدس انه يبرد الاورام والخراجات العارضة فى ظاهر البدن اذا استعمل مع مرهم الزفت والشمع قال روفس ينفع من القروح والبثور اذا خلط بدهن الورد والورد وطلى عليهما نفعهما وادملهما قال ارجيجانس ينفع من القروح والاورام الحارة والنفاخات طلاوه بدهن الورد العتيق

قال ديسقوريدس يسود الشعر اذا خلط مع اخلاط اجزا تشاكله واذا شرب يابسا قمع الصفرا وينقى المعدة ويحبس الطبيعة وينشف الرطوبات الرديه فى المعده قال جالينوس ينقى الاخلاط الغليظة من البدن وينفع من دا الثعلب ودا الحية اذا طلى عليهما من خارج وينبغى ان يشرط الموضع قبل ذلك ثم يدلك عليه قال روفس ينفع من المغص الشديد وينقى المعدة من الاخلاط البلغمية الردية

ومنها محلل وهو الدوا الذي من شانه ان يفرق ويبدد الخلط بتنجيره واخراجه اياه عن موضعه الذي اشتبك

اسما الادوية بالعربية	بالفارسية	بالسريانية	بالرومية	باليونانية	ماهيتها	مختارها	طبايعها	منافعها	مضرتها	اصلاحها
آذريونه	بخخروس مريم	عقار اعرطيثا	بيقوفكاالوفن	فوطيلوفين	هو اصل العرطيثا وقيل انه اصل نبات آخر	الابيض الحديث منه	اسحق حار يابس في الثالثة	من السموم ولدغ الهوام وداء الثعلب	بالمثانة والآلات البول	ببزر القثا وبقلة الحمقا
الرامال	مشهور	ارماليل	فوتيهيج	الفنده	حشيشة يجلب من اليمن يشبه القرفة	الحديث الطيب الرايحة	اسحاق سخونة وقبض وتخفيف	يطيب النكهة ويقوي الدماغ والقلب جدا	يثقل الطبيعة	بالجلاب والقطونا
الارز	برنج	ارزي	الايريزين	مروفن	من الحبوب المعروفة ابيض اللون واحمر	الابيض النامي في الطبخ	عيسى حار في الاولى يابس في الثانية	من لدغ المعدة وباللبن يزيد في شهوة الباه	ردي لاصحاب القولنج	بالعسل والسكر الاحمر
الارنب	خرگوش	مشهور	لاغعون	مرلبسهون	حيوان معروف بري وبحري	البري الصيد الكلاب	غير الطعام يابس	دمه ينفع من السحج مقلوا ويجلو البصر	اكل لحمه يورث السهر	بالابازير الكبار اللطيفة
الازادرخت	كنار	معروف	ابيلدارون	ذيازوين	شجرة معروفة كبيرة لها ثمر يشبه النبق	فقاحه اذا كان طريا	فقاحه حار في الثالثة يابس في الاولى	يفتح سدد الدماغ وينقي الراس من البلغم	ثمره رديه للمعدة	بالبنفسج المربى والانيسون
الاسطوخودوس	معناه موافق الارواح	مشهور	سنحاس	اسطوخودوس	نبات بلا نور حريف مع مرارة يسيرة	الاخضر الحديث منه	الرازي حار في الاولى يابس في الثانية	من المرة السوداء وينقي الدماغ من الاخلاط الردية	بالرية ويورث الغثيان	بالصمغ العربي والكثيرا
الاسارون	بادرين دارشيشي	نردين دبرا	اساروين	سرانيوس	خشب فوفيري طيب الرايحة لذاع اللسان	ما يميل الى الصفرة الذكي الرايحة	جالينوس حار يابس في الثالثة	من وجع المفاصل كذلك ينفع من عرق النساء	يجفف الاعصاب	بالزبيب المنقوع ودهن اللوز
الاسقيل	بيازموش	بصلا ذيبا	افيقطون	بالفونيس	بصل بري لونه اصفر يميل الى البياض	ما في طعمه حلاوة مع حدة	حنين حار يابس في الثالثة	من الصرع والربو والسعال العتيق	يصدع ويورث الدوار	بالسكنجبين السكري
الاسفيداج	سپيداب	اسباذاج	فسيميثين	مرسيثي	هو رماد الرصاص او رماد الآنك	الابيض الصلب النقي	روفس بارد يابس في الثانية	يلين الاورام الصلبة وينفع من بثور العين	بالاعصاب وما يليها	بالسكر والصمغ العربي
الآس	مورد	اسا	مرسينن	الطيقوفيس	شجر معروف فيه مرارة مع عفوصة	الخسرواني المستدير الورق الغض	عيسى بارد في الاولى يابس في الثانية	يقوي القلب والمعدة ويذهب الخفقان	يجفف الطبع ويولد السهر	بالبنفسج السكري

ANNA CONTADINI

THE ZOOLOGICAL-MEDICINAL MATERIAL IN THE ARCADIAN LIBRARY MANUSCRIPT

Although the manner of presentation is quite different, the zoological material in the twelfth-century *Kitāb al-Musta'īnī* of Ibn Baklarish in the Arcadian Library is clearly capable of being related to the more specifically zoological-medicinal literature of the period.[1] However, its affiliations are difficult to establish, and the following notes must be viewed as a preliminary contribution. They attempt to characterize the nature of this material, and to compare it to the equivalent *manāfi'* material found in the manuscripts of Ibn Bakhtishu''s *Kitāb Manāfi' al-ḥayawān* (*The Book on the Usefulness of Animals*).

'Ubayd Allah ibn Jibra'il ibn Bakhtishu' was a member of an illustrious family of physicians who ran the school of medicine at Jundishapur and later were personal physicians to a number of Abbasid Caliphs.[2] The last known member of this line, he lived in the eleventh century, and it is likely that the material preserved in his zoological-medicinal writings represents the culmination of a lengthy experimental and textual tradition. Ibn Bakhtishu''s *Book on the Usefulness of Animals* is extant in several copies in Arabic and Persian, and three of the Arabic ones are illustrated.[3] The earliest known copy, in the British Library, has the title *Kitāb Na't al-ḥayawān* (*The Book of the Description of Animals*). In this work the discussion of each animal is divided into two parts. The first is a general introduction, in which the principal characteristics of the animals are treated, as well as their habits and their reactions to different situations. This part, according to the earliest extant copy, derives from Aristotle's *De animalibus*. The second part, attributed to Ibn Bakhtishu' himself, deals with the different parts of the animal and how they may be used to beneficial effect, principally to cure various human illnesses.[4]

As for the compilation of simples made by Ibn Baklarish, although plants provide the majority of the entries, there are a considerable number of zoological entries (and also, incidentally, some mineral ones), and in this respect it is akin to Dioscorides' *Khawāṣṣ al-ashjār* (*The Properties of Plants*; *De materia medica*), which contains a smal-

1. Ibn Baklarish, Yusuf ibn Ishaq al-Isra'ili, a Judaeo-Arab physician who lived and operated in Almería where he wrote the *Kitāb al-Musta'īnī* for his patron, the Hudid ruler of Saragossa, al-Musta'in bi-llah Abu Ja'far Ahmad ibn Yusuf al-Mu'tamin bi-llah, who reigned between 1085 and 1109 (478–503); see Albert Dietrich, 'Ibn Biklāri<u>sh</u>', *Encyclopedia of Islam*, new edition, Suppl. p. 383. Hitherto scholarly attention has focused on the importance of the *Kitāb al-Musta'īnī* for the Romance words that it contains, while Reinhardt Dozy used it for his *Supplément aux dictionnaires arabes*, Leiden 1881.

2. Ibn Abi Usaybi'a, *'Uyūn al-anbā' fī ṭabaqāt al-aṭibbā'*, ed. August Müller, Cairo 1882–4, I, pp. 123–48; see also Anna Contadini, 'The Ibn Baḫtīshū' Bestiary Tradition: the Text and its Sources' in: *Medicina nei secoli: arte e scienza*, 6.2, 1994, pp. 349–64.

3. For a list of manuscripts see Anna Contadini, '*The Kitāb Na't al-ḥayawān* (BL Or. 2784) and the So-called Ibn Bakhtīshū' Illustrated Bestiaries', School of Oriental and African Studies, University of London, 1992 (unpublished PhD thesis), pp. 149–50 and p. 152.

4. Ibn Bakhtishu', *Kitāb Na't al-ḥayawān*, London, British Library, MS Or. 2784, datable to *c.* 617–22/1220–5, fols. 94a–95b. For this manuscript in general and its Aristotelian connection see Anna Contadini, 'A Bestiary Tale: Text and Image of the Unicorn in the *Kitāb Na't al-ḥayawān*', *Muqarnas*, 20, 2003, pp. 17–33 (see pp. 19–20); eadem, 'The *Kitāb Manāfi' al-ḥayawān* in the Escorial Library', *Islamic Art*, 3, 1988, pp. 33–57.

Fig. 42.
Top: Hippopotamus (*al-faras al-baḥrī*); middle: Beaver (*al-qasṭāriyūn*); bottom: Weasel (*ibn ʿirs*). Dioscorides, *Khawāṣṣ al-ashjār* (*De materia medica*), Samarkand, 475 A.H./1083 A.D. Leiden, University Library, Cod. Or. 289, fol. 61b

ler section (varying in size depending on the version) dealing with animals and their parts [Figs. 42–4].[5] The verso side of the folio (the even-numbered page, right-hand) of the Ibn Baklarish manuscript has the beginning of the entries, the recto side (odd-numbered, left-hand page) the continuation, so that the text has to be read horizontally across the double spread. Typically, there are six entries per page, separated by thin red lines. The verso side comments on the name, often giving equivalents in other languages, while the recto is devoted to the medicinal uses [Figs. 45, 46].

The number of animals touched upon in the *Kitāb al-Mustaʿīnī* is some 58, and includes man, woman and child (see list below), as in the *manāfiʿ* literature, where human beings are generally considered as part of the animal kingdom.[6] One obvious difference from the *manāfiʿ* texts, however, is in organization. In the *Kitāb al-Mustaʿīnī* the same animal may reappear at various points throughout the tables, as the text (in alphabetical *abjad* order) is arranged according to individual components and not, with few exceptions, by animal. The logic of the alphabetical organization thus means that the various organs of a given animal are dispersed and scattered. The *manāfiʿ* literature, on the other hand, deals globally with each animal, discussing its characteristics and then listing the properties of various organs. Furthermore, the animals are presented within groups according to a zoological taxonomy. A typical order is: man, domestic mammals, wild mammals, domestic birds, wild birds, reptiles, fish, crustaceans and insects.[7]

The alphabetical arrangement of the *Kitāb al-Mustaʿīnī* often produces a group of entries where the initial term provides the common feature of a single body part or substance. Thus, for instance, under urine (*bawl*) we have the following series of entries (pp. 68–71):

~ urine of a man (*insān*)
~ children (*aṭfāl*)
~ a pig (*khinzīr*)
~ cows (*baqar*)
~ buffaloes (*jawāmīs*)
~ a goat (*māʿiz*)
~ camels (*ibil*)
~ sheep (*ḍaʾn*)

5. Among the manuscripts of Dioscorides, for Leiden University Library, Cod. Or. 289, dated 475/1083, and Istanbul, Topkapı Saray Library, Ahmet III, 2127, dated 626/1229, both of which have a section on animals, see Mahmoud M. Sadek, *The Arabic Materia Medica of Dioscorides*, Quebec 1983; for Istanbul, Süleymaniye Library, Aya Sofya 3703 (dated 612/1224), see Alain Touwaide, *Farmacopea araba medievale: codice Ayasofia 3703*, 2 vols., Milan 1992. For Dioscorides in general see Albert Dietrich (ed. and trans.), *Dioscurides Triumphans: ein anonymer arabischer Kommentar (Ende 12. Jahr. nach Chr.) zur Materia Medica*, 2 vols., Göttingen 1988; Michael Rogers, 'The Arab Contribution to Botany and Pharmacology', *Arab Affairs*, 6, 1988, pp. 71–86 and idem, 'Text and Illustrations. Dioscorides and the Illustrated Herbal in the Arab Tradition' in: Anna Contadini (ed.), *Arab Painting. Text and Image in Illustrated Arabic Manuscripts*, Leiden 2007, pp. 41–7; Minta Collins, *Medieval Herbals. The Illustrative Traditions*, British Library Studies in Medieval Culture, London – Toronto 2000, chapter 2.
6. This is the case for all manuscripts in the Ibn Bakhtishuʿ tradition as well: see Contadini, 'The Ibn Baḫtīshūʿ Bestiary Tradition'.
7. Contadini, 'The Ibn Baḫtīshūʿ Bestiary Tradition', pp. 349–50.

اسب آبی

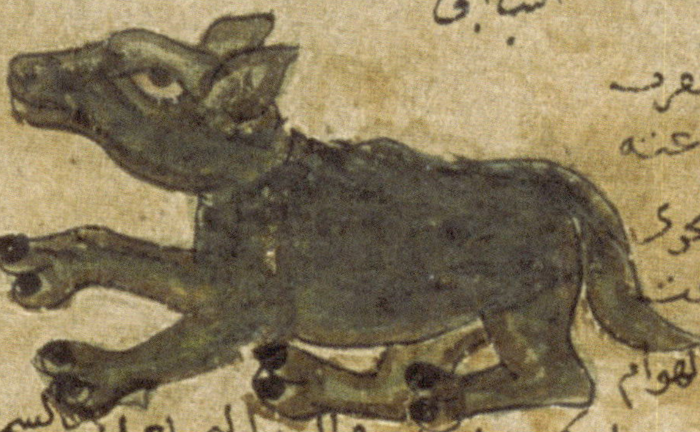

علا لسع النمل البحري والعقرب
والعكوس البحريه نفع من ساعته
العطوما وهو الفرس البحري
خصى هذه اذا ابست ودق
وشربت بطلا نفع من لدغ الهوام

جند بيدا ستر

هو حيوان يكون ويعيش في البر والبحر يعدو على السمك
والسراطين يوخذ خصاه ويسحق
ويشرب منه مثقال لسع الهوام
والسموم والادويه القتاله وهو
معطش واذا شرب منه وزن مثقالين
مع الفوتنج البري ادر الطمث و

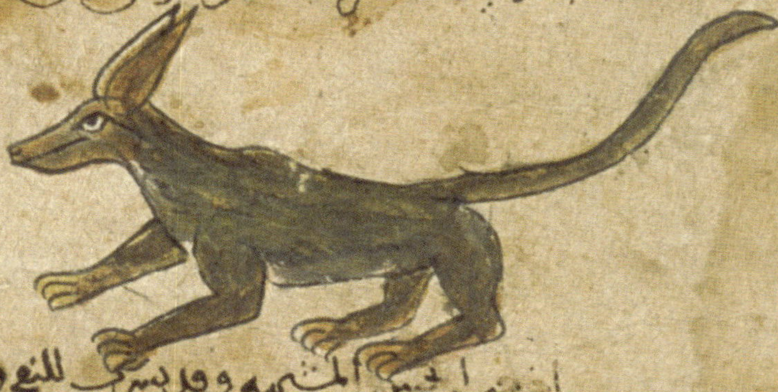

اخرج المشيمه وقد يشرب للنفخ والمغص والفواق واذا خلط بخل ودهن
ورد ومسح به الراس او اشتم من به نسيان او سبات نفعه وكذلك يفعل اذا
شرب به واذا شرب او تمسح به وافق الارتعاش والوجع المسمى اسيموس وجميع
اوجاع الاعصاب ... والمختار منه المزدوجه اعني
الملتصقه ... في حجاب ... واحد وما في داخلها
يشبه الموم ... الطعم ... متقشر يحجب ...
... بالشواء والصمغ ... الحديد ...
... هذه الدابه اذا لحقها الصيادون تسل خصيتها فتلقيها
... محال ولان خصيتها لاصقه بموضعها مثل خصي الخنزير و...
ان ... الخصي مع الحجاب الذي يحويها وهي رطوبه شبيهه بالعسل
و... ذلك ...

ابن عرس بري

اذا سلخ واخرج بطنه وطرح به ثم
... والطاو...
منه وزن ... مثقالين ... نفع من نهش

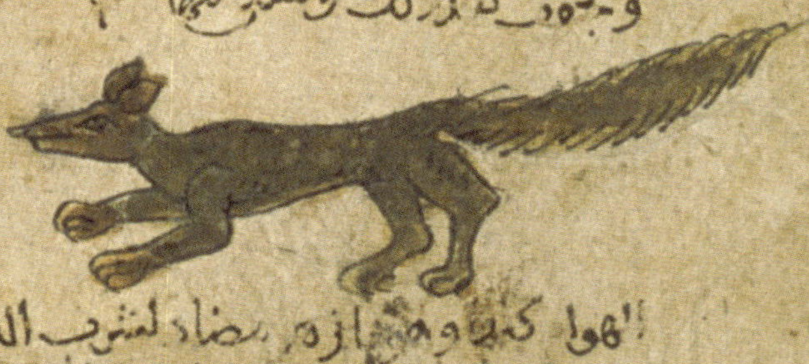

الهوام ... لشرب الدوا القتال الذي ... اذا
شرب ... بعسل ... ونطبخ ثم يشرب منه

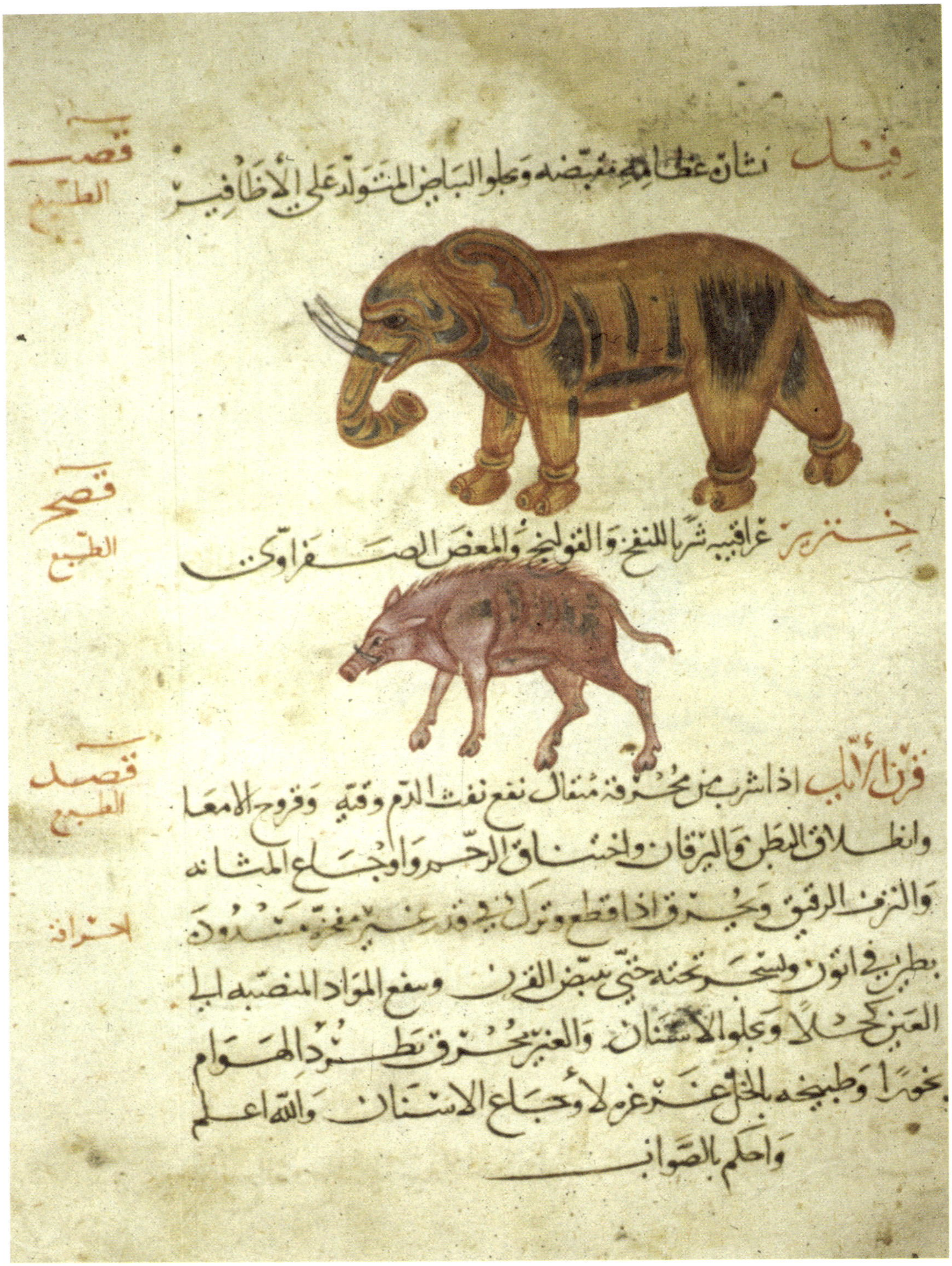

Fig. 43.
Elephant (*al-fīl*) and Pig (*al-khinzīr*). Dioscorides, *Khawāṣṣ al-ashjār* (*De materia medica*), Northern Iraq or Syria, 626 A.H./1229 A.D. Istanbul, Library of the Topkapı Saray, MS Ahmet III, 2127, fol. 67a

Fig. 44.
Rooster (*al-dīk*). Dioscorides, *Khawāṣṣ al-ashjār* (*De materia medica*), Samarkand, 475 A.H./1083 A.D. Leiden, University Library, Cod. Or. 289, fol. 63b

NEXT OPENING
Fig. 45.
Ibn Baklarish, *Kitāb al-Musta'īnī*, The Arcadian Library manuscript, pp. 88–9: hedgehog and lamb brain (*dimāgh al-qunfudh wa-l-ḥamal*)

FOLLOWING OPENING
Fig. 46.
Ibn Baklarish, *Kitāb al-Musta'īnī*, The Arcadian Library manuscript, pp. 262–3: crow (*al-ghurāb*)

من الفزع من الما ويعرض لمن يأخذه فوم ناب الكلب الكلب اذا عض انسانا فا
يجعلونه في قطعة من جلده ويشدونه في العضد ليحفظ من يشد عليه من
الكلاب الكلبة ❁ ذنب الايل اذا دق وسحق وشرب
نفع من نهشة الافعي ❁ حوافر الجواميس اذا احرقت وشرب
منها انا ما كثره درهمين ونصف في كل يوم نفعت المصروعين واذا
خلطت بزيت ووضعت على الخنازير حللتها واذا تضمد بها ابرات الشقاق
العارض من البرد ❁ لبخراوس وهي زوائد عدد طاهرة
قرب ركب الخيل وعند الحوافر اذا دقت وسحقت وشربت بخل
ابرات من الصرع وكذلك حوافرها ❁ اظلاف الماعز
اذا احرقت وخلطت بخل ولطخ بها موضع دا الثعلب ابرات منه ❁
النعال الخلقان التي للخف اذا احرقت وسحقت وذرت على حرق
النار وعلى السحج العارض من الخف ابراته ❁

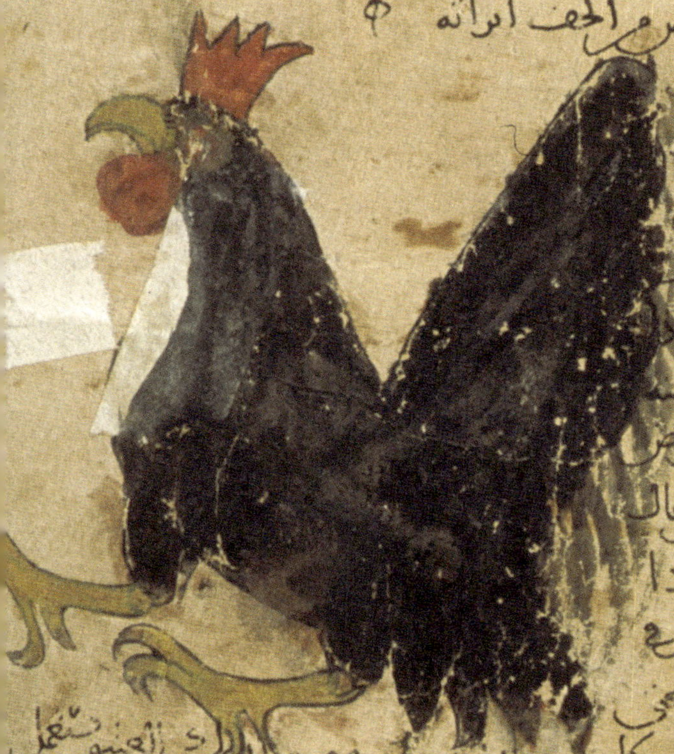

قطوريس وهو الديك
اذا شقق ووضعت
وهي سخنة على نهش الهوام
ابرات منه وينفع ارسل
وكذا دون ودماغها اذا
شرب بشراب نفع ايضا منه
ووضع نزف الدم العارض
من حجاب الدماغ الذي يقال
له مننجس والديك اذا
احرق واخذ الحجاب الذي في
داخل الحوصلة وجفف وسحق
وشرب بشراب وافق من كانت معدته بارده ومن الديك العتيق يستعمل
لاسهال البطن ... يخرج اخلاطها وتصير مذاقها ... ويطبخ
... هو طولي ما ... منه بلت هو طولي ويحم ... ومن الناس من يطبخ معه
... حجري اذا النبات المسمى ... وطه ...

المعروف بالخلام ومضر بالامتنان والله الزايله عن الاعتدال الى البرودة امام طبعها — وامام عرضها
فانه عرمضر بغلاحه ان اللبن اذا اخرج من الضرع فبحسب طول مدته وبعد
الغليه فلمنع من الفولج ويطلق البطن لا سيما اذا طبخت بالسنبلة

٨٩

منافعها وخواصها ووجوه استعمالها

يقلع من الحمرة والاورام الحاره اذا طلي عليها واذا خلط بماء عنب الثعلب او ماء حي العالم كان فعله اقوى ومن خلط بدقيق الشعير وحمل على الاورام التي في التربيز والخصوتين

يقطع حرارة الصفرا ويبرد المعده والكبد ويقطع العطش وينفع حرارة الرحم ويقوي المعده وليسط الطبيعه ۞

وهو نافع للقروح الحادثة في الغلاه والدبر ويدمل القروح الخبيثه المنتشره في البدن واذا خلط نفع البلغم او فيروطي خلل الزيلان ويقلع من قروح العمر ان استعمل وحده او مع العسل المنزوع الرغوه ويقلع من مداواة الخوانيق وقوة الرمروحس بانضه بجبيه منفيه له قوة بجلاء ويقطع اللحم الزائد في القروح ۞

اذا شرب من بحكه شارب السم نفعه نفع النفع واذا حمل على مواضع لدغ العقارب سكنها وان محو منه شي ودس بالخل ودلك به موضع القوابي الحادثه في الجسد من المره السوداء اذهبها ويقلع من النسعفه في الراس وجميع الجسد ۞

اذا استعمل نقلو انفع من قرحة الامعاء ويقطع الاسهال المزمن واذا شرب بخمر نعلى مثل ذلك عن بعول الطين واذا اكلت بالزنجبيل والبصل هيجت شهوة الجماع وزادت في الطبيعه من شرب منه مع ماء الجبل مسهال بالخل والعسل نفع من عشا البصر

اذا اشوى ووضع على نهش الهوام ونهود في جبن ليشف نفع منه ويجب ان يوانز وضعها على نهش الهوام ولسع العقارب المره بعد المره ودلكه يختلفه ليشوكل واحد منهما والرضاحيه والرجاح ليفعل مثل ذلك وقبل جميع الطين اما خاصه واذا اشرب منه ماع الروب نفع من نهش الهوام ويقطع الدم العارض من نحب الرماع ۞

والربو ووجع المفاصل ويعج المعده ومن يطبخ بالارنب او الفراطم او الشبث والكمون

— ونفعه من سائر ذلك وخاصه النفع من القولنج — سنفعه عجيب ۞

٨٨

اسجق اما اللبن الحامض بارد يابس بطيء الانهضام بعيد الانحدار ثقيل في المعدة مولد للخلط المر
وكثيرا ما يولد الضرس في من كانت معدته حارة واما متى كانت الاسنان واللثة بلغمية فيحال اصلاحه
عمره بالخروج من الضرع كان لنقصان جودة غذائه وكثرة فساده. واما من الربوط

الاسم	طبائعها بالدرجة	تفسيره باختلاف اللغات	ابداله
دردي الخل	حار يابس في الثالثة	هو عكار الخل وهو الذي يرسب بقعر القليان وهو ارضيه عكر العنب	[illegible]
دوغ	بارد يابس في الثانية	هو مخيض البقر ويعرف بالبربرية اغودو ومعناه لبن محمض. اسجق. هو الرايب. ابن ماسويه هو اللبن الحامض المنزوع الزبد المتخذ من لبن البقر	الرايب
دهنج	حار يابس في الثانية	هو اصناف صنف يعمل من المرقشيثا بان يصبغ اللون ويقطع عنده انه لم يجد يطبخ الكحل فاذا صار في لون المغرة رفع وقد يعمل من حجارة النحاس ومنه صنف يكون اجنبيس	اقليميا [illegible]
دهنج	حار يابس في الثانية	هو حجر اخضر في لون الزبرجد وذلك ان ان يكون به يكون في معادن النحاس وقال ابن الجلاس في معرفة الاحجار الحجار يقع له بخار من الكبريت المتولد فيه فيرتفع ذلك البخار مثل الزنجار فاذا صار الى موضع نضجه ادى لكل انه	[illegible]
دماغ العصفور	حار رطب في الثانية	الدماغ بالفارسيه مغز ويعرف المخ بالفارسيه ايضا مغز وبالسريانية مخا وقيل فيه	ادمغة العصافير
ديك	حار رطب في الاولى	يعرف بالفارسيه خروس ومعناه جعل الزنط وبالبربرية تايزت	[illegible]

وانه يخرج عنه ذلك كموسى الزجاج غليظا ويوافق الحميات المزمنة ولا ان يعرض

fex

dichrous ٥

emathitis: petra turcisca

cerebellu

Galus alector

وصمغ ماال الى الحلاوة يقرب من حلاوة عروق السوس مع قبض يسير ومرارة خفيفة ومن الفلسطيني وهو ينبت في الصيف دقيق الورق مجتمع الاغصان كـ ... ارانبه مما يخلف في كل سنة واما الاول الكبير فيسقا العام كله والاسماء المواضع الرطبة والمروج

منافعها وخواصها ووجوه استعمالها

نافع من اوجاع الكبد محلل للحمى بمائها ويفتح السدد العارضة فيهما وورق هذا النبات اذا دق فانعما وخلط بشحم الخنزير العتيق ووضع على القروح العسرة الاندمال ابراها ... العافية نافع من الجذام المتقادمة والخانيه حمى الربع وحمات الحسار وقد يجعل الروم نواره ومقوا اخضر في ذبر الرجاجة فتبسط كل يوم ه ومن غيره لام اصلاحه ما لا تبسوه

اذا عمل منه حسو وشرب نفع من نفث الدم والقيح عن اسحق قال غيره اذا عمل منه حسو ويجسى فانه لمعتاد اوفيه ونصف واقي نفث الدم واذا تضمد به كان له قوة تغري وتنضج

المستعمل من عزره الشوكة جميعا وهو قابض يقطع الطبيعة ويعمل منه سويق كما يعمل من النبق ويشرب للاسهال وذكر ان هذا النبات كثيرا بالتراب في بلاد البربر ونواحيه الغيروان وهو معروف مشهور هنالك ه

ما عمل منه في جلود البقر فانه اذا ذيب بالخل ولطخ به نفع من القوبا ويقشر الجرب المتقرح الذي ليس بغابر وينفع من حرق النار واذا حل بالماء الحار واذا حل بالعسل والخل نفع الجراحات وعن الشمع يصلح ان يخلط في مراهم الراس وادوية الجرب ه ه

الطين في تاخير الغراب وهو حار يابس كما هو في انا حار بدو ويصب عليه ثلاث سكر جات خل ويترك اياما حتى يعفن ثم يخرج ويسحق على ملائه من اسرب ويخضب به الشعر فانه يسوده وقال ونقل انه ينفع به التردد فيو حار الرود ويسحق ويطلى به الراس فيسوده ه

الشين على بركة الله وتاييده

السواد كور ... الزيتون فيه ماده ... ابرة منه صنف ... الذي تعرفه العامة بشجـ ... نزرود ... اخضر وتعنصر ... يعمل ... منه

... ومعرفة ... والكمان ... النقادة ... من البحر ... سرد ... ما ... ينا

الغافث اربعة اصناف منها صنف كبير الورق ولونه الى الغبرة يلزق بالبر وله نوار ... اصفر
منها النوع يصنع العطارة لانه ارطب انواع الغافث واكثر ما به ومنه صنف ثاني يعرف بالغافث
اصل الحسن الرقيق الورق احمر الورق نواره صغير ورائحته كرائحة الكبير وطعمه مثل طعمه وهو

الاسما	الطبايع والدرج	تفسيرها باختلاف اللغات	الابدال منفعتها
عاقرقرحا	حار في الثالثة ... 17	يقال له بالعجمية مشكنه ار ديابي من طريق انه يلتصق بالبر وبالعربية الغرار ويسمى بالعجمية ايضا البارده وبالبربرية الترملاين وبالعجمية ايضا البلفيره وهي حشيشة البراغيث ه	...
غبار الرحى	حار يابس في ...	هو غبار يجتمع على حيطان الرحى مما يتطاير عند الطحن ومنه يعمل غرا المعقرين ليلصق به الكتب ه	...
غبيرا	بارد يابس ...	قيل هي شجرة مشوكة لا ارتفاع لها اغصانها حمر وورقها يشبه ورق الكمثرى البري ولها حب مدور اغبر اللون ولذلك قيل لها غبيرا وهو الجوذر بالبربرية ه	...
غرا	حار ...	يراد معنا بالغرا ما يصنع من جلود البقر الذي يلزق به المواعين وغير الحوت الذي يستعمله القواسون وصناع الغيران وهو اصلب ما يلزق به ه	بعضها من بعض
غراب	حار يابس ...	الغراب هو الغراف وهو ابو المرقال وهو الاعرج لانه يحجل كانه مقيد ومن اسمائه حاتم ويقال له الحور تفاولا وابن دانه لوقوعه على دابة البعير ... ويقال ان الغراب هو اسود الحجم منها ويقال للصغير الجر	الاطلية التي يصلح ...
تم	جز	الغين على بركة الله ه	جز

ومنه صنف ثالث على النبات ... عواده قليلة الورق ...
البراغيث ويقال ... رائحة ...
ما وصفنا ...

قل

We have, in all, twelve such groups:

~ rennet (*infiḥa*): of hare (*arnab*); cows; deer/stag (*ayyil*); camel and antelope (*jamal wa-ẓaby*); horses (*khayl*); dog (pp. 46–7)
~ droppings (*ba'r*): of sheep; goat (pp. 68–9)
~ urine (as above)
~ skin (*jild*): of hedgehog (*qunfudh*); ram and billy goat (*kabsh wa-tays*) (pp. 78–9)
~ blood (*dam*): of snake (*thu'bān*, pp. 84–5); man; bear (*dubb*); lambs (*khirfān*); turtle-doves (*shafānūn*); doves (*fawākhit*); billy goats; kid (*jady*); hare; dog; bull (*thawr*); frogs (*ḍafādi'*); pigeons (*ḥamām*) (pp. 90–3)
~ dung (*zibl*): of man; boy (*ṣabī*); cows; sparrows (*'aṣāfīr*); pigeons; chickens (*dajāj*); mice (*fa'r*); Egyptian vulture (*rakham*); lizard (*ḍabb*); donkeys (*ḥamīr*); horses; pig; elephant (*fīl*); dog; wolf (*dhi'b*) (pp. 116–17)
~ spleen (*ṭiḥāl*): of pig; goat; fox (*tha'lab*) (pp. 146–7)
~ liver (*kabid*): of goat; hedgehog; pig; donkey; bear; dog (pp. 162–3)
~ milk (*laban*): of cows; sheep; goat; women (*nisā'*); horses; she-asses (*utun*) (pp. 170–1)
~ meat (*laḥm*): of chameleon (*ḥirbā'*); vipers (*afā'ī*); donkeys; mice; cows; hedgehog (pp. 172–3)
~ gall-bladder (*marāra*): of sheep; goat; bull; pig; bear; chickens; wolf; partridge (*ḥajal*); fish (*samak*); hyena (*ḍab'*); crane (*kurkī*); doves; eagle (*'uqāb*); sea scorpion (*'aqrab al-mā'*); turtle (*sulaḥfāh baḥrī*); gazelles (*ẓibā'*);[8] elephant (pp. 184–9)
~ fat (*shaḥm*): of sheep; goat; stag; bear; fox; donkey; duck (*baṭṭ*); chickens.

There is, as one might expect, an emphasis on domestic species, birds as well as mammals, but, as the above inventory shows, there are also a number of other animals. As a further group entry we may mention eggs:

~ eggs (*bayḍ*): egg white (*bayāḍ al-bayḍ*); boiled eggs (*bayḍ maslūq*); soft eggs (*bayḍ nīmrasht*); very lightly cooked eggs (*bayḍ khafīf jiddan*)

In addition, there are a few other body parts or secretions for which there is only a single entry. In order of occurrence these are:

~ spittle (*buṣāq*, pp. 68–9)
~ old skins (*julūd 'atīqa*, pp. 80–1)
~ hedgehog and lamb brain (*dimāgh al-qunfudh wa-l-ḥamal*, pp. 88–9)
~ ear wax (*wasakh al-ādhān*, pp. 102–3)
~ hoof (*ḥāfir*, pp. 140–1)
~ bone marrow (*mukhkh al-'iẓām*, pp. 188–9)
~ sweat (*'araq*; pp. 212–13)
~ charred bones (*'iẓām muḥraqa*, pp. 212–13)
~ goat penis (*dhakar al-tays*, pp. 260–1)

8. The manuscript has *ḍ·bāh*, but since *ri'm* and *shādin* are given as equivalents, it may be read as a plural of *ẓaby*.

~ human hair (*sha'r al-insān*, pp. 270–1)
~ various fats (*shuḥūm mukhtalifa*; the animals mentioned are fish, lion, goose and pigs, pp. 272–3).

Finally, there are a number of entries devoted to particular animals, in order of occurrence:

~ hare (pp. 48–9)
~ snail (*ḥalazūn*, pp. 142–3)
~ swallow (*khuṭṭāf*, pp. 257–8)
~ Spanish flies (*dharārīḥ*, pp. 260–1)
~ flies (*dhubāb*, pp. 260–1)
~ crow (*ghurāb*, pp. 262–3)
~ scorpion (*'aqrab*, pp. 212–13)
~ spider (*'ankabūt*, pp. 212–13).

When we turn from these differences in formal arrangement to consider what is said about the properties of each organ, extruent or species, we enter a familiar world. The means of preparing the remedies, with the animal part being variously cooked, stirred into a potion or paste, crushed and ground, and the liquids, plants and other substances used in conjunction with it, can all be matched in the *manāfi'* literature, as can the conditions and diseases for which they are most frequently prescribed, ranging from, among many others, curing blisters and inflammations, stopping nosebleeds, alleviating toothache and the pains of childbirth, to stimulating sexual desire and potency and conception. One would expect, accordingly, to find a considerable amount of common material, reflecting a consensus among doctors in the Islamic world about the particular virtues of a given body part, enshrined in what might be described as a common body of knowledge with a related teaching syllabus expressed through a common textual tradition. The material selected by Ibn Baklarish might then be expected to represent this common tradition.

But things are not quite that simple for, as I have observed elsewhere, the appearance of familiarity conveyed by these texts is often deceptive.[9] Typological similarities certainly abound, but when one moves from the general to the specific, the uses different texts describe for a given ingredient are frequently not the same. This warns us that the relationship between Ibn Baklarish and the other *manāfi'* texts may be far from straightforward, that lines of affiliation may be difficult to detect, and that common sources may only occasionally be established with confidence.

This is not to say that there are no clear instances of congruence, and it is possible, indeed, to find one or two cases of virtual identity. A particularly clear example of shared material may be shown by juxtaposing the texts of Ibn Baklarish and Ibn Bakhtishu', as represented by the *Kitāb Na't al-ḥayawān*, concerning one of the bizarre processes to which the crow [Figs. 47 and 48] is subjected:

9. A fuller discussion of this point is found in Contadini, 'The *Kitāb Na't al-ḥayawān* (BL Or. 2784)', pp. 73–4. See also Remke Kruk, 'Elusive Giraffes: Ibn abi l-Ḥawāfir's Badā'ī al-akwān and Other Animal Books' in: Anna Contadini (ed.), *Arab Painting*, pp. 49–64.

Ibn Baklarish [Fig. 46]:

الطبري تاخذ الغراب وهو حي ويصيره؟ كما هو في إناء جديد ويصب عليه ثلاثة سكرجات خل وترك أياما
حتى يعفن ثم يخرج ويسحق على صلاية من اسرب ويخضب به الشعر فإنه يسوده

Ibn Bakhtishuʿ:

وإن أخذ غراب وطرح كما هو حي في إناء مقير جديد ويصب عليه ثلاثة سكرجات خل وترك أياما حتى
يعفن و يخرج ويسحق على صلاية من رصاص ويطلى به الشعر فإنه يسوده

You take a crow while still alive. It is put [?] *just as it is into a new vessel and three saucers of vinegar are poured over it. It is left for some days until putrid, and is then taken out and pounded on a lead pounding block and the hair is dyed with it: it will turn black.*

In the Escorial version of Ibn Bakhtishuʿ's *Book on the Usefulness of Animals*, an almost identical passage occurs [Fig. 48].[10] Considered in isolation, this passage provides strong grounds for assuming access to a common source, and suggests that much of the material in Ibn Baklarish dealing with animals may be related to corresponding passages in *manāfiʿ* texts. This assumption is reinforced by one of the uses to which human hair is put, where Ibn Baklarish's text is again virtually identical to that of the *Naʿt*:

Ibn Baklarish:

إذا بل بالخل ووضع على عضة الكلب الكلب برأ من ساعته

Ibn Bakhtishuʿ:

إذا بل بالخل ووضع على عضة كلب كلب نفع من ساعته

When wetted with vinegar and applied to a rabid dog bite it will cure/help instantly.[11]

A further point of congruence is provided by another use of human hair, but here the *Naʿt* is more specific about the condition to be treated:

Ibn Baklarish:

إذا بخرت المرأة بالشعر منع من وجع الرحم

Ibn Bakhtishuʿ:

إذا دخن به امرأة منع من الورم المعروف بخناق الرحم

When a woman is subjected to the smoke of [*burning*] *hair it prevents pain in the womb/the inflammation known as 'suffocation of the womb'.*

10. *Kitāb Manāfiʿ al-ḥayawān*, San Lorenzo del Escorial, Biblioteca Real, MS ar. 898 (dated Rabīʿ al-awwal 755/March 1354); see Contadini, 'The *Kitāb Manāfiʿ al-hayawān* in the Escorial Library'.
11. The comparable section of the Escorial text is missing.

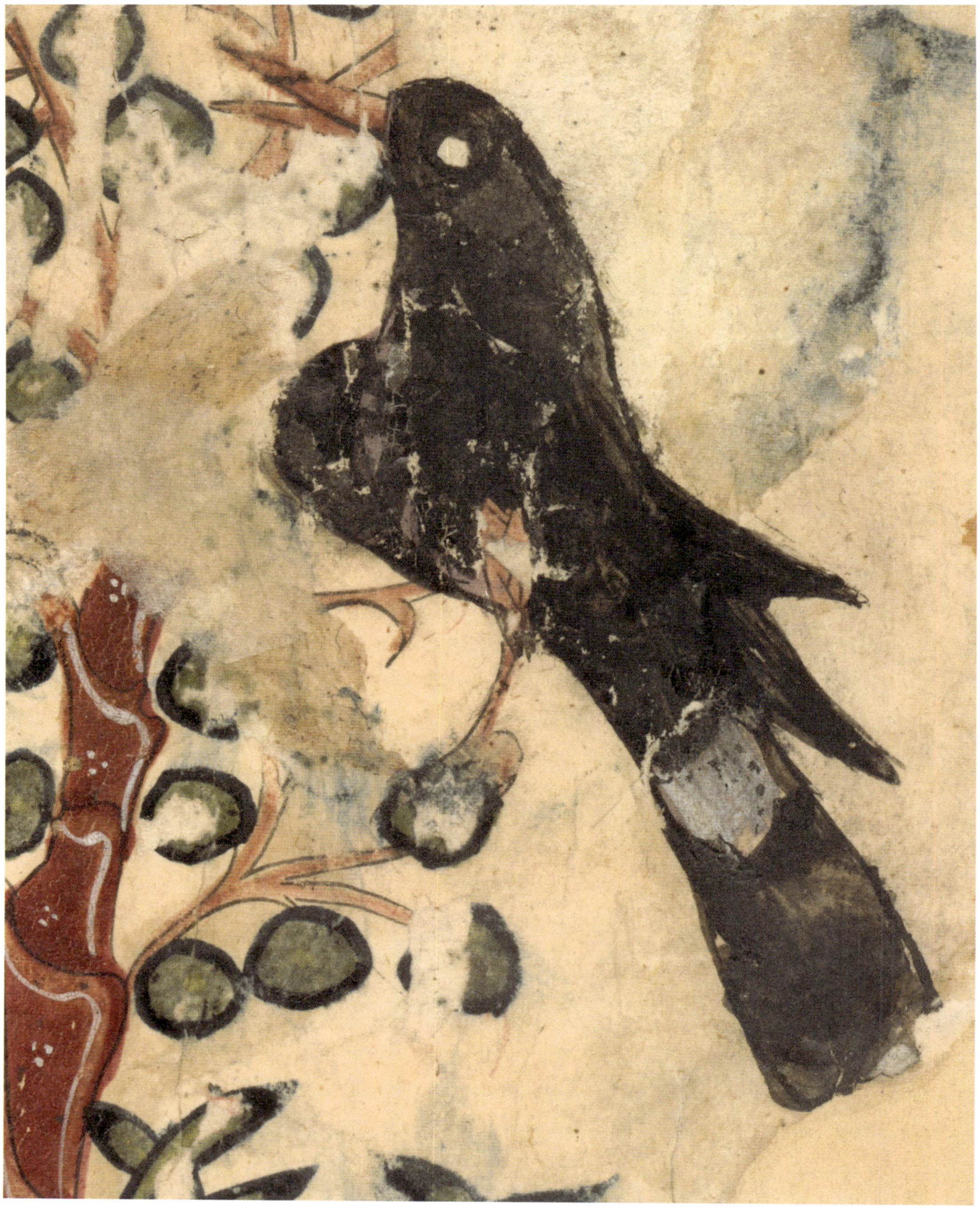

Fig. 47.
Crow (*al-ghurāb*). *Kitāb Naʿt al-ḥayawān*, North Jazīra, dateable *c.* 617–22/1220–5. London, British Library, MS Or. 2784, fol. 40b (detail)

OPPOSITE
Fig. 48.
The crow (*al-ghurāb*), the raven (*al-ghudāf*), the magpie (*al-ʿaqʿaq*). *Kitāb Manāfiʿ al-ḥayawān*, Syria, probably Damascus, dated Rabīʿ al-awwal 755 A.H./March 1354 A.D. San Lorenzo del Escorial, Biblioteca Real, MS ar. 898, fol. 101b

NEXT OVERLEAF
Fig. 49.
Hedgehog (*al-qunfudh*). *Kitāb Manāfiʿ al-ḥayawān*, Syria, Probably Damascus, dated Rabīʿ al-awwal 755 A.H./ March 1354 A.D. San Lorenzo del Escorial, Biblioteca Real, MS ar. 898, fol. 58a

FOLLOWING OVERLEAF
Fig. 50.
Hedgehog (*al-qunfudh*). *Kitāb Naʿt al-ḥayawān*, North Jazīra, dateable *c.* 617–22/1220–5. London, British Library, MS Or. 2784, fol. 202a

Thus, whereas Ibn Baklarish refers to a generalized pain in the womb, Ibn Bakhtishuʿ speaks specifically of 'suffocation of the womb'. Similarly, the conclusion of Ibn Baklarish's text on the crow إنه نفع فيه الدود فيؤخذ الدود وسحق ويطلى به ا لرأس فيسوده ('it is useful with worms in: the worms are taken, pounded and applied to the head, turning [the hair] black')—is clearly to be identified as a shorthand version of a complicated and lengthy process detailed in both the *Naʿt* and the Escorial text of Ibn Baktishuʿ. But there is also a significant difference: in the *Naʿt* (fol. 42a) and the Escorial text (fol. 102b), the resulting concoction, which includes sesame oil, is used to treat something wholly unrelated: instead of a means of turning hair black it is a remedy for leprosy (and, in the *Naʿt*, also palsy).

In the event, the degree of congruence exhibited by the first passages quoted is the exception rather than the rule. Generally, we find something quite different. For when it comes to specifics there is actually very little common material: if in Ibn Baklarish *x* is prepared in manner *y* and is used to cure *z*, in Ibn Bakhtishuʿ's *Naʿt* and the Escorial text it is likely to be prepared in manner *p* and used to cure *q*. In short, what seems to be universal is not agreement upon a particular treatment for a particular condition, but rather what might be categorized as a treatment syntagm: condition > choice of body part > manner of preparation > specification of dosage > result, where the 'body part > preparation > dosage' sequence calls upon a set of conventional (paradigmatic) choices that nevertheless allow for a myriad of combinations. This would seem to give a rather negative answer to the question of possible textual affiliations, despite the existence of certain common elements: the processes described are the same, but the ingredients and the conditions treated may well not coincide.

The difference between Ibn Baklarish and the *manāfiʿ* literature is further underlined when one compares coverage. For, despite the much wider range of animals and hence accumulated body parts in, say, Ibn Bakhtishuʿ's *Naʿt* and the Escorial text, there are several entries in Ibn Baklarish for which they contain no equivalent. It is striking, for example, that the first set of six animal part entries relate to *infiḥa* (rennet), a term only mentioned in the *Naʿt* in relation to the dog. When we turn to other parts that are mentioned by both Ibn Baklarish and the Ibn Bakhtishuʿ texts we find, for example, that the *Naʿt* fails to mention the blood of the hare, dog and bull; and the Escorial text, likewise, has nothing on the gall bladder of sheep and goats. To take a fairly average animal in terms of the number of times it appears in Ibn Baklarish—the hedgehog [Figs. 49 and 50]—we find that, of the four body parts cited (skin, liver, meat and brain), the *Naʿt* mentions only one, while in the lengthy account in the Escorial text, which includes such specifics as the right eye and left testicle, two fail to appear. When we turn to the items that are held in common we find that, of the several uses for hedgehog meat listed in the *Naʿt* and the Escorial text, not one appears in Ibn Baklarish, while the account of the liver in the Escorial text likewise has nothing in common with that of Ibn Baklarish. On the other hand, there are instances of partial overlap. For example, among the four uses proposed in

12. See Anna Contadini, 'The Horse in Two Manuscripts of Ibn Bakhtīshūʿ's *Kitāb Manāfiʿ al-ḥayawān*' in: David Alexander (ed.), *Furusiyya. The Horse in the Art of the Near East*, 2 vols., Riyadh 1996, I, pp. 142–7, where a full translation of the section on the horse in the Escorial manuscript is given and the original text is reproduced.

انه فان اراد انسان أن يعلم أيهما تحلق الشعر وأيهما
تنبته فليكسر البيضة ويدخل فيها ريشة فان خرجت مختلفة قد
انتثر بعضها فهي التي تحلق وان خرجت سليمة صحيحة فهي التي
تنبت الشعر **الغراب والغداف والعقعق**

Pica Graculus Corvus montanus Cornix

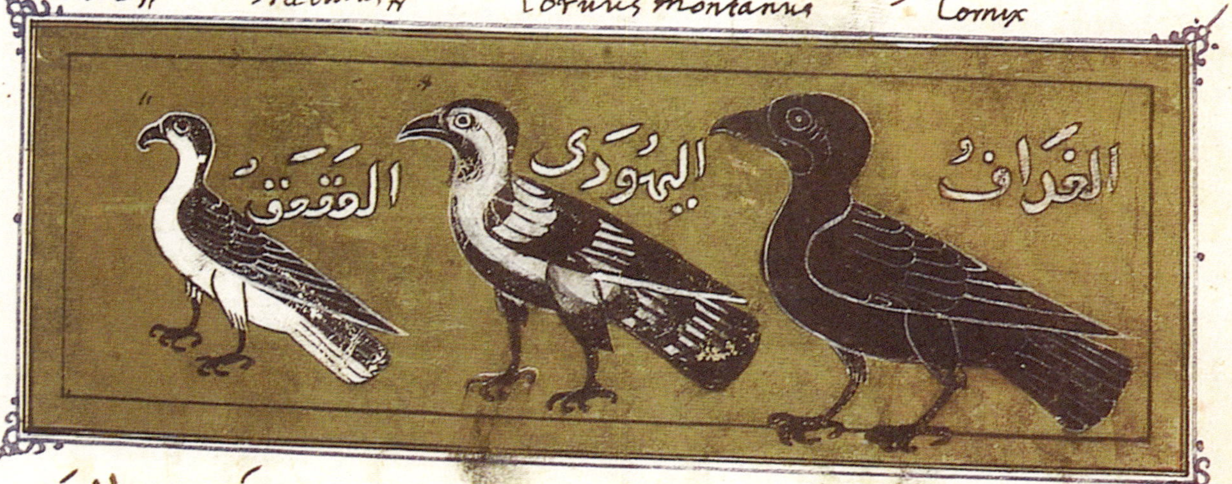

من طبيعة الغراب الاستتار عند السفاد لا يفرخ في السنة
اكثر من فرخين وله حذر شديد وفطنة عجيبة وفيه تناصر
اذا صاح احدهما مستنجدا وافوه من كل ناحية
تناصرا له وشبه وبين طيور الليل عداوة شديدة
ومن طبيعة الغداف الابيض ولا يفرخ من سفاد بل من

التزاق

حتى يكون سطرا طويلا فحين تغيب الشمس ينهض اولها من الطرف
الايمن فيمشي وراء ظهورها حتى يقعد الى الاقصى في الطرف
الايسر فاذا قعد صاح فنهض الذي كان يليه من الطرف
الايسر فيفعل مثل فعله فيفعل ذلك ليلتها اجمع فيبيت في ارض
ويصبح في اخرى ومن منافعه ان قلبه اذا شوي وجفف
وشرب منه وزن درهم مسحوق بمثله عسل عتيق نفع من الخفقان
وسقوط النفس وشجع الجبان ويزيد في جودة الذهن وينفع من
الصداع

القنفذ

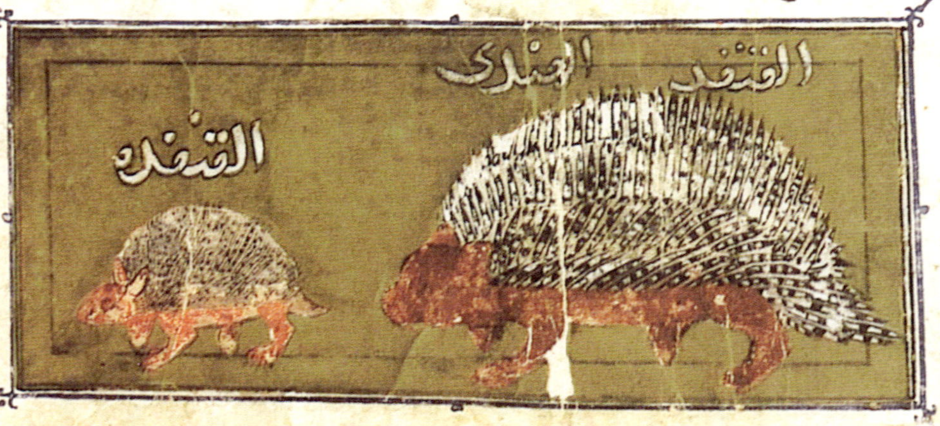

من طبعه ان يجعل لجحره الذي ياويه بابين احدهما من ناحية

ليلا يأتيه الذئب فيأكلها

نعت القنفذ الهندي وصورته

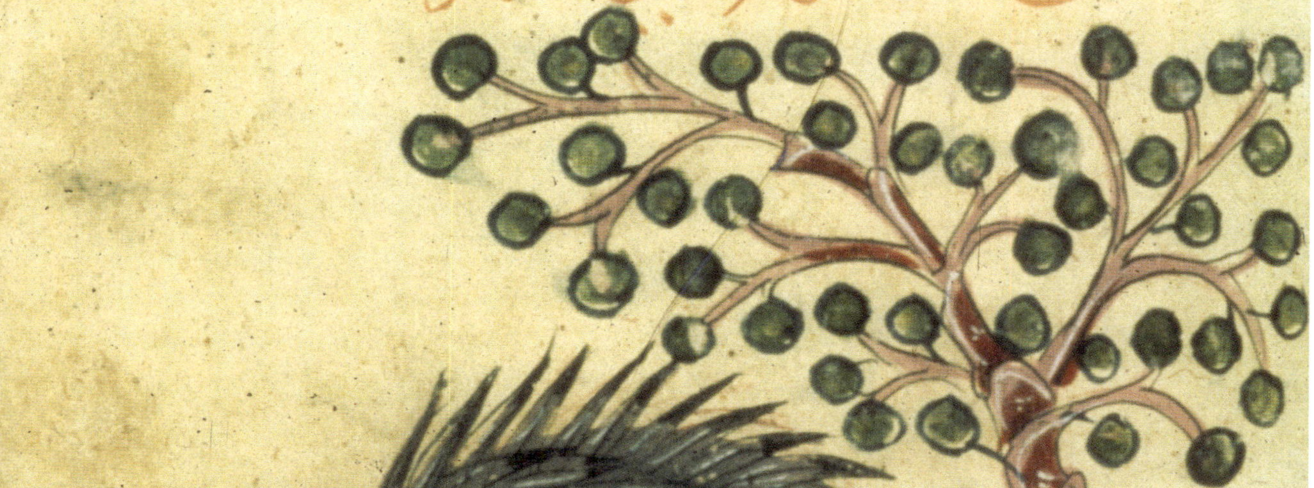

من طبعه أن يجعل الجحر الذي يسكن

the *Kitāb al-Mustaʿīnī* for horse dung and the five in the Escorial text,[12] two match exactly: used as fumigant, it brings forth the foetus (alive or dead, Ibn Baklarish grimly adds); and drops of the expressed juice, mixed with rose oil, alleviate earache. But it is equally important to note that the others do not match, so that we remain faced with tantalizing hints of contact emerging out of a body of material that points to a general cultural agreement about methods of treatment, but all too frequently fails to agree on specifics. This general picture also emerges clearly from other *manāfiʿ* texts. Indeed, in the manuscripts examined by Remke Kruk approximately half the uses mentioned in each text are unique to it.[13]

It is relevant in this context to note that the sources mentioned in these texts fail to match also. The three cited by Ibn Baklarish in his zoological entries are Ishaq ibn Sulayman, al-Tabari and al-Masihi. The first, Ishaq ibn Sulayman al-Isra'ili (*c.* 855–*c.* 955 / 243–343), was a court physician to the Aghlabids of Qayrawan and later to the first Fatimid caliph ʿUbayd Allah al-Mahdi, and the author of several medical treatises that were used within the Jewish and medical community in general. The degree to which his works were influential is indicated by the fact that they were translated not only into Hebrew but also into Latin, and were esteemed throughout the Middle Ages.[14]

The al-Tabari mentioned by Ibn Baklarish may be identified with a certain ʿAli ibn Rabban al-Tabari, a ninth-century Christian (probably Nestorian) physician who converted to Islam and wrote several medical works while serving Abbasid caliphs in Samarra and Baghdad.[15] ʿIsa b. Yahya al-Masihi al-Jurjani was also a Christian physician, and was a teacher of Ibn Sina (Avicenna), who dedicated some of his works to him. He lived between the end of the tenth and the beginning of the eleventh century, and was active in Baghdad, Khurasan and Khwarazm. Among his medical writings the best-known is a comprehensive encyclopedia, the *Kutub al-mi'a fī al-ṣināʿa al-ṭibbiyya* (*The Hundred Books on the Medical Art*).[16]

As for the sources mentioned in the Ibn Bakhtishuʿ manuscripts,[17] we have Aristotle and, even if they do not call upon Galenic medicine, there is a reference to Galen.[18]

13. See Kruk, 'Elusive Giraffes'.
14. Constantine the African and Gerard of Cremona translated works of Ishaq Isra'ili into Latin; see Alexander Altmann, 'Isḥāḳ b. Sulaymān al-Isrā'īlī', *Encyclopedia of Islam*, new edition, IV, p. 111, Carl Brockelmann, *Geschichte der arabischen Litteratur*, 2 vols., Weimar 1898–1902, I, pp. 235–6, no. 10 and *Supplementband* I (1937), p. 421, no. 10; Fuat Sezgin, *Geschichte des arabischen Schrifttums*, 9 vols., Leiden 1967–2000, III (1970), pp. 295–7 and V (1974), p. 413.
15. See David Thomas, 'al-Masīḥī al-Djurdjānī', *Encyclopedia of Islam*, new edition , X, p. 17, Brockelmann, *Geschichte der arabischen Litteratur*, I, pp. 414–15, no. 1a, Sezgin, *Geschichte des arabischen Schrifttums*, III, pp. 236–40 and VII (1979), pp. 237–40.
16. See Albert Dietrich, 'Ṭabarī ʿAlī b. Rabban', *Encyclopedia of Islam*, new edition, VI, p. 726, Brockelmann, *Supplementband* I, pp. 423–4, no. 20, 2nd edition (1943), I, pp. 273–4, no. 18, and Sezgin, *Geschichte des arabischen Schrifttums*, III, pp. 326–7 and V, pp. 336–7. For the manuscript in Oxford, Bodleian Library, MS Hunt. 202, dated Shaʿbān 592/July 1196, see Emilie Savage-Smith, 'Between Reader and Text: Some Medieval Arabic Marginalia' in: Danielle Jacquart and Charles Burnett (eds.), *Scientia in Margine: études sur les marginalia dans les manuscrits scientifiques du moyen âge à la Renaissance*, Geneva 2005, pp. 75–101 (at pp. 86–92).
17. I include here not only the *Na't* and the Escorial text, but also the *Kitāb Manāfiʿ al-ḥayawān* in Paris, Bibliothèque nationale de France, MS ar. 2782, dated 700/1300: see Contadini, 'The *Kitāb Na't al-ḥayawān* (BL Or. 2784)', pp. 166–70.
18. See Brockelmann, *Geschichte der arabischen Litteratur*, I, p. 205, no. 7; Manfred Ullmann, *Die Natur- und Geheimwissenschaften im Islam*, Leiden 1972, pp. 12–14.

Similarly, Dioscorides[19] is mentioned, and also Kasuqratis, probably to be identified as Xenocrates of Aphrodisias who lived in the first century A.D.[20] Other sources mentioned are: Ahrun, probably to be identified with Ahron (otherwise known as Aaron), a Christian priest who lived in Alexandria in the sixth/seventh century and wrote medical treatises, especially the *Pandectae Medicinae*, which was translated from Syriac into Arabic;[21] al-Ahwazi, an unidentified figure whose name suggests that he originated from Ahwaz, a town situated on the Khuzistan plain;[22] Yanis ibn Istifan al-Turjuman, possibly to be identified with Istifan ibn Basil, the first translator of the *Materia medica* of Dioscorides;[23] Shaykh Abu al-Hasan, probably a learned figure of the circle of Mayyafariqin;[24] Muhammad ibn Musa al-Munajjim, cited as the author of a *Kitāb al-mamālik* and evidently one of the Banu al-Munajjim, the famous translators, as well as copyists and binders, employed in the Bayt al- ḥikma;[25] and ʿIsa ibn ʿAli, a Nestorian physician educated at Jundishapur, a pupil of Hunayn ibn Ishaq and physician to the Caliph al-Muʿtamid (reigned 256–72/870–90). He wrote a *Kitāb al-Manāfiʿ allatī tustafādu min aḍāʾ al-ḥayawān* (*The Book on the Usefulness of the Organs of Animals*) of which several manuscripts survive.[26]

19. For Dioscorides, see n. 5 above; also Brockelmann, *Geschichte der arabischen Litteratur*, I, pp. 206–7, *Supplementband* I, pp. 369, 370–1; Ullmann, *Die Natur- und Geheimwissenschaften*, pp. 11–12.

20. Carmen Ruiz Bravo-Villasante, *Libro de las utilidades de los animales*, Madrid 1980, p. xvi, already suggested this identification. Sezgin, *Geschichte des arabischen Schrifttums*, III, p. 57, says that the Arabic name for Xenocrates occurs either as 'Iksānuqrāṭis' or 'Kisānūqrāṭis'; see also Ullmann, *Die Natur- und Geheimwissenschaften*, pp. 10–11.

21. Ibn al-Nadim reports under this name a priest: 'Ahron the Priest. Living in the first part of the regime [of Islam] he wrote in Syriac his book which Masarjis translated. Among his books there was The Pandect. He wrote it in thirty sections and Masarjis added two more sections to it': Ibn al-Nadim, *Fihrist*, trans. Bayard Dodge, 2 vols. (continuous pagination), New York and London 1970, p. 698. See Max Meyerhof, '*The Book of Treasure*, an Early Arabic Treatise on Medicine', *Isis*, 14, 1930, pp. 55–76 (at p. 55). Ibn al-Qifti, *Tārīkh al-ḥukamāʾ*, Leipzig 1903, p. 126 records that ʿUbayd Allāh wrote a 'missive' (*risāla*) on Galen based on the historical work of a monk called 'Hārūn ibn ʿAzzūn'. Ibn Abi Usaybiʿa, *ʿUyūn al-anbāʾ fī ṭabaqāt al-aṭibbāʾ*, I, p. 72, calls him 'Hārūn ibn ʿAzzūr'. Max Meyerhof, 'An Arabic Compendium of Medico-Philosophical Definitions', *Isis*, 10, 1928, pp. 340–9 (at p. 343, n. 17), suggests that this could be the Ahron ibn Aʿin the priest, who lived in Alexandria, or possibly the Nestorian historian Ahron mentioned in J. Baumstark, *Geschichte der syrischen Literatur*, Bonn 1922, p. 241. The Ahron cited in the *Naʿt* is more likely to be the Alexandrian priest who wrote on medicine. For this identification see also Sezgin, *Geschichte des arabischen Schrifttums*, III, pp. 166–8.

22. See Laurence Lockhart, 'Al-Ahwāz', *Encyclopedia of Islam*, new edition, I, p. 305.

23. Originally the *Materia medica* of Dioscorides was translated from Greek into Syriac, and the latter provided the basis for the Arabic version. This was made by Istifan ibn Basil, with the original text in front of him, and corrected by Hunayn ibn Ishaq in Baghdad in the ninth century; see César Emil Dubler, 'Diyusḳuridīs', *Encyclopedia of Islam*, new edition, II, pp. 348–50.

24. Sezgin, *Geschichte des arabischen Schrifttums*, III, p. 351; Ullmann, *Die Natur- und Geheimwissenschaften*, p. 22.

25. See Dominique Sourdel, 'Bayt al-Ḥikma', *Encyclopedia of Islam*, new edition, I, p. 1141.

26. See the list in Ullmann, *Die Natur- und Geheimwissenschaften*, pp. 21–2. Ibn al-Nadim, *Fihrist*, p. 699, writes: 'ʿIsa ibn ʿAli. He was one of the pupils of Hunayn [ibn Ishaq] and an excellent man. Among his books there was The Benefits Made Use of from the Organs of an Animal.' Ibn Abi Usaybiʿa, *ʿUyūn al-anbāʾ fī ṭabaqāt al-aṭibbāʾ*, I, p. 203, mentions this book on animals (*Kitāb al-manāfiʿ allatī tustafād min aʿḍāʾ al-ḥayawān*). See also Sezgin, *Geschichte des arabischen Schrifttums*, III, pp. 259 and 377. He is confused with ʿAli ibn ʿIsa al-Kahhal (e.g. in Brockelmann, *Geschichte der arabischen Litteratur*, I, p. 233, no. 8, *Supplementband* I, p. 417, no. 8), who lived in the eleventh century and never wrote, as far as I could ascertain, treatises on zoology. See also Eugen Mittwoch, 'ʿAlī ibn ʿĪsā', *Encyclopedia of Islam*, new edition, I, p. 388; Sezgin, *Geschichte des arabischen Schrifttums*, III, pp. 337–40; George Sarton, *Introduction to the History of Science*, 3 vols., Baltimore 1927–48, I, p. 731.

Of these, only the classical sources, Aristotle, Galen and Dioscorides, are shared with Ibn Baklarish (they are mentioned in the Introduction of the *Kitāb al-Mustaʿīnī*[27]). Given that the obeisance to classical authorities may be ritual, material derived from them having been consulted in later works, it might be concluded that we are confronted with textual (and human) lines of transmission that had for some time lost contact with each other. If that were so, it was only to be expected that Ibn Bakhtishuʿ should fail to be mentioned by Ibn Baklarish (and likewise by al-Ghafiqi, his younger contemporary, whose *Kitāb al-Adwiya al-mufrada* cites both the *Kitāb al-Mustaʿīnī* and the same sources mentioned by Ibn Baklarish).[28] But, although most of Ibn Bakhtishuʿ's authorities seem to have had primarily Iraqi connections, the notion of self-contained, geographically separate schools is hardly sustainable. Doctors travelled vast distances to study with eminent authorities, and it is in any case clear that the sources cited by Ibn Baklarish hailed from far and wide. One of them, indeed, ʿAli ibn Rabban al-Tabari, may reasonably be assumed to have had contacts with some of Ibn Bakhtishuʿ's forebears during his time at the Abbasid court.

Nevertheless, at this stage in our knowledge of the corpus it is not possible to be specific about the textual affiliations of the zoological element of the *Kitāb al-Mustaʿīnī*. Although the passages that can be matched in other works clearly demonstrate, if not the existence of a common stock of material, then at least access to other texts, they provide insufficient evidence to identify specific sources. With time we may hope to say rather more about the contents of this particular segment of the *Kitāb al-Mustaʿīnī*, but even if much still remains obscure at present, it is at least obvious that it provides a substantial supplement to the zoological literature, and one eminently worthy of further study.

27. See Henri Paul Joseph Renaud, 'Trois études d'histoire de la médecine arabe en occident', *Hespéris*, 10, 1930–1, pp. 135–50 (see pp. 148–9).
28. Albert Dietrich, 'al-G͟hāfiḳī', *Encyclopedia of Islam*, new edition, Suppl. pp. 313–14. In the same way we may note that Ibn Bakhtishuʿ is mentioned by al-Marwazi (b. *c.* 1050, d. after 1120) as a source in his *Kitāb Ṭabāʾiʿ al-ḥayawān*: Contadini, 'The *Kitāb Naʿt al-ḥayawān* (BL Or. 2784)', pp. 72–3.

BIBLIOGRAPHY

ʿABD AL-SALAM AL-ʿALAMI, *ʿAbd al-Salām Ibn M. al-ʿAlamī*, Rabat 1986.

AHMAD IBN QASIM AL-HAJARI, *Kitāb Nāṣir al-dīn ʿalā ʾl-qawm al-kāfirīn (The supporter of Religion against the Infidels)*, historical study, critical edition and annotated translation by P.S. van Koningsveld, Q. al-Samarrai and G.A. Wiegers (Fuentes Arábico-Hispanas, 21), Madrid 1997.

ALEXANDER, David (ed.), *Furusiyya. The Horse in the Art of the Near East*, 2 vols.,Riyadh 1996.

ALONSO, A., 'Correspondencias arábigo-españolas en los sistemas de sibilantes', *Nueva Revista de Filología Hispánica*, 8, 1946, pp. 12–76.

AMMAR, Z., and Y. SERI, 'Ibn Biklarish, One of the Greatest Sefarad Physicians', *Korot*, 15, 2001, pp. 79–91 (in Hebrew).

ARBERRY, A.J., *The Chester Beatty Library. A Handlist of the Arabic Manuscripts*, VI, Dublin, 1963.

ASBAGHI, Asya, *Persische Lehnwörter im Arabischen*, Wiesbaden 1988, p. xviii.

ASHTOR, Eliyahu, *The Jews of Moslem Spain*, 3 vols., Philadelphia 1973–84.
—— 'The Number of the Jews in Muslim Spain', *Zion*, 28, 1963, pp. 34–56 (Hebrew).

ASIN PALACIOS, M., *Glosario de voces romances registradas por un botánico anónimo hispano-musulmán (siglos XI–XII)*, Madrid–Granada 1943.

BARCELÓ, Carmen, 'Mozárabes de Valencia y "lengua mozárabe"', *Revista de Filología Española*, 77, 1997, pp. 253–79.
—— 'Romance Lexicon in Pharmacological Treatises Written in Muslim Spain: Its Origin and Transmission', *Journal for the History of Arabic Science*, 12, 2001, pp. 111–30.

BAUMSTARK, A., *Geschichte der syrischen Literatur*, Bonn 1922.

BELLAMY, James A., 'Qasmuna the Poetess. Who was she?', *Journal of the American Oriental Society*, 103, 1983, pp. 423–4.

BERNABÉ PONS, Luis F., 'Una nota sobre Aḥmad ibn Qāsim al-Ḥaŷarī Bejarano', *Sharq al-Andalus*, 13, 1996, pp. 123–8.

BRAVO-VILLASANTE, Carmen Ruiz, *Libro de las utilidades de los animales*, Madrid 1980.

BRIQUET, Charles M., *Les filigranes: dictionnaire historique des marques du papier dès leur apparition vers 1282 jusqu'en 1600. A Facsimile of the 1907 Edition with Supplementary Material Contributed by a Number of Scholars*, ed. Alan Stevenson, Amsterdam 1968.

BROCKELMANN, Carl, *Geschichte der arabischen Litteratur*, 2 vols., Weimar 1898–1902.
—— *Geschichte der arabischen Litteratur. Supplementbände*, 3 vols., Leiden 1937–42.
—— *Lexicon Syriacum. Editio Secunda Aucta et Emendata*, Halle 1928.

BUONAZIA, Lupo, 'Biblioteca Nazionale di Napoli: codici arabi' in: *Cataloghi dei codici orientali di alcune biblioteche d'Italia*, 7 fascicles, Florence 1878–1904.

BUSTAMANTE, J., F. CORRIENTE and M. TILMATINE: *Abulhayr Alʾišbīlī, Kitābu ʿumdati ṭṭabīb fī maʿrifati nnabāt likulli labīb (Libro base del médico para el conocimiento de la botánica por todo experto)*, I, Madrid 2004.

BUSTO, J.C., review of Niederehe's work in *Aljamía*, 12, 2000, pp. 210–12.

CARMEN PEÑA A. Diaz, and C. ALVAREZ DE MORALES, 'Corpus medicorum arabico-hispanorum', *Awrāq*, 4, 1981, pp. 79–111.

COHEN, Mark R., *Under Crescent and Cross. The Jews in the Middle Ages*, Princeton 1994.

COLBERT, Edward P., 'John of Biclaro' in: *New Catholic Encyclopedia*, New York etc. 1967, VII, p. 1036; 2nd edition, 2003, VII, p. 965.

COLIN, Georges S., and Henri P. J. RENAUD, *Ibn al-H'achcha (13e siècle), Glossaire sur le Mans'uri de Razès (10e siècle): texte arabe établi sur plusieurs manuscrits et publié avec une introduction*, Rabat 1941.

COLLINS, Minta, *Medieval Herbals. The Illustrative Traditions*, British Library Studies in Medieval Culture, London–Toronto 2000.

COLOMINA I CASTANYER, Jordi, *Llengües en contacte als regnes de València i de Múrcia (segles XIII–XV)*, Alicante 1995.

COLON, Germán, 'Les relacions del lèxic aragonès medieval amb el lèxic català', *Estudis de filologia catalana i romànica*, Valencia and Barcelona 1997.

CONTADINI, Anna, (ed.), *Arab Painting. Text and Image in Illustrated Arabic Manuscripts*, Leiden 2007.
—— 'A Bestiary Tale: Text and Image of the Unicorn in the *Kitāb Naʿt al-ḥayawān*', *Muqarnas*, 20, 2003, pp. 17–33.
—— 'The Ibn Baḫtīshūʿ Bestiary Tradition: the Text and its Sources', *Medicina nei secoli: arte e scienza*, 6.2, 1994, pp. 349–64.
—— 'The *Kitāb Naʿt al-ḥayawān* (BL Or. 2784) and the So-called Ibn Bakhtīshūʿ Illustrated Bestiaries', School of Oriental and African Studies, University of London, 1992 (unpublished PhD thesis).
—— 'The *Kitāb Manāfiʿ al-ḥayawān* in the Escorial Library', *Islamic Art*, 3, 1988, pp. 33–57.

COROMINAS, Juan, *Diccionario crítico-etimológico de la lengua castellana*, 4 vols., Madrid–Berne 1958.
—— 2nd edition, *Diccionario etimológico castellano e hispánico*, 6 vols., Madrid 1980–91.

COROMINES, Joan, *Diccionari etimològic i complementari de la llengua catalana*, 9 vols., Barcelona 1983–91.

CORRIENTE, Federico, *A Dictionary of Andalusi Arabic*, Leiden 1997.
—— *et al.*, *Las lenguas prevalencinas*, Alicante 1986.
—— 'El romandalusí reflejado por el glosario botánico de Abulxayr', *Estudios de dialectología norteafricana y andalusí*, 5, 2001, pp. 93–241.

DAVIDSON, Herbert A., *Moses Maimonides. The Man and his Works*, Oxford 2005.

DE JONG, Piet, and DE GOEJE, Michael Jan, *Catalogus Codicum Orientalium Bibliothecae Academiae Lugduno Batavae*, vol. III, Leiden 1865.

DERENBOURG, Hartwig, 'Notes critiques sur les manuscrits arabes de la Bibliothèque Nationale de Madrid' in *Homenaje a D. Francisco Codera*, Saragossa 1904.

DERENBOURG, Hartwig, and Henri P.J. RENAUD, *Les manuscrits arabes de l'Escurial*, Paris 1941.

DIETRICH, Albert (ed. and trans.), *Dioscurides Triumphans: ein anonymer arabischer Kommentar (Ende 12. Jahr. nach Chr.) zur Materia Medica*, 2 vols., Göttingen 1988.

DOZY, Reinhardt, *Catalogus Codicum Orientalium Bibliothecae Academiae Lugduno Batavae*, vol. I, Leiden 1851.
—— *Supplément aux dictionnaires arabes*, 2 vols., Leiden 1881; 2nd edition, Paris 1927.

DUCROS, M. A. H., *Essai sur le droguier populaire arabe de l'inspectorat des pharmacies du Caire* (Mémoires présentés à l'Institut d'Égypte, 15), Cairo 1930.

EFROS, Israel, 'Maimonides' Arabic Treatise on Logic. Introduction', *Proceedings of the American Academy for Jewish Research*, 34, 1966, pp. 155–60 (English section) and Judaeo-Arabic text, pp. 9–42 (Hebrew section).

ELKHADEM, Hosam, *Le 'Taqwīm al-ṣiḥḥa' (Tacuini sanitatis) d'Ibn Buṭlān: un traité medical du XIe siècle. Histoire du texte, édition critique, traduction, commentaire*, Louvain 1990.

Enciclopedia universal ilustrada europeo-americana, 70 vols. in 72, Barcelona 1907–30.

Encyclopedia of Islam, new edition, Boston 1998.

AL-FARUQ ʿUMAR AL-ʿASLI, '*Kitāb al-Mustaʿīnī fī l-ṭibb* li Ibn Buklārish', *Al-Ṣaydalī* (Tunis), 40, 1991, pp. 52–54; 41, 1991, pp. 56–59, 42, 1991, pp. 46–51 and 44, 1992, pp. 49–51.

FERRANDO, Antoni, 'La configuració lingüística del País Valencià després de la conquista jaumina', in: Federico Corriente *et al.*, *Las lenguas prevalencinas*, Alicante 1986, pp. 81–91.

FRAGO GRACIA, Juan A., 'Castellano y aragonés en el Antiguo Reino de Valencia', in: Federico Corriente *et al.*, *Las lenguas prevalencinas*, Alicante 1986, pp. 45–63.

GALMÉS DE FUENTES, Álvaro, *Dialectología mozárabe*, Madrid 1983.
—— *Las jarchas mozárabes. Forma y significado*, Barcelona 1994.

GARIJO, Ildefonso, 'Ibn Buklāriš' in: *Enciclopedia de al-Andalus. Diccionario de autores y obras andalusíes*, vol. I, Granada 2002.

GLICK, Thomas F., *Islamic and Christian Spain in the Early Middle Ages. Comparative Perspectives on Social and Cultural Formation*, Princeton 1979.

GOITEIN, Shlomo D., *A Mediterranean Society. The Jewish Communities of the Arab World as Portrayed in the Documents of the Cairo Geniza*, Berkeley etc., 6 vols., 1967–93.

GUILLÉN ROBLES, Francisco, *Catálogo de los manuscritos árabes existentes en la Biblioteca Nacional de Madrid*, Madrid 1889.

HAJJI KHALIFA, *Kashf al-ẓunūn*, Teheran 1967.

HAMARNEH, Sami Khalaf, and Glenn SONNEDECKER, *A Pharmaceutical View of Abulcasis al-Zahrāwī in Moorish Spain*, Leiden 1963.

HAMMER-PURGSTALL, Joseph von, *Literaturgeschichte der Araber*, Vienna 1855.

HEAWOOD, Edward, *Watermarks Mainly of the 17th and 18th Centuries*, Hilversum 1950.

HERRERA, M.ª Teresa (ed.), *Diccionario español de textos médicos antiguos*, I, Madrid 1996.

HOTTINGER, Joh. Henricus, *Promtuarium sive bibliotheca orientalis exhibens Catalogum, sive, Centurias aliquot, tam Authorum, quam librorum Hebraicorum, Syriacorum, Arabicorum, Aegyptiacorum, Aethiopicorum etc.*, Heidelberg 1658.

HOUTSMA, Martijn Theodor, *Uit de Oostersche correspondentie van Th. Erpenius, Jac. Golius en Lev. Warner. Eene bijdrage tot de geschiedenis van de beoefening der Oostersche letteren in Nederland* (Verhandelingen der Koninklijke Akademie van Wetenschappen, Afdeeling Letterkunde, vol. 17, pt. 3), Amsterdam 1887.

IBN ABI USAYBIʿA: *ʿUyūn al-Anbāʾ fī ṭabaqāt al-aṭibbāʾ*, ed. August Müller, 5 vols., Cairo 1882–4, reprinted Beirut 1955–6.
—— *ʿUyūn al-Anbāʾ fī ṭabaqāt al-aṭibbāʾ. Sources d'informations sur les classes des médecins*, ed. and trans. Henri Jahier and Abdelkader Noureddine, Algiers 1958.

IBN AL-JAZZAR, *The Reliable Book on Simple Drugs (Kitāb al-Iʿtimād fī'l-adwiya al-mufrada)*, Frankfurt-am-Main 1985 (facsimile edition).

IBN JULJUL, *Die Ergänzung Ibn Gulgul's zur Materia medica des Dioskurides*, ed. and trans. Albert Dietrich, Göttingen 1993.
—— *Libro de la explicación de los medicamentos simples tomados del libro de Dioscórides*, ed. and trans. Ildefonso Garijo, Córdoba 1988.
—— *Maqāla fī adwiya al-tiryāq. Tratado sobre los medicamentos de la tríaca*, ed. and trans. Ildefonso Garijo, Córdoba 1992.
—— *Maqāla thāmina. Tratado octavo*, ed. and trans. Ildefonso Garijo, Córdoba 1992.
—— *Tafsīr asmāʾ al-adwiya min kitāb Diyusqūrīdūs*, ed. and trans. Ildefonso Garijo, Córdoba 1992.

IBN AL-NADIM, *Fihrist*, trans. Bayard Dodge, 2 vols., New York and London 1970.

IBN AL-QIFTI, *Tārīkh al-ḥukamā'*, Leipzig 1903.

IBN WAFID, *Kitāb al-adwiya al-mufrada (Libro de los medicamentos simples)*, ed. and trans. Luisa F. Aguirre de Cárcer, 2 vols., Madrid 1995.

IFRAH, Georges, *Histoire universelle des chiffres*, Paris 1994.

KHAN, Geoffrey, 'Inventing Tradition and Constructing Identity: the Genealogy of ʿUmar ibn Hafsun between Christianity and Islam', *Al-Qantara*, 23, 2002, pp. 269–97.
—— 'The Medieval Karaite Transcriptions of Hebrew into Arabic Script', *Israel Oriental Studies*, 12, 1992, pp. 157–76.
—— 'On the Question of Script in Medieval Karaite Manuscripts: New Evidence from the Genizah', *Bulletin of the John Rylands Library*, 75, 3, 1993, pp. 132–41.
—— 'The Orthography of Karaite Hebrew Bible Manuscripts in Arabic Transcription', *Journal of Semitic Studies*, 38, 1, 1993, pp. 49–70.

AL-KHATTABI, M. al-ʿArabi, *Al-aghdhiya wa-l-adwiya ʿinda mu'allifī al-gharb al-islāmī. Madkhal wa-nuṣūṣ*, Beirut 1990.
—— *ʿUmdat al-ṭabīb fī maʿrifat al-nabat li-Abī l-Khayr al-Ishbīlī*, 2 vols., Rabat 1990; new edition, Beirut 1995.

KRAUS, Paul, 'Hebräische und syrische Zitate in Isma'īlitischen Schriften', *Der Islam* 19, 1931, pp. 243–63.

KRAUSS, Samuel, *Griechische und lateinische Lehnwörter im Talmud, Midrasch und Targum*, Berlin 1898–9.

KROTKOFF, Georg, 'Studies in Neo-Aramaic Lexicography' in: Ann Kort and Scott Morschauser (eds.), *Biblical and Related Studies Presented to Samuel Iwry*, Winona Lake 1985, pp. 131–2.

KRUK, Remke, 'Elusive Giraffes: Ibn abi l-Ḥawāfir's Badāʾī al-akwān and Other Animal Books' in: Anna Contadini (ed.), *Arab Painting. Text and Image in Illustrated Arabic Manuscripts*, Leiden 2007, pp. 49–64.

LABARTA, Ana, 'La farmacología de Ibn Buklāriš: sus fuentes' in: *Actas del IV Coloquio Hispano-Tunecino (Palma de Mallorca, 1979)*, Madrid 1983, pp. 165–74.
—— 'Ibn Buklāriš' in: Carmen Peña *et al.*, 'Corpus medicorum arabico-hispanorum', *Awrāq*, 4, 1981, pp. 79–111.
—— *Libro de dichos maravillosos (miscelàneo morisco de magia y adivinacíon)*, Madrid 1993.
—— 'El prólogo de *al-Kitāb al-Mustaʿīnī de Ibn Buklāriš* (texto árabe y traducción anotada)' in: Juan Vernet (ed.), *Estudios sobre historia de la ciencia árabe*, Barcelona 1980, pp. 181–316.
—— 'El prólogo de 'al-Mustaʿīnī' de Ibn Buklāriš según los manuscritos de Madrid y Nápoles. Transcripción, traducción y estudio', Universidad de Barcelona 1972 (unpublished Tesis de licenciatura).

LANGERMANN, Y. Tzvi, *The Jews and the Sciences in the Middle Ages*, Aldershot 1999.

LECLERC, Lucien, *Ebn al-Beïthār: Traité des simples. Notices et extraits des manuscrits de la Bibliothèque Nationale; traduction française*, Paris, 1877–83; new edition, *Ibn al-Baytār: Traité des simples, traduction de L. Leclerc*, Paris 1987.

LEVEY, Martin, *Early Arabic Pharmacology. An Introduction Based on Ancient and Medieval Sources*, Leiden 1973.
—— 'The Pharmacological Table of Ibn Biklarish', *Journal of the History of Medicine*, 26, 1971, pp. 413–21.
—— 'The Pharmacology of Ibn Biklārish in the Introduction to his *Kitāb al-Mustaʿīnī*', *Studia Islamica*, 6, 1969, pp. 98–104.

LEVEY, Martin, and Noury AL-KHALEDY, *The Medical Formulary of al-Samarqandī and the Relations of Early Arabic Simples to those Found in the Indigenous Medicine of the Near East and India*, Philadelphia 1967.

LEVEY, Martin, and Safwat S. SOURYAL, 'The Introduction to the Kitāb al-Mustaʿīnī of Ibn Biklārish (fl. 1106)', *Janus*, 55, 1969, pp. 134–66.

LÉVI-PROVENÇAL, Evariste, *Catalogue de la Bibliothéque Génerale du Protectorat français au Maroc*, Paris 1913.

LEWIS, Bernard, *The Jews of Islam*, Princeton 1984.

LOEW, Immanuel, *Die Flora der Juden*, 4 vols., Vienna–Leipzig 1924–34; reprint 1967.

MAHFUZ, Muhammad, *Tafsīr mufradāt al-Anṭakī bi-l-lahja al-tūnisiyya*, ed. Ibrahim ben Mrad, Beirut 1996.

MAIMONIDES, Moses, *Sharḥ asmā' al-ʿuqqār (l'explication des noms de drogues): un glossaire de matière médicale*, ed. Max Meyerhof, Cairo 1940; English trans. Fred Rosner, *Moses Maimonides' Glossary of Drug Names, Translated from Max Meyerhof's French Edition* (Memoirs of the American Philosophical Society, 135), Philadelphia 1978.

MÉLIKOFF, Irène, 'Dānishmendids', *Encyclopedia of Islam*, new edition, II, pp. 110–11.

MENÉNDEZ PIDAL, Ramón, *Orígenes del español. Estudio lingüístico de la Península Ibérica hasta el siglo XI*, Madrid 1926; 3rd edition, Madrid 1950.

MENSCHING, Guido, *La sinonima delos nombres delas medeçinas griegos e latynos e arauigos*, Madrid 1994.

MEYERHOF, Max, 'An Arabic Compendium of Medico-Philosophical Definitions', *Isis*, 10, 1928, pp. 340–9.
—— 'The Book of Treasure, an Early Arabic Treatise on Medicine', *Isis*, 14, 1930, pp. 55–76.

MIELI, Aldo, *La science arabe et son rôle dans l'évolution scientifique mondiale*, Leiden 1966.

MORAG, Shlomo, 'The Pronunciations of Hebrew', *Encyclopaedia Judaica*, XIII, p. 1133.

MUTZAFI, Hezy, *The Jewish Neo-Aramaic Dialect of Koy Sanjaq*, Wiesbaden 2004.

New Catholic Encyclopedia, New York etc. 1967; 2nd edition 2003.

NICHOLS, J. M., 'The Arabic Verses of Qasmuna bint Isma'il ibn Baghdala', *International Journal of Middle East Studies*, 13/2, 1981, pp. 155–8.

NIEDEREHE, Hans-Josef, *Bibliografía cronológica de la lingüística, la gramática y la lexicografía del español desde los comienzos hasta el año 1600*, Amsterdam–Philadelphia 1995.

NUTTON, Vivian (ed.), *The Unknown Galen* (Bulletin of the Institute of Classical Studies, Suppl. 77), London 2002.

PEÑARROJA TORREJÓN, Leopoldo, *El mozárabe de Valencia*, Madrid 1990, p. 433.

PORMANN, Peter E., 'Yūḥannā ibn Sarābiyūn: Further Studies into the Transmission of his Works', *Arabic Sciences and Philosophy*, 14, 2004, pp. 233–62.

PREUSS, Julius, *Biblisch-talmudische Medizin. Beiträge zur Geschichte der Heilkunde und der Kultur überhaupt*, Berlin 1911; trans. Fred Rosner, *Biblical and Talmudic Medicine*, New York 1978.

RABIN, Chaim, 'Hebrew and Arabic in Medieval Jewish Philosophy' in: *Studies in Jewish Religious and Intellectual History Presented to Alexander Altmann on the Occasion of his Seventieth Birthday*, ed. Siegfried Stein and Raphael Loewe, Birmingham, Alabama, and London 1979, pp. 235–45.

RENAUD, Henri P. J., 'Trois études d'histoire de la médecine arabe en Occident: I. Le Mustaʿīnī d'Ibn Beklāreš', *Hespéris*, 10, 1930, pp. 135–150.
—— 'Un problème de bibliographie arabe: le *Taqwīm al-Adwiya* d'al-ʿAla'i,' *Hespéris*, 16, 1933, pp. 60–98.

RENAUD, Henri P. J., and Georges S. COLIN (eds.), *Tuḥfat al-Aḥbāb. Glossaire de la matière médicale marocaine*, Paris 1934.

RIBERA, Julián, *Bibliófilos y bibliotecas en la España musulmana*, Saragossa 1896; reprinted in idem, *Disertaciones y opúsculos*, Madrid 1928, vol. I, pp. 181–228.

RICORDEL, Joëlle, 'Le catalogue médical

d'Ibn Biklārish: une formulation nouvelle pour les connaissances pharmaceutiques andalousiennes' (in press).
—— 'Le médicament composé: théories andalouses sur l'évaluation de son degré (XIIe siècle)', *Revue d'Histoire de la Pharmacie*, 49, nr. 330, 2001, pp. 135–48.
—— 'Les "pierres" dans les tables médicales d'Ibn Biklārish (fin 11e / début 12e s.)' in: 'Identité culturelle des sciences et des philosophies arabes: auteurs, œuvres et transmissions', Colloque International, Namur–Brussels, 15–18 January 2003 (unpublished).
—— 'Les Tables des medicaments simples d'Isḥāḳ ibn Biklarish. Édition, traduction française et analyse (des lettres alif à zāy), 3 vols., November 2004, Université Paris VII-Denis Diderot' (unpublished thesis).

ROGERS, Michael, 'The Arab Contribution to Botany and Pharmacology', *Arab Affairs*, 6, 1988, pp. 71–86.
—— 'Text and illustrations. Dioscorides and the Illustrated Herbal in the Arab Tradition' in: Anna Contadini (ed.), *Arab Painting. Text and Image in Illustrated Arabic Manuscripts*, Leiden 2007, pp. 41–7.

RUSKA, Julius, *Das Steinbuch des Aristoteles. Mit literargeschichtlichen Untersuchungen nach der arabischen Handschrift der Bibliothèque Nationale*, Heidelberg 1912.

SADEK, Mahmoud M., *The Arabic Materia Medica of Dioscorides*, Quebec 1983.

SÁENZ-BADILLOS, Angel, and Judit TARGARONA BORRAS, *Diccionario de autores judíos (Sefarad. Siglos X–XV)*, Córdoba 1988.

SANCHIS GUARNER, Manuel, 'Las hablas del Alto Mijares y de Fanzara (Provincia de Castellón)', *Boletín de la Real Academia Española*, 47, 1967.

SARTON, George, *Introduction to the History of Science*, 3 vols., Baltimore 1927–48.

SAVAGE-SMITH, Emilie, 'Between Reader and Text: Some Medieval Arabic Marginalia' in: Danielle Jacquart and Charles Burnett (eds.), *Scientia in Margine: études sur les marginalia dans les manuscrits scientifiques du moyen âge à la Renaissance*, Geneva 2005, pp. 75–101.
—— 'Galen's Lost Ophthalmology and the *Summaria Alexandrinorum*' in Vivian Nutton (ed.), *The Unknown Galen* (Bulletin of the Institute of Classical Studies, Suppl. 17), London 2002, pp. 121–38.
—— *Islamic Medical Manuscripts at the National Library of Medicine* (www.nlm.nih.gov/hmd/arabic).
—— *A New Catalogue of Arabic Manuscripts in the Bodleian Library, Oxford*, vol. 1: *Arabic Manuscripts on Medicine and Related Topics*, Oxford forthcoming.

SCHMIDT, Jan, *The Joys of Philology. Studies in Ottoman Literature, History and Orientalism (1500–1923)*, 2 vols., Istanbul 2002.

SEZGIN, Fuat, *Geschichte des arabischen Schrifttums*, 9 vols., Leiden 1967–2000.

SIMONET, Francisco Javier, *Glosario de voces ibéricas y latinas usadas entre los mozárabes*, Madrid 1888; reprinted Madrid 1982.

SOKOLOFF, Michael, *A Dictionary of Jewish Babylonian Aramaic of the Talmudic and Geonic Periods*, Ramat-Gan and Baltimore 2002.

STEINGASS, Francis, *Persian–English Dictionary*, London 1892.

STEINSCHNEIDER, Moritz, *Die arabische Literatur der Juden*, Frankfurt-am-Main 1902.
—— *Hebraeische Bibliographie*, Berlin 1880.

STERN, Samuel M., 'Contributions to the History of Samuel Hanagid', *Zion*, 15, 1950, pp. 135–45 (Hebrew).
—— *Hispano-Arabic Strophic Poetry. Studies by Samuel Miklos Stern*, selected and edited by Leonard Patrick Harvey, Oxford 1974.
—— 'Les vers finaux en espagnol dans les muwaššahs hispano-hébraïques: une contribution à l'histoire du muwaššah et à l'étude du vieux dialecte espagnol "mozarabe"', *Al-Andalus*, 13, 1948, pp. 299–346.

TOUWAIDE, Alain, *Farmacopea araba medievale: codice Ayasofia 3703*, 2 vols., Milan 1992.

TÜRKER, Mubahat, *Mūsā b. Maymūn'un Makala fī Sinā'at al Mantik'i, Review of the Institute of Islamic Studies*, Publications of the Faculty of Letters, Istanbul University, III, Parts 1–2, 1959–60.
—— 'Mūsā ibn-i Meymūn'un *Al-Makāla fi Sinā'at al-Mantik*' in: Arpaca Asli, *Türk Tarih Kurumu Basimevi*, Ankara 1961.

ULLMANN, Manfred, *Die Medizin im Islam*, Leiden–Cologne 1970.
—— *Die Natur- und Geheimwissenschaften im Islam*, Leiden 1972.

VAN KONINGSVELD, Pieter Sjoerd, 'Andalusian-Arabic Manuscripts from Christian Spain: a Comparative Intercultural Approach', *Israel Oriental Studies*, 12, 1992, pp. 75–110.
—— 'Christian Arabic Literature from Medieval Spain: an Attempt at Periodization' in: *Christian Arabic Apologetics during the Abbasid Period (750–1258)*, ed. Samir Khalil Samir and Jürgen S. Nielsen, Leiden 1994, pp. 203–24.
—— 'Christian-Arabic Manuscripts from the Iberian Peninsula and North Africa: a Historical Interpretation', *Al-Qantara*, 15, 1994, pp. 423–51.
—— *The Latin–Arabic Glossary of the Leiden University Library. A Contribution to the Study of Mozarabic Manuscripts and Literature*, Leiden 1997.

VILLAVERDE AMIEVA, Juan Carlos, Review article, *Aljamía*, 3, 1990, pp. 62–3.
—— Review article, *Aljamía*, 9, 1997, pp. 143–4.
—— 'Sobre el estudio del mozárabe en fuentes árabes: a propósito de Ibn Buklāriš' in: *Homenaje a Álvaro Galmés de Fuentes*, vol. III, Oviedo–Madrid, 1987, pp. 703–21.

VOORHOEVE, Petrus, *Handlist of Arabic Manuscripts in the Library of the University of Leiden and other Collections in The Netherlands*, 2nd edition, The Hague 1980.

WASSERSTEIN, David J., 'An Arabic version of Abot 1:3 from Umayyad Spain', *Arabica*, 34, 1987, pp. 370–4.
—— 'Encore une fois Abot 1:3 dans l'Espagne omeyyade', *Arabica*, 38, 1991, pp. 275–7.
—— 'Inventing Tradition and Constructing Identity: the Genealogy of 'Umar ibn Hafsun between Christianity and Islam', *Al-Qantara*, 23, 2002, pp. 269–97.
—— 'The Language Situation in al-Andalus', in: *Studies on the Muwaššah and the Kharja*, ed. Alan Jones and Richard Hitchcock, Reading 1991, pp. 1–15.
—— 'Langues et frontières entre juifs et musulmans en al-Andalus' in: *Judíos y musulmanes en al-Andalus y el Magreb. Contactos intelectuales*, ed. Maribel Fierro, Madrid 2002, pp. 1–11.
—— 'The Muslims and the Golden Age of the Jews in al-Andalus' in: *Israel Oriental Studies*, 17: *Dhimmis and Others. Jews and Christians and the World of Classical Islam*, ed. Uri Rubin and David J. Wasserstein, 1997, pp. 179–96.
—— *The Rise and Fall of the Party-Kings, Politics and Society in Islamic Spain, 1002–1086*, Princeton 1985.
—— 'Samuel Ibn Nagrila ha-Nagid and Islamic Historiography in al-Andalus', *Al-Qantara*, 14, 1993, pp. 109–25.

WIEGERS, Gerard, *A Learned Muslim Acquaintance of Erpenius and Golius: Aḥmad b. Ḳāsim al-Andalusī and Arabic Studies in The Netherlands*, Leiden 1988.

WÜSTENFELD, Ferdinand, *Geschichte der arabischen Ärzte und Naturforscher*, Göttingen 1846.

YUSUF AL-HAKIM, 'Ali B., *al-Ḍawḥa al-mushtabika fī ḍawābiṭ dār al-sikka*, ed. Husayn Mu'nis, *Revista del Instituto de Estudios Islámicos en Madrid*, 6, 1958, pp. 63–204 (reprinted separately, Madrid 1960).

AL-ZAHRAWI, *Kitāb al-taṣrīf*, facsimile ed. F. Sezgin, Frankfurt-am-Main 1986.

INDEX

١

كتاب الادوية المفردة للاسرائيلي

صمغ ... شقشقة ... رقيب ... نحل

... الثوب ... زبل الدجاج ...

[illegible]

... قاضي ... الحكيم ...

[illegible]

... الله ... والقدرة

رطل هو اثني عشر اوقية ... هو نصف قسط رطل

... اربع اسباع ... عشر

[illegible]

... يحك ويعمل فتيل وليقطع دم المقعدة لوبان وزعفران ...
... ويحك ويصيره ... مستوية غير منعقدة ويعمل فتايل طول ...
... البدء عند عملها يدهن بدهن ورد ومما يقطع افواه العروق ويسقي
دم الطمث ودم البواسير ان يوخذ عصاره فقا الحمار والعفص
ورد ... السعير من كل واحد اربعه مثاقيل ومن ورق السذاب ...
... المر يدق كل واحد على حدته ويجمع الجميع بمراره ثور ثم يستعمل
لذلك ما يحتمل السره والمتين نافع ان شا الله صفه ... ينزل
الحار حلبه وشحم حنظل وشحم كلا عشر والوزن من كل واحد جزو
... البدن ... والشحم ... ويحلل الجميع ويستعمل ...
... ويقطع باذن الله من اوجاع الوركين والمثانه وعرق النسا ومن
... وجع يوخذ من الحلبه مقدار الكفايه فيصير في قدر جديد
ويصب عليه من الخل فيصير في قدر جديد ويصب عليه من الخل الممزوج
... ويطبخ على جمر حتى تتهرا الحلبه ثم يصير عليها رطل عسل
او ... على قدر الحلبه ويطبخ حتى ينعقد ثم يصب في صلابه ويسحق
حتى يصير ... الطلا دهن ورد ان كان الوجع شديدا مسخن
بدهن شيرج او ... انها لم يظهر الحر علامه ويحمل على
... الوجع بعداد ...

[illegible] والادويه [illegible]

ومن البقول الجرجير [illegible] وافسنتين [illegible] والجزر [illegible] الجوز [illegible] الماء [illegible]

اليحموري والحمص [illegible] الحار [illegible] البقلة [illegible] الفلفل [illegible] والشقاقل [illegible]

والخولنجان والكبابه والبهمنين الاحمر والابيض وبزر الجزر [illegible] والزنجبيل وبزر الجرجير [illegible] وبزر الجزر [illegible]

وبزر الكتان [illegible] وبزر [illegible] وبزر الفجل [illegible] وبزر البصل والسلجم [illegible]

[illegible] والسنبل والعود [illegible] والزرنباد والكروبه [illegible] والقرنفل [illegible] والجوز [illegible]

والنمل الاسود اذا اخذ منه [illegible]

[illegible] صفه [illegible] من قلوب [illegible]

[illegible] العسل [illegible]

[illegible]

[illegible] رطل [illegible] واذا [illegible]

قلوب العنصل [illegible] معطش [illegible]

[illegible] في الشمس [illegible] الحنظله [illegible]

وقد ذكروا [illegible] ارهاد [illegible]

[illegible] واذا [illegible] الذي [illegible]

[illegible] علكيه [illegible]

[illegible] فقطع [illegible]

[illegible] الحلو [illegible]

[illegible] العسل [illegible]

الشربه منه [illegible]

والله الشافي [illegible]

صماذ اخر لوجع الورك، يوخذ اصل الكبار فيدق دقا ناعما ويسحق وينخل

يعجن بخل خمر ممزوجا بالما ويلزم الورك فانه يسكن الوجع ولمثل ذلك ايضا

مزيا جارا يوخذ من لباب الخبز خمسة اجزا ومن التمر المنزوع النوى جزو

في خل ممزوجا بما ومن ورق البنج الرطب جزا ومن دهن الورد

يدق ورق البنج نعما ثم يخلط بالخبز والتمر حتى يعتصر [illegible]

وقع الوجع [illegible] علته [illegible]

بسم الله الرحمن الرحيم وبه استعين وعليه اتوكل

الحمد لله الذي تفرد بالكمال و[illegible] من النقصان ذي العزة والجلال و
القدرة والسلطان خالق الانسان ومعلمه البيان وجاعله مميزا على جميع الحيوان بما خصه به
من نور العقل وابانه من المزية والفضل حمدا يقضي حق الايه وتوجب المزيد من نعمائه

قال المولف [illegible] ان كان المتقدمون قد الفوا ودونوا وصنفوا واحسنوا فلم يبق لمن
جاء لهم دور من باخر زمانه لكنه مما يلزم من يوثق علمه واحسانه فواجب على من علم ان
ان يرون ويصح وحقيق من جاء بالحكمة ان ينشر ويبيح لمن اتى علما لزمه بيانه ولم يجز له كتمانه
لكن عليه ان يجزأ به اهله ولا يودعه غير مستاهله وان يشح عليه كل ضنين ولا يرتعه
لدى جاهل باضاعته ضنين حتى يضعه في مكانه ويجعله في ميزانه فقد قيل حوافة المقصر
من طرح الدر بين ارجل الخنازير. ولما رايت المستعين بالله ابا جعفر احمد بن المومنين
بالله بن [illegible] ادام الله امره واعز نصره اوحد زمانه واوحد في علمه وبيانه قد حاز
الفضل [illegible] بازمته مخلص في الفخر حلو الاريز ونزع لمودة غايه التبريز
خلد [illegible] دام على الايام نعمته ولا زال الزمان مشرفا بدوام سلطانه وتمكين
سعده و[illegible] جعلت وسيلة اليه وذريعة لديه احسن الهدى وافضل ما عرضه
الاخبار على [illegible] لحضرته الرفيعة وروحانيته الشريفة الذي فضل الله بها
اهل عصرنا و[illegible] انا ادمغرنا من ان اخصه ادام الله تاييده ووصل نصره وتسعيده
بكتاب جمعت فيه ما [illegible] من فوائد الحكماء ونظمت فيه ما انتثر من جواهر العلماء الملتقطة
في عرصات الزوايا المستخرجة من [illegible] المكنون في الاذوله المفردة لك في الهمة في علاج
الابدان على تقلب الايام وتغير الازمان وطرزته باسمه العالي اعلى الله كلمته وبره ووصل
افضاله وسعده فسميته المستعيني ليشرف به وينفق سوقه بسببه واستشعرت فيما
اوردته واصدرته وجمعته وحضرته الاذعان لفهمه الراجح والاستسلام لمن يرضى علمه
البارع علما باني كمن جلب التمر الى هجر واهدى الى جهينة الخبر وسلكت فيه طريقة المنقر بين
وصنعته على عادة المتقدمين وذلك انهم ذكروا ان التاليف لا يتم حتى يتضمن احدى ثلاثة
[illegible] ما جمع متفرق والثاني اختصار مطول والثالث ايضاح مشكل وكتاب مفرد

[illegible] الخصال و[illegible] فقط [illegible] لمن تقدمني من كتب الادوية المفردة جميع
ما جمعته في هذا الكتاب لان جميع [illegible] وطبعه وفي اي درجة هو من الحرارة والبرودة والرطو
واليبوسة ثم جعلت ما له من الاسماء الشاذة وغير الشاذة على حسب الالسنة منها سريانية
ومنها فارسية ومنها يونانية ومنها عربية ومنها رومية ومنها عجمية عامية وجليت
على كل واحد من هذه الاسماء بقدر ما وجدت متفرقا في كتب جمة لان [illegible] الضرورة داعية
الى ذلك لتحير الناس فيها وضلالهم بسببها متى وقعت في نسخة من النسخ [illegible] من هذه الاسماء
وربما بطلت النسخة على صاحبها بالجملة لذلك التغيير فقد كان واتفق ان هذه الخطة [illegible]
هذا وهي من اعظم الاشياء منفعة لقاريه والصيادلة [illegible] جميع المفترقات [illegible] وأجل منفعة
وذلك انه جعلت في اكثر هذه الاسماء الابدال منها اذا عدمت وقل ما رايتها مجتمعة في كتاب من كتب
من كتب الادوية المفردة بل رايت جل هذه الكتب خالية عن ذلك فذكرت البدل على كل دوا
لان الضرورة في هذا الموضع مثل الضرورة في ذكر الاسماء من بطلان النسخ [illegible] عن تركيبها
لان كثيرا ما تعدم بعض الادوية في وقت دون وقت وفي بلد دون بلد [illegible]
لتتم العلاج فقد كملت الخطة الاولى على احسن ما امكن ان يكون من [illegible] في
اثر الابدال منافعها وخواصها ووجوه [illegible] ونبهت على ما منها رديه القاتلة غير
مامونة العاقبة واصلاحها بالجيد ومقدار الشربة منها لان هذا الباب [illegible] عظيم ٢
الخطر لانه قد يجر شيئا كثيرا فمنها ادوية كثيرة رديه القاتلة [illegible] لا يجب [illegible]
وربما كانت اوزانها فوق المقدار المحتمل فاضرت [illegible] ضرر عظيمة واورثت اسقاما
جسيمة وقد شاهدت ذلك لرجل يدعي صناعة الطب [illegible] غير عارف بها قد سقى
انسانا دوا مسهلا فيه من شحم الحنظل وزن درهمين واجاب [illegible] ووقعه في مغص وعصار
واوجاع المعيرة والامعاء ولولا انه اكثر من شرب السمن والعسل مع الكثيرا والقمح [illegible]
لقتله على المقام ولو علم هذا الرجل الجاهل ان الشربة من شحم الحنظل ما بين ثلاث قراريط الى ستة
قراريط بغير اصلاحه لم تقدم ان يسقي منه في شربة واحدة وزن درهمين والقيراط عندهم ثلاث
حبات . فهذا باب كبير يجب ان يتحرى ويستقصى [illegible] الغلط فيه وجليت على كل غير
اقاويل المتقدمين ونسبت كل قول الى قايله وجعلت [illegible]

وعوض من جا البنوس جيم وعوض من ار سقط لسقوط القرا وكتب الحرف من اسم [illegible]
لتسميتها فقد بان من هذا أيضا صحيح نص الخصلة [illegible] به على الفصل [illegible] تنبيها [illegible]
جميع ذلك باختصار وإيجاز وجعلت جميع ما ذكرت في هذا الكتاب مع العقاقير على حروف
أبجد هوز حطي في كلمن سعفص قرشت ثخذ ضظغ ليسهل على الطالب مطلوبه منها
وأدخلتها في جدول حتى يخف طلبها وليسهل أيضا التبيين عنها وليسقط تكرارها وذلك أني أدخلت
كل عقير في [illegible] مقسوم على خمسة أقسام وضعت في القسم الأول اسمه وفي الثاني طبعه
ودرجته وعوضت من الدرجة الأولى بألف وعوضت من الدرجة الثانية بباء ومن الدرجة الثالثة
بجيم ومن الدرجة الرابعة بدال وفي القسم الثالث تفسيرها باختلاف اللغات وفي القسم الرابع
الأبدال منها وفي القسم الخامس منافعها وخواصها ووجوه استعمالها وجعلت في أعلى الجدول
وأسفله [illegible] لتسميتها على كل عقير من عقاقيره وربما اقتصرت على القليل منها دون الكثير
أو على [illegible] على حسب الاتساع فيها لأن منها أدوية اكتفيت بما ذكرت عليها
في آخر الجدول [illegible] وبه فصل الجدول عن وصف جميع قواها وقد ذكرت منافعها فوصفتها
فوق الجدول [illegible] تكمل الفائدة بذلك . فليقرأ من أول الجدول إلى آخره فإذا فرغ من قراءة
ما فوق الجدول [illegible] ما في أسفله إذ هو أصله ثم متصل عنه . وأما الهواء فقد بينت قبل
على الجدول الوجوه التي بها عرف الأوائل طبائع الأدوية المفردة ومنها استخرجوا الدرج
لمعرفة طبائع المركبات [illegible] وكيف ينبغي أن تركب والداعية إلى تركيبها لم تكن على
قوى الأدوية المشتملة على [illegible] ووضعت ما يحتوي من ضروبها إذ المركب على ما ينبغي
ويفرق ما يجب أن يعرفه قبل [illegible] الترجمة [illegible] ثم ذكرت العلة التي دعت الأوائل
إلى إبدال العقاقير وكيف [illegible] معرفة ذلك ومنها كملت الخصلة الثالثة التي هي
إيضاح مشكل لأن معرفة الأشياء مع ما هي [illegible] في كتب القدماء الأجلاء فهي لباب العلم غامضة
وعبارة وأعزة لعسيرة عن فهم من لم يجر له حنكه ولا معرفة متقدمة وقراءة ممن له بالشيخ
بما أغلقه القدماء وليتبين له تشبيها ما أبهمه العلماء فوضعته منها بالبسط ما يكون
من القول وأوضح دون العلل الخبيث ليفهمه جميع من قرأه ويعلمه كل من طالعه فيربح لنا ويظهر
البناء لأن الثلاث الخصال متضمنة كتابنا هذا على ما شرطناه فيها فلنبدأ بعون الله وحسن

[illegible] بجميع ما وعدناه وشرح كل ما ضمّناه فصار فصلا لا يخالطه علم سواه ولا ٧
يشوبه شي خاشاه لتقرب مقاصده وينجلي [illegible] ولا يحتاج في ذلك الى ان يتعب النفس
ويجهد الفكر وبالله التوفيق وهو حسبنا ونعم الوكيل

القول في تعرف قوى الادوية المفردة قال المؤلف

الوجوه التي منها عرف الاوايل قوى الادوية ومنها استنبطوا الدرج [illegible] احدها الطعوم
والثانية الروايح والثالث بايرادها على البدن المعتدل وبهذا الوجه [illegible] وهو اعلى
طبايع الاغذية ⁂ واضعف هذه الوجوه عندهم ما يعرف منها بالطعوم والروايح [illegible]
المعروف عندهم يعرف بالقياس واضعفها عندهم واثبتها في معتقدهم [illegible] يعرف منها بايرادها
على البدن المعتدل لانه يعرف بذلك بالتجربة والمعاينة واما استخراجهم قوى الادوية المفردة
واستنباطهم لدرجاتها من قبل طعومها فقالوا كلما اجتمع اللسان في الغاية فهو في الدرجة
الرابعة من البرودة وبالضد في الاول وما بينهما اما قريب من الاول ففي الثانية وما قريب من
الرابعة ففي الثالثة مثل ان تعالى الخل وعلى الحنطة والارباق في [illegible] مثلهما
حال البنوم والقراط الفاضل اجعاله الاسفل ضد الاعلى لم يعلم الله من باب [illegible] ويعتبر امثالا
يقيس عليه لذي فهم فان توهم متوهم في قولهم بالضد في الاول وقال انه صحيح
قلنا له اعلم ان الاسفل ضد الاعلى وكانه في هذا كله يختلط كلام [illegible] تشبيه
تا سلم المعلومين في صناعة الطب الذي اخفى عليهم حال البنوم [illegible] مثلا بالضد
في الاول ضد الغاية فقط لانك قلت كلما اجمع اللسان في الغاية فهو في الدرجة الرابعة من البرد
وبالضد في الاول لان الغاية من الانتها وضدها على الحقيقة الابتدا وان كان من [illegible] هذا الضد
وتعلق باضداد الطبيعيات فقط ولم يعلم خارج ساير الاضداد قلنا له قد اعاب وهو قولنا
ضد الغاية لا غاية ولو وجدنا المعنى اللفظة لعين الغاية لفظة ثانية تحت القسمة لم يلتبس هذا الضد
على من يتوهم مثل هذا الوهم كما نجد للحر لفظة ثانية تضادها وهي البرد فالبرد ضد للحر
كما ان الغاية ضدها لا غاية فقد صار صورة لا غاية ضد للغاية لان لا رفع الغاية كما رفع المبرد
للحر فصار ضده كذلك لا غاية رفع الغاية فصار ضدها وعلى هذا المثال اجعل قياسك على ساير
الاقسام الباقية وما يحرد اللسان ويقبضه واحزاوه في الغاية فهو في الدرجة الرابعة من الحرارة

٦

وبالضد في الاول وما بينهما اما اقرب من الاول ففي الثانية واما اقرب ففي [illegible]
واما استخراجهم قوانينها واستنباطهم رسمها من قبل الروائح فقالوا ما كان منها ينفذ في الدماغ
بسرعة عند الشم ويصدع غاية الصداع ويسخن ويلهب الدماغ فذلك عندهم في الدرجة
الرابعة من الحر وبالضد في الاول وما بينهما اما اقرب من الاول ففي الثانية واما اقرب من
الرابعة ففي الثالثة وما يسكن عند الشم ويخدر الحواس وينوم نوما ثقيلا ويولد سباتا
فذلك عندهم في الدرجة الرابعة من البرد وبالضد في الاول وما بينهما اما اقرب من الاول
ففي الثانية واما اقرب من الرابعة ففي الثالثة والمعتدل عندهم على مجرى القياس هو ما ورد
على اللسان ولم يحس منه حاسة الذوق ولا عمل فيه ولا اخرج اللسان ولا فرق بعض اجزائه على
ما يفعله المر ولا غسله على ما يفعله الحريف ولا نول فيه حرارة على ما يفعله المالح والحامض
ولا جمعه ولا عفصه على ما يفعله القابض والعفص والعفص في ذلك اقوى فعلا من القابض لكن
المعتدل عندهم ما ورد على اللسان ولا يفعل فيه شيئا من هذه الاعراض المذكورة بل تحسه
حاسة [illegible] لذاذة قليلة وقال بعض الاطباء ان الطعام الحلو هو المعتدل لانه ليس بحار
فيحرق اللسان ولا بارد فيجمعه لكنه معتدل لكسبه حاسة ولذاذة فقط ومنهم
من قال ان الحلاوة الظاهرة دالة على الحرارة وعلى قدر الحلاوة تكون الحرارة . ومنهم من قال
ان الدسم هو من انواع المعتدل لانه دون الحلاوة ۝ ۝ واما الوجه الثالث الذي هو من
الوجوه واوضحها وابينها فهو الماخوذ من تاثيرها وافعالها في الابدان المعتدلة لانه اذا دوا
او غذا او ورد على البدن لا يخلو ان يفعل فيه من ان يوثر فيه في الغاية فيحكم على ذلك الدوا والغذا
انه في الدرجة الرابعة او يوثر فيه تاثيرا يحتاج معه الى زمان فيحكم عليه انه في الدرجة
الاول وما بينهما اما اقرب من الاول ففي الثانية واما اقرب من الرابعة ففي الثالثة فيحصل
لكل كيفية مطلقة اربع درجات مثال ذلك انك تقول حار في الدرجة الاول وحار في الدرجة
الثانية وحار في الدرجة الثالثة وحار في الدرجة الرابعة فيحصل الكيفية الحرارة اربع درجات
ولانها لها [illegible] وغايته [illegible] قسمت الاوائل كل درجة من هذه الدرجات على ثلاثة اقسام
وذلك انه يقال حار في اول الدرجة الاول وحار في اخرها وحار في وسطها وفي سائر الكيفيات
كذلك وذلك على التقريب والمجاز لا على التحقيق والبرهان لان القسمة ابدا ممكنة الى ما لا

٩

في مراتب الدرجات لانا لو شئنا ان نقسم كل جزء من هذه الثلاثة اقسام على ثلاثة
اقسام ايضا لو جرت كل قسم منها فيما خالف صاحبه في الحرارة والبرودة او الرطوبة او اليبس
على حسب الدرجة التي قسمناها ولو شئنا ايضا ان نفعل ذلك الى ما لا نهاية له لجرت لنا القسمة و
وثبتت التجربة اذ يخالف كل قسم منها صاحبه في الزيادة والنقصان لكن القسمة الاولى
لقربها هي المستعملة في صناعة الطب لانا اذا قلنا دواء في اول الدرجة الاولى كان قربه من
الاعتدال قريبا اكثر منها اذا قلنا دواء في وسط الدرجة الاولى وما كان … في … الدرجة الاولى
اقرب الى الاعتدال مما كان في آخرها لان ما كان في آخرها الدرجة الاولى فهو قريب من الدرجة الثانية
وتباعد من الاعتدال وعلى هذا القياس اجمل قياسك في سائر الدرجات ولم ير بعض الاطباء زيادة
في هذه القسمة وصفة ثالثة في هذا المعنى الذي في استخراج قوى الادوية المفردة واستنباطهم
درجاتها وذلك ان الدواء اذا لقي البدن المعتدل فانه اما ان يكون شبيها لمزاج البدن الذي يلقاه
في السخونة والبرودة والجفوفة والرطوبة فيدل ذلك على ان الدواء معتدل بين … الكيفيات
والعلوية كيفية تعرف لها ولا نسب الى بها فليس يجب مما هذا سبيله ان يسمى … ولا رطبا
ولا يابسا ايضا ولا يسمى ايضا حارا ولا باردا وانما يجب ان يسمى معتدلا فقط و[illegible] يكون
ذلك الدواء غير شبيه بالبدن الذي يلقاه فيكون اسخن منه او اشد حرا منه او ابرد او ارطب
فان ذلك يسمى باسم مشتق من الكيفية الغالبة عليه ولهذا تحدث الاوائل عن امر الادوية
وجعلوا لكل واحد مما يغلب عليه شيء من هذه الكيفيات الاربع اربع درجات ولكل
درجة ثلاثة مواضع كما بيناها انفا وقالوا ما غير البدن المعتدل ولم يبالغ في تغييره ولا تبين
ذلك التغيير بيانا ظاهرا ولا علم الا ببرهان فذلك الدواء في الدرجة الاولى وما غيره تغييرا
بينا وليس بالشديد فهو في الدرجة الثانية وما غيره تغييرا شديدا ظاهرا الا انه ليس في الغاية
ولا المفسد جملة فهو في الدرجة الثالثة وما غيره تغييرا في الغاية القصوى وافسده جملة
فهو في الدرجة الرابعة . اما البارد فانه يخدر ويسحك ويثبت . واما الحار فانه يحرق ويجفف
ويلهب ان شاء الله تعالى وانا قد بلغنا الى ما اردناه من تحقيق الوجوه التي منها وقف الاوائل
على طبائع الادوية المفردة وكيفية استنباطهم لدرجاتها باختصار والحاجز … يحتاجون
الان الى معرفة طبائع المركبات واذ ذاك لما بحث قوانين الدرجات ومن الاسم ولا يخفف …

الا بغير معرفة طبائع المفردات ويحفظون ذلك انما هو بالقياس والتجربة على ما يبين من اقاويل
الاوائل ومن الناس كثير من يدعي تركيب النسخ ويتبعها وافرقة البرهان على طبائعها ودرجاتها
فلذا سألوا عن ما هي ذلك قالوا من الرؤيا يسخن ويبرد ومن الجفيف ومن الرطب بالاطلاق
فقط دون ان يعلموا عن درج كل واحد منهما ولا يحفظوا ما بينهما من المباعدة وكان يجب
كيفية [illegible] بسيطة لان اشياء كثيرة تكون حارة وتختلف في الحرارة من قبل اختلاف درجاتها
اختلاف [illegible] كثيرة تكون باردة او رطبة او يابسة وتختلف ايضا في اختلاف درجاتها فاذا
تركب على غير [illegible] ولا نظام لم يكن لذلك التركيب دوام بل كان خبطا ومن بيان مثال الادوية
المسخنة في الدرجة الاولى افسنتين اسطوخودوس اذخر بابونج اكليل الملك
سنبل ساذج شاهترج شاه شبرم سنا ونحو هذه ومثال الادوية
المسخنة في الدرجة الثانية بادروج برنجمشك اظفار الطيب علك
زراوند ابرنج ريباس زعفران عنبر عود مسك ونحو هذه ومثال الادوية
المسخنة في الدرجة الثالثة افثيمون انيسون انجدان بسبايج بل وفل وشل
دارصيني وشونيز زوفا حرمل قرنفل ونحو هذه ومثال الادوية المسخنة في
الدرجة الرابعة فربيون بلادر يتوع فلفل قطران شيطرج
خردل ثوم ونحو هذه ومثال الادوية المبردة في الدرجة الاولى اقاقيا اسه
املج الاملجات آس بلوط برد بسر ورد شعير معنبرا اسفانا
ونحو هذه ومثال الادوية المبردة في الدرجة الثانية بزرقطونا امبرباريس
لسان الحمل سماق عفص عنب الذيب قثا خيار قرع دلاع خس
رباس ونحو هذه ومثال الادوية المبردة في الدرجة الثالثة دم الاخوين طباشير
فوفل كافور صندل تمر هندي بقلة حمقا حي العالم عصا الراعي ونحو هذه
ومثال الادوية المبردة في الدرجة الرابعة خشخاش اسود جوز ماثل افيون
بنج اسود رامط جرير المر ربق ونحو هذه وعلى هذا المثال تصنيف الادوية
المرطبة والميبسة اولا [illegible] حتى ينتهي الى الدرجة الرابعة التي هي الغاية والنهاية في درجات
الادوية وما ادخلنا هنا من معرفة الادوية لم ندخلها الا على سبيل المثال ولم نقصد الا استقصا

بـ... ...وقوف على اكثرها واجب ان يلتمس من كتبها انها و... درجاتها بالتحرير
والتفصيل فليعتمد على قراءة الجدول الموضوع لهذا المعنى فمنه يقف على ذلك ان شاء الله

القول في معرفة طبائع المركبات وكيف ينبغي ان يركب ...

ينبغي لمن اراد تركيبها ان يعرف الحاجة الى تركيبها ٥ قال المؤلف الذي يحتاج ان يتحكم
فيه اولا وينبغي تركيب المعتدل اذ هو اشرف التراكيب لما يرفع منه الى الخارج عن
الاعتدال وهو اعظم فايدة واجل منفعة واغمض صناعة لان المعتدل وان كان اشرف
التراكيب فمعلوم يكاد لا يجهل تركيبه كما ان الخارج عن الاعتدال يجهلوا يكاد الا
يعلمه الا من تدرب في قراءة الكتب المخصوصة بذلك وارتاض في درس قوانين المسائل
ويعرف معرفة طبائع المفردات وحقق مواضعها من الدرجات وما في كل درجة من الاجزاء
الحارة والباردة واليابسة والرطبة فحينئذ يمكنه علم تركيب الادوية الخارجة عن الاعتدال
وهو علم لا يستغنى احد ممن يتزيا بهذه الصناعة عنه ومن كان منهم خاليا عن هذا العلم
لم يوثق بعلاجه لانه اذا جهل هذا التركيب في الادوية فقد جهل المرض ولا يعلمه البتة لان
المرض هو شيء خارج عن الاعتدال وقد قلنا ان الاعتدال معلوم وهو لكثرة ... واستواء
والصحة معلومة ايضا وهي لكثرة الطباع واستواء الاخلاط وتناسبها في الاعتدال وان يكون
الانسان لا ينقصه شيء من اموره المعتادة الطبيعية كانت او غير طبيعية فالطبيعية
مثل قوام الهضم واعتدال اليقظة والنوم وان تكون جميع الحواس على استواء من افعالها
المعتادة والغير طبيعية هي الارادية مثل التصرف في جميع الحركات نحو القيام والقعود
وجميع الارادات التي يحتاج الانسان فيها الى الفكرة فاذا كانت هذه كلها على قوام
واعتدال سمي الانسان صحيحا وهو الاعتدال الانساني وهذا الاعتدال المعلوم غير مجهول
فاذا دخلت آفة ما على هذا الاعتدال غيرته وابطلت بعض هذه الاشياء الارادية او
الطبيعية وربما ابطلتها جملة او جلها او القليل دون الكثير ولا يكون ذلك الا عن خروج
احدى الطبائع بزيادة او نقصان وهذا هو ضد الصحة كما ان الصحة ضد المرض والمرض لا يكون
الا بفساد الاخلاط وخروجها عن الاعتدال فيجب للطبيب ان يعلم اولا درجة كان البدن
المعتدل من الحر والبرد واليبوسة والرطوبة حتى يكون مقابلته بالادوية صحيحة فان قال قائل

ان هذا امر يعسر الحكم لا نقدر احد على معرفته فلذلك ان ابطلنا هذا الباب ...
نبطل معرفة تحقيق قوى الادوية المفردة اذ لم نعلم الا حتى جربت وامتحنت في الابدان المعتدلة
لان كل دوا ... هذا اذا ورد على البدن المعتدل لا يخلو طبيعته من ان تؤثر فيه اما في الغاية
واما يسير من الغاية واما في ما بينهما فاذا اسلفنا هذا وحققنا عندنا فليس بالعسير اذا اغلب
واحد من الاخلاط على البدن المعتدل ان نعمل فيه هذا القياس اذ كان الاخلاط منحصرة تحت الاربع
درجات ... الادوية ايضا منحصرة تحت الاربع درجات فما العسير من هذا التعرف ومعنا
... النظر للطبيب الماهر اليقظان والمعرفة الوجود ووجوه اخر كثيرة يستخرج
منه ... وان تخطى القياس فيها ولولا الذي تضمنت الاختصار والايجاز لطولت
... فيما ذكرت منها الكتاب لمن فهم فاذا صح عند الطبيب ان البدن المعتدل خرج
عن الاعتدال بجزء واحد من الحر لزمه ان يقابله بدوا يكون في جزء واحد من البرد فقط حتى
يقاوم الجزء من البرد لجزء الغالب من الحر ويصرفه الى الاعتدال الطبيعي الذي كان عليه
اولا وكذلك ... ان يفعله في سائر الاجزاء الباقية وهذا يعسر شاق على كثير من الاطبا
لا سيما من لم يتعلم منهم طبيب حتى بلغ الاوائل في تحصيل درجات الادوية المفردة والمركبة
ايضا لانهم لو امعنوا النظر واجهدوا الفكر لوجدوا الامر واحدا لا فرق بينهما اذ لا
في كل واحد منهما البدن المعتدل وانا اقول ان الدوا المعتدل هو الذي تساوت اجزاؤه و
اعتدلت طبيعته فاذا صح ذلك فيه قيل له معتدل على الحقيقة والمعتدل المتساوي الطبيعة
هو ان يكون فيه من الحر بقدر ما فيه من البرد ويكون فيه من الرطوبة بقدر ما فيه ايضا من
اليبوسة فما كان على هذا السبيل من التركيب سمي معتدلا لان الطبائع فيه معتدلة
لم يعل بعضها بعضا وكذلك انا لما جعلنا الحار الذي لا يتبين الا بعد زمان وتحقيق نظر في الدرجة
الاولى وجعلنا ما ظهرت حرارته ولم تضر لامسه في الدرجة الثانية وجعلنا ما لذع لامسه
ولم يحرق في الدرجة الثالثة وجعلنا ما احرقت حرارته وقرحت اجزاء لامسه في الدرجة
الرابعة . وبالضد في الدرجات الباردة وجب ان يكون المعتدل فيما بين الذي في الغاية من الحرارة
وهو الذي يحرق اجزاء لامسه ويقرحها وبين البارد هو ضده لذلك وهو الذي يجمع اجزاء لامسه ويقمعها
لان الذي في غاية الحرارة يعبر عن الاعتدال باربع درجات والذي في غاية البرد يعبر عن الاعتدال

ايضا بأربع درجات فالاعتدال اذا متساوي الطبيعيات لا يعلو واحدة منهما فيلتبس النقصا
ويعرف فهذا مثال ذلك انا لو اخذنا جزوا من ماء مغلي وجزوا مثله من جليد وخلطناهما لألفيناه
معتدل القوام ولم نسمه لا بحار ولا بارد ولا برطب ولا يابس لان ما فيه من حر مثله بعينه
فيه من البرد ومثال ما فيه من الرطوبة مثله فيه من اليبوسة لان الجليد لم يبلغ الى ان يكون
الا ما اليبس الداخل عليه . ومثال ثان في هذا المعنى وهو اغمض من هذا […] انا لو اخذنا
جزوا من الخردل الذي هو في الدرجة الرابعة من الحر واليبس وجزا مثله من […] هو
في الدرجة الرابعة من البرد والرطوبة لكان من مزج الخلطين خلطا معتدلا و[…]
باسم ثان غير الاعتدال فقط اذ تساوت فيه الاجزاء . ومثال ثالث في تركيب المعتدل […] ابعد
من هذا واغمض جدا وذلك انا لو اردنا ان نركب دوا معتدلا من حار في الدرجة الرابعة […] بارد في
الدرجة الاولى اخذنا درهما من عقير في الدرجة الرابعة وخلطناه بخمسة عشر درهما من عقير
في الدرجة الاولى من البرد فيعتدل التركيب بمقارنة ذلك ان في الدرهم في العقير الحار الذي في الدرجة
الرابعة ستة عشر جزوا من اجزاء الحر […] الوسيط واحدا ابدا لسبب الجزو المقا[…] البرد لان كل
عقير يكون في الدرجة الرابعة في الدرهم منه ستة عشر جزوا من اجزاء الحار وجزو واحد من برد
فلهذا نطرحه ابدا فيبقا خمسة عشر جزوا فاحفظها ثم اعلم ما في الدرهم من العقير الذي في
في الدرجة الاولى من البرد فيخرج لك جزوين فتسقط من ذلك واحدا ابدا فيبقى واحد لان كل
عقير يكون في الدرجة الاولى من البرد جزوان من برد وجزو واحد من حر فلهذا السبب يسقط
الواحد ابدا فافهم علته المحفوظ فيخرج لك خمسة عشر فهو عدد الدراهم التي تحمل من العقير
البارد في الدرجة الرابعة على الدرهم الواحد من العقير الذي في الدرجة الرابعة من الحر فيعتدل
التركيب وعلى هذا المثال افعل في سائر الدرجات عند تركيبك المعتدل فيصح لك التركيب
ان شا الله . واما التركيب المنحرف عن الاعتدال الى احد الطبيعيات فاصعب من هذا واغمض
وان كان لا يعلم الا بعد علم الاعتدال ضرورة لانه علم لا يستغنى عنه كل من تناول اشيا
من علم الابدان غير انهم لما راوا ما فيه من المشقة والصعوبة فعدوا عنه وتكلموا على نسخ
الكتب وقلدوها ولم يعلموا انها قد مرت على ايدي كثير ممن لم يحسن نقلها ولا عرف وضعها
وربما الصحيفة اكثرها او زاد فيها او زال عنها شيا او نقص من مقاديرها و ربما سقط منها عقير

١٤

أو عفونات أو أمثال أو أكثر ولم يتبين ذلك إلا بعد النضج وحصل أوزانها وتبين من طبيعتها
وأضاف عقاقيرها بعضها إلى بعض ثم أضاف جملتها إلى الوزن المعتدل المخرج به درج ذلك
الدواء المركب فعند ذلك يصح المقابلة به والمقدار الذي يجب متى وقف على حقيقة ذلك الدواء
والدواء فإن يخرج واخرج درجة بإضافته إلى الوزن المعتدل أن يحصل أيضا منافعه التي وجدت له
ويقابلها [illegible] المفردة التي في تلك النسخة فإن وجدت على شروطها ورتبتها ازداد يقيننا
في [illegible] فلا فلاح لذلك إلا أيضا من الوقوف على حقيقة طبيعة المرض الذي أعدت
له [illegible] ومقدار الشربة منها حتى يحتمل الطبيعة ولم لا زادة ومن كان على خلاف
ذلك [illegible] جميع ما يتناوله من المعاجين على غرر وتوقع. وأنا أقدم في ذلك مقدمة تخصها
من أقاويل [illegible] أن يكون [illegible] دستورا للتركيب وذلك أن ما كان في الدرجة الأولى من الحر
فيه من الحر جزءان وجزء واحد من البرد وما كان في الدرجة الثانية من الحر فيه أربعة أجزاء
وجزء واحد من برد. وما كان في الدرجة الثالثة من الحر فيه ثمانية أجزاء حارة وجزء واحد من برد
وما كان في [illegible] الرابعة من الحر فيه ستة عشر جزءا حارة وجزءا واحدا من برد وفي كل
واحد منها من اليبس بقدر ما فيه من الحر إن كان يابسا في الدرجة التي فيها الحر وكذلك الرطوبة
وما كان في الدرجة الأولى من البرد فيه من البرد جزءان وجزء واحد من حر وما كان في الدرجة
الثانية من البرد فيه من البرد أربعة أجزاء وجزء واحد من حر وما كان في الدرجة الثالثة
من البرد فيه من البرد ثمانية أجزاء وجزء واحد من حر وفي كل واحد منها من الرطوبة بقدر
ما فيها من البرودة إن كانت رطوبتها في درجة بردها فإن تجاوزت رطوبتها أو يبسها
درجة البرودة أو الحرارة زدت في أجزائها على قدر ما تجاوزت من الدرج وإن نقصت عن الدرجة
التي فيها الحرارة أو البرودة نقصت منها على قدر ذلك. فإذ قد علمت ما أصل في الحر والبارد فإن
أردت أن تعلم في أي درجة يقع دواء مركب من عدة أدوية مفردة مختلفة الطبيعيات
حصلت ما فيه من الأدوية الحارة في الدرجة الرابعة وحصلت أوزانها فإن كانت اليبوسة
مع الحرارة في درجة واحدة أخرجت لكل درهم منها ستة عشر جزءا من حر وستة عشر جزءا
من يبس وجزءا واحدا من برد وجزءا واحدا من رطوبة ولتكتب الأجزاء الحارة تحت الحار
و[illegible] تحت البارد واليابسة تحت اليابس ثم تعلم ما فيه أيضا من الأدوية الباردة في الدرجة

الرابعة

وتحصل [illegible] كانت الرطوبة مع البرودة في تلك الدرجة اخرجت لكل درهم ستة عشر
جزوا من برد وستة عشر جزوا من رطوبة وجزو واحد من حر وجزوا واحد ايضا من يبوسة
وتكتبه ايضا تحت كل كيفية . ثم تعلم ما فيهما من الادوية الحارة في الدرجة الثالثة وتحصل
اوزانهما فان كانت اليبوسة معهما في درجة واحدة اخرجت لكل درهم ثمانية اجزا حارة وثمانية
اجزا يابسة وجزوا واحدا باردا وجزوا واحدا ايضا رطبا وتكتب ايضا تحت كل كيفية على
على مراتبها . ثم تعلم ما فيهما من الادوية الباردة في الدرجة الثالثة وتحصل [illegible] فان كانت
الرطوبة معهما في درجة واحدة اخرجت لكل درهم ثمانية اجزا باردة وثمانية [illegible]
واحدا حارا وجزوا واحدا يابسا وتكتب كل كيفية تحت الكيفية المذكورة [illegible] ثم
ما فيهما من الادوية الحارة في الدرجة الثانية وتحصل اوزانهما فان كانت اليبوسة [illegible] في
درجة واحدة اخرجت لكل درهم اربعة اجزا حارة واربعة يابسة وجزوا واحدا باردا وجزوا
واحدا رطبا وتكتب ذلك ايضا تحت كل كيفية ثم تعلم ما فيهما من الادوية الباردة في الدرجة الثانية
وتحصل اوزانهما فان كانت الرطوبة معهما في درجة واحدة اخرجت لكل درهم [illegible] اربعة اجزا
باردة واربعة اجزا رطبة وجزوا واحدا حارا وجزوا واحدا يابسا وتكتبه ايضا تحت كل كيفية
ثم تعلم ما فيهما ايضا من الادوية الحارة في الدرجة الاولى وتحصل اوزانهما فان كانت اليبوسة معهما
في درجة واحدة اخرجت لكل درهم جزوين حارة وجزوين يابسة وجزوا واحدا باردا وجزوا
واحدا رطبا . ثم تعلم ما فيهما من الادوية الباردة في الدرجة الاولى وتحصل اوزانهما فان كانت الرطوبة
معهما في درجة واحدة اخرجت لكل درهم جزوين باردة وجزوين رطبة وجزوا واحدا حارا
وجزوا واحدا يابسا . ثم تضم جميع ما كتبت الحار مع الحار والبارد مع البارد واليابس مع
اليابس والرطب مع الرطب وتحصل جميع الاجزا فان غلب الحار على البارد بجزوين كان الدوا
حارا في الدرجة الاولى . وان غلب الحار على البارد بثمانية اجزا . باربعة اجزا كان الدوا حارا
في الدرجة الثانية وان غلب الحار على البارد بثمانية اجزا كان الدوا حارا في الدرجة الثالثة
وان غلب الحر على البارد بستة عشر جزوا كان الدوا حارا في الدرجة الرابعة وكذلك فافعل
في سائر الكيفيات تجد مطلبك ان شا الله ○ ومن الاطبا من يسمي معرفة الاجزا اعداد فمتى سمع
ان البزر المعتدل خرج عن الاعتدال باربعة اعداد علم انه في الدرجة الثالثة وكذلك [illegible]

في سائر الاجزاء والاعراض هذا عوضا من الاجزاء فالفرق بين قولهم اعداد او بين قولهم اجزاء
ولو امكن لنا ان نداوي جميع ما يحدث في البدن من [illegible] ات العلل بادوية مفردة لم نحتج البتة
في كل وقت من الاوقات الى دواء مركب لاكن الضرورة تبعثنا على ذلك لانه قد يخرج المعتدل
عن الاعتدال باعداد ما ولا نعدم دواء مفردا في تلك الاعداد فتدعوا الضرورة الى تركيب
دواء من عدة ادوية مفردة حتى تقاوم المرض الذي حتى تقاوم تلك الاعداد التي خرج بها
البدن المعتدل مثال ذلك ان البدن المعتدل اذا خرج عن الاعتدال باربعة اعداد الى الحر
والبرد [illegible] انا نحتاج ان يكون الدواء الذي نداوي به هذا المرض قد خرج عن الاعتدال الى البرد
بمثل [illegible] ان لم نقدر على دواء مفرد يكون برده بهذا المقدار ووجدنا دواء من احدهما
في [illegible] اعداد من البرد والاخر في خمسة اعداد من البرد وخلطناهما جميعا بلغنا ما اردنا
وجدنا به والمطلوب في نصف هذا المركب وهو الشربة منهما المعدة العلة وكذلك يجب ان نفعل
في الاعداد الباقية وفي الادوية المفردة ادوية كثيرة لا يمكن ان يستعمل دون ان نخلط بادوية
غيرها لدفع غائلتها وضررها مثل خلطنا بالسقمونيا الانيسون والزوفا وبعض الاصماغ
كيلا يضر بالمعدة وبالكبد ومثل خلطنا بشحم الحنظل الكثيرا والصمغ العربي كيلا يسحج المعا
ومثل خلطنا الافيثمون بدهن اللوز كيلا يورث غما وغشيا ومثل خلطنا ايضا التربد بدهن اللوز
ليمنعه عن فساد المعدة والمعا وقد نخلط به ايضا الهليلج كيلا يضر بالمعا ومثل خلطنا المصطكي مع الصبر
ليمنعه عن ضرر المعدة وقد نخلط به ايضا كيلا يضر بالاسفل وقد نغسل الادوية لنرفع ضرره
عن مفاصل العضوين ونحو ذلك وقد نخلط مع الادوية البشيعة الكريهة ادوية طيبة كيما
يسهل على الانسان شربها وتقوى المعدة على ضبطها وتثبت فيها حتى تفعل جميع افعالها لان
كثيرا من الادوية التي تشرب تبلغ من بشاعتها وكراهية طعمها ان يكون ساعة تشرب
يعرض في شاربها الغثيان حتى تتقيا في ذلك الوقت دون ان تمكث وربما مكث بعضها مدة يسيرة
لا ينتفع بها فيجب لذلك ان نخلط بادوية لتمنع عن هذه الافات كلها لان ما كان من الادوية
يلذ لشاربها وتقبلها المعدة كان فعلها احسن واخف على الطباع وما كان على خلاف ذلك
فبالضد وقد نخلط الادوية ايضا ليقوى بعضها ببعض بمنزلة اصول الايرسا والوج والعقار يعوق
في الـ... ونحوها ومنها ما نخلط ايضا ليمنع قوة الادوية عن النفوذ بسرعة مثل الافيون

في المعجون الحارة ومثل عجيننا بعض الأدوية المسهلة بالمركبات المحسورة لبطول مخلطها في
المعدة فلستوفي فعلها ومثل هذه وأشباهها

القول في قوى الأدوية المسهلة على رأي جالينوس قال

المؤلف إن إنسانا لو شرب دواء مخصوصا بإخراج خلط من الأخلاط لا يعتاد لذلك الدواء إن
كان ضعيف الفعل لطيفا سهلا على الطباع يستفرغ أولا الفضل الذي هو مخصوص به
بسهولة ولين من غير كرب ولا عنف ولا مشقة و[illegible] وإن
صار كان يتوقع من ذلك الخلط الذي قصد إخراجه فإن كان ذلك الدواء [illegible] قوته
في البدن بعد استفراغه الخلط المخصوص به استفرغ بعده الخلط الذي [illegible] و
واللطافة بصعوبة ومشقة لأن استفراغه له إنما هو لقوة فعل الدواء وقهره له [illegible] مخصوص
بإخراجه فيحدث ذلك كربا والحالا في جميع البدن وربما أعقب استفراغا [illegible] البدن لأنه
أخرج ما لم يكن في طبيعته ولا قصد إخراجه فهذان وجهان يجب من أجلهما أن ينفع البدن في
في أمراض ردية فإن بقيت قوة الدواء بعد ذلك في البدن أخرج أيضا ما [illegible] الخلط في
الخفة واللطافة فإن كان الفعل ذلك الدواء إلى أن ينتهي إلى أخلط الأخلاط وأثقلها جرما وأبعدها
انقيادا الفعل ذلك الدواء فيستفرغه لشدة قوته وصعوبة عظيمة لأنه لم يبلغ إلى إخراج
ذلك الخلط الغليظ الثقيل والدواء غير مخصوص بإخراجه إلا حتى فنيت جميع رطوبات البدن
فهلك الإنسان من قوته ولم يمكث حتى يستحكم فيه العلل مثال ذلك أن لو شرب دواء ما
مخصوصا بإخراج المرة الصفراء لو جزنا الدواء إذا كان لطيفا ضعيف الفعل يسيرا في طبيعته
وكميته يستفرغ المرة الصفراء أولا بسهولة ولين لأنه مخصوص بإخراجها لم يسكن وينقطع
من غير كرب ولا مشقة ولا يعقب سقامة لا سيما إن كان البدن ممتليا من المرة الصفراء الخالصة
أو كان الزمان صيفا لأنه إذا كان البدن ممتليا من مرة صفراء وأدخل عليه دواء مخصوصا بإخراجها
أعانت الطبيعة على دفعها من البدن لقلقها بها ومجاهرتها لها لأن البدن إذا كان ممتليا من
خلط كان خلت الطبيعة عن تدبيره لها لخصوص بها وانصرفت إلى مجاهرة ذلك الخلط ومصارعته
كي تغلبه ولتعارقه وتنقي البدن منه فإن وافى البدن دواء مخصوصا بإخراج ذلك الخلط
ووجد من الطبيعة عونا على ذلك قوي كل واحد منهما بصاحبه وأثر في ذلك الخلط تأثيرا ب

والطبيعة في الصيف ايضا تحتاج الى اخراج المرة الصفرا من الابدان وان حفظها في الشتا
المشاكلة المرة الصفرا لمزاج فصل الصيف لان الصفرا في ذلك الوقت تقوى بسبب الحر
واليبس الذي يعينها من خارج ولمزاحا فتحتاج الطبيعة حينيذ الى ان تستخرج الحرّ الذي اما
تسكن الهوا المحيط بنا واما تسكين غلبه المرة الصفرا من داخل واما حفظها البلغم في الشتا
فلمخالفه مزاجها لمزاج الشتا وموافقتها لبرودته ورطوبته فان كان الدوا قويا وثبت قوته
في البدن بعد استفراغه للمرة الصفرا الذي هو مخصوص باخراجها كما ذكرنا استفرغ
بعدها البلغم لانه اخف الاخلاط الباقيه فيكون استفراغه له لسلسه وصفوته ولم يكن بها
وزلها فيه لانه استفرغ ما لم يكن من خصوصيته ولا من طبيعته ولا سيما ان كان الزمان صيفا
فيكون ذلك لفضل قوة الدوا او عنفه على الطبيعة لا من شان الطبيعة ان تحامى من كل خلط
من الاخلاط وترفع عنه ولمنع عن اخراجه من البدن في الزمان الذي هو يخالف لطبيعة الخلط
ومزاجه لحاجته الى مقاومته كل زمان لما يضاده وهي لذلك لمنع عن خروج البلغم وتحفظه
في الابدان في فصل الصيف وتسهل خروجه في الشتاء لحاجتها الى مقاومه حر الصيف ولييسه
ببرد البلغم ورطوبته وكذلك تفعل في ساير الاخلاط مع ساير الفصول فان ثبتت قوه الدوا
وتلبث في البدن بعد استفراغه للبلغم استفرغ بعد المرة السودا لمشقه اكثر وبليه الا
ان الدوا غير مخصوص باخراجها وانما استفرغها لفضل قوة الدوا مع ان الدوا لم يقو عليها
الا بعد ان فنيت رطوبات البدن لانها لغلظها ولبعد انفرادها تتأخر حتى يقوى الدوا عليها
لقوته وقهرها فيتولد من اخراج ذلك من العلل والاسقام ما ان لم يتدارك هلك الانسان
من قرب فان ثبتت قوة الدوا في البدن بعد ذلك وكان فيه من القوة ما يقهر الطبيعة اختلس
منها الدم واستفرغه من البدن وتولد حينيذ من الطبيعة والدوا مجاهدة ومصارعة
حتى يحدث عن ذلك الغشي والكرب وضروب من البلايا فان دام ذلك لم يومن على الطبيعة
ان تضعف وترجع عن جميع ما كانت تتناوله وتخلي تدبيرها للخصوم بها فيهلك الانسان
بكامله ومن قبل ان الطبيعة تدفع عن الدم دايما ولا يمكن الدوا اخراجه الا عن غلبتها وقهرها
لفضل قوه وعنف والسبب في دفع الطبيعة عن الدم دايما وحمايتها له دون ساير الاخلاط
طيبه وعذوبته فلنتزه من اجل ذلك مع قربه من مزاج بدن الانسان وحاجتها اليه

يعيرها أيضا وتربيه البدن ألا ترى لو عدمت الدم لما وجدت في غيرها من الأخلاط العوض
منه لبشاعة سائرها وكراهة طعمها ولبعدها من مزاج بدن الإنسان وحاجتها إليه في
تغذية الأعضاء ومخالفتها له بالطبع وذلك أن المرة الصفراء حارة يابسة مرة حريرة في
يحرقه والبلغم يشبع الطعم تفه مبرد لبدن الإنسان مرخ له لا طعم فيه ولا لذاذة والمرة
السوداء باردة يابسة حامضة عفصة معفنة قطاعة ولهذه الأسباب كرهتها الطبيعة ولم
تستعملها في تغذية البدن وأعدت لكل واحد منها موضعا تحصرها فيه حتى تمنعها من الجولان
على جميع البدن لئلا تضر بالأعضاء فتضربها بإفراط مخالفتها لها وقد ذكرت في رسالة التمييز
والترتيب التي لي في تقديم الأغذية بعضها على بعض صفة هذه المواضع وكيف تحصر الأخلاط فيها
وتحصل بها بما يجانس من القول. وأما الدم فبسبب عذوبته ولذاذته ومشاكلته لبدن الإنسان
قبلته الطبيعة وصيرته جولا معها على جميع البدن. فإن قال قائل ألم تقل الأطباء أن جميع
الأخلاط محمولة في الدم غير مفارقة له. وقولهم أيضا إنا احتجنا استفراغ البدن من
جميع الأخلاط أخرجنا من الدم على حسب الحاجة والقوة إذ الأخلاط كلها محمولة فيه وخارجة
بخروجه مما اتكال لجولانها معه على جميع البدن. قلنا له إن الأخلاط وإن كانت محمولة في الدم
وغير مفارقة له فإن الذي تحجبه منها مقدار يسير للمعونة من القوة والقدرة ما لغير طبيعته
ولم تعب بلذاذته بل تجول منها معها بمقدار حاجة الطبيعة إليها لتمد بها القوى الطبيعية
الأربع التي في كل واحد من الأعضاء أولها القوة الجاذبة وطبيعتها الحرارة واليبوسة ولا بد لهذه
القوة أيضا من مادة ليستعملها على حال النماء الطبيعية وهي المرة الصفراء والثانية القوة الماسكة
وطبيعتها البرودة واليبوسة ولا بد لهذه القوة أيضا من مادة ليستعملها على حال النماء الطبيعية
وهي المرة السوداء والثالثة القوة الهاضمة وطبيعتها الحرارة والرطوبة ولا بد لها أيضا من مادة
ليستعملها على حال النماء الطبيعية وهي الدم والرابعة القوة الدافعة وطبيعتها البرودة والرطوبة
ولا بد لها أيضا من مادة ليستعملها على حال النماء الطبيعية وهي البلغم. واعلم أن كل عضو من الأعضاء
ما كبر منها وما صغر لا بد له من هذه القوى الأربع. وقد شرحنا ذلك شرحا كافيا في رسالة
التمييز والترتيب فإذا كان لا بد لكل عضو من أعضاء البدن من هذه القوى الأربع ليتم
ذلك العضو بها فعله من جذب وحصر وهضم ودفع وكل واحد من هذه القوى لا بد لها من مادة

لطبيعة تفهم معرفة القوى على احوالها الطبيعية فليست تبلغ من لطفها الى تقدير الزمن بحسب تلك
الاحوال لان الذي يجول منها على جميع البدن لمعرفة الضرورات انما هو الطفها وارقها واسلمها
من الآفات المذمومة ولعسر منعها في احتباسها اغلظها واثقلها واشرها حرافة وحموضة
واكثرها مرارة وحدة . واما قولهم ايضا ان احتجنا الى استفراغ البدن من جميع الاخلاط
اخرجنا من الدم على حسب الحاجة والقوة بالفصد اذ الاخلاط كلها محمولة فيه وخارجة بخرو جه
فما يكون ذلك الا في فصل الربيع فقط لان هذا الفصل معتدل من جميع الكيفيات لا تغلب تدب
فيه كيفية على كيفية وان يكون البدن ايضا لم يظهر عليه غلبة الاخر الاسطقسات الثالثة اعني
المرة الصفراء والمرة السوداء والبلغم فحينئذ يجب ارسال الدم على حسب الحاجة والقوة
والسن فيخرج مع خروجه من جميع الاخلاط بقدر ما ينتفع به البدن فان مال البدن الى الطبيعة
او الطبيعة غلط من الاخلاط جعلنا اكثر عنايتنا وقصرنا استفراغ ذلك الخلط الذي مال اليه
البدن واعلم ان الادوية المسهلة تسهل اولا من الخلط الذي يقصد اخراجه ثم من غيره لم يعرف لك
تخرج ما هو غلط الى ان يتم فعل ذلك الدواء في ذلك الخلط وجالينوس في قوى الادوية المسهلة
فصل قال فيه ان الادوية التي شانها ان تنقي المرة السوداء يسهل منها اولا الماء المرار الاسود وكذلك
وكذلك المسهلة للمرة الصفراء والبلغم الا ان الفضل بين ما يسهله كل واحد منها وبين الاخر b
هو ان الاسهال اولا يكون لما هو من كل خلط لم يعرف لما هو غلط وذلك ان كل دواء يسهل خلطا
ما انما يجذب منه اولا الارق الخلط الملائم له الا انه على طول الزمان يجذب الاخلاط واما الادو د
تستفرغ الدم من البدن لقوة جذبها له من العروق المتصلة بالمعدة والامعاء دون سائر الاخلاط ط
فهي ادوية قتالة لم يوجد استعمالها في شيء من الاشياء ولذلك سكت المتقدمون عن ذكرها في
كتب الطب لئلا يبلغ بها اشرار الناس الى قتل من يريدون قتله وقال جالينوس لي كتبه في بلاد برافي+
نبوتيه وانا صبي وسمعت بها عن رجل وجدته والذي ان ناوله الانسان اسهله اولا الدم ثم قتله + paracomnia
يعرف لك فعلمت ان به خلفا كثيرا على هذا المثال بحثت عنه باستقصاء فوجدت المستعمل له من
اتاه الى الحاكم فاستقصى عليه الحاكم واراد ان يكون قتله له فقط بل العبرة ان كان اوقعه على ذلك
الدواء او تعلمه منه . فزعم انه لم يعرفه اياه انسان لكنه هو وجده في بعض الاوقات كبير خنزير
ليصرفه الى بعض الكهوف فخرج بطنه للخلا فوضعها على تلك الحشيشة فلما قام واحد

ونثر الحبر على تلك الحشيشة رشح دم فرسال من جميع الحبر محروس من ذلك على تلك
الحشيشة بجزء الزئم واسقا منها لبعض من لقيه ليمتحنها فلما وجدها على ما قد ذكر استعملها
له للشر منذ ذلك الوقت وانه قد قتل به خلقا كثيرا فلما سمع السلطان قوله وكان فهما قال
في وصف ذلك السم انه ينبت في كل موضع تكثر فيه امراض تسر عيناه ونساق الى القتل كيما
لا ينتشر النبات في طريقه لاحد فيعرفها وقال في ابن معرفة الفضة فقد توجد ان الادوية كثيرة
فوتها معرفة القوة اعني جزء الزئم منذ اول الامر الا انه يجب الامساك عن ذكرها كما يجب ايضا
الامساك عن ادويته فتاله على جميع من له عقل وذلك انه قد كان قوم يتخرصون بقول في امثال
معرفة الادوية القتالة الا انه لا يوجد احد ممن له عقل يخرج انسانا من مقاوي

قال المؤلف ٥ واذ قد بلغنا الى ما اردنا من قوى الادوية المسهلة فيجب علينا
ان نعلم كيفية اخذها ونقدم ما ينبغي ان نقدم قبل اخذها وما يجب التزامه بعد اخذها. فاقول
انه ينبغي لمن قصد شرب دوا مسهل ان يقوم غذاه قبل اخذه بيومين او ثلاثة ويقال منه ايضا
والمكون حبرا ونقص فيه الى ما يلين الطبيعة لسهوله وتحرزه على حسب المستعمل للدوا
في مزاجه والاخلاط الغالبة عليه ويجتنب الجماع قبل شرب الدوا بثلاثة ايام او اربعة والتعب
والنصب والبردخل الحمام في كل يوم ان كان الزمان حريفا ويستعمل صب الماء الفاتر على بدنه
والجلوس فيه والتمدد في الحمام مرة اطول من عادته قليلا حتى ترق الاخلاط وتنحل المسام
فيجد الدوا سبيلا الى اخراج الخلط المقصود دون عنف على الطبيعة فان كان الفصل شتا
فليعمل فيه مثل ذلك وان كان صيفا فليقرب الحمام البتة وان كان ربيعا فليتحرز فيه اقل
من زمنه الخريف قليلا ويشرب ايضا في جميع الفصول خلا الصيف الاشربة الملطفة كشراب
الافسنتين والسكنجبين وطبيخ الاصول وشراب الاذخر ونحوها على حسب الخلط المقصود
اليه لانا ان قصدنا اخراج خلط غليظ اخذنا قبل شرب الدوا المسهل ان نقدم من الادوية ما
تلطف الفضول ويرققها ويفتح سدد البدن اكثر مما يحتاج اليه متى قصدنا اخراج خلط
لطيف على هذا المثال اعمل فيما بينهما فان كانت الفضول في البدن كثيرة فجه فليقدم
هذا التدبير قبل شرب الدوا المسهل بايام كثيرة على حسب فجاجة الاخلاط وغلظها ليلطف
غلظ تلك الفضول ويحل لزوجتها ويتسع المسام على خروجها فتخرج الاخلاط بسهوله

وليس يجوز ذلك طريقا للدوا المسهل وعونا له ولاسيما ان كان الدوا محتاجا الى اخراج ذلك
الخلط وقد قال ابقراط في كتاب الفصول كل بدن تريد تنقيته فينبغي ان تجعل ما تريد اخراجه جه
منه يجري بسهولة . قال المؤلف قد اقتصرنا على جميع ما قلناه في هذا المعنى ومن لم تكن
اخلاطه بدنه غليظة ولا بنه ولا لزجة فيقتنع من التدبير قبل شربه الدوا المسهل لما تقدم من
تدبير الحمام وصب الماء الفاتر على البدن وتليين الطبيعة بالاغذية الملطفة فقط وبالجملة فيجب
ان يدبر من اختار الاخراج خلط حار يابس بالتدبير المرطب المبرد وبالضد بضده وما بينهما
على حسب ذلك ويجب ايضا لشارب الدوا ان يمتنع اخذه في وقت اهتمامه واغتمامه والفكرة القوية
لكي يحتاج الى استخراج معانيها من فنون العلم ولا عند الفرح الشديد والزيادات لكثير من الاطباء
يقولون انه يجب ان يستعمل الدوا المسهل عند الحركات الشديدة القوية من حركات النفس
كانت او من حركات البدن وينبغي ان يؤخر اخذ دوا كان من الادوية المسهلة على خلو من المعدة
لا على شدة الجوع ونكايته لانه ربما اجتذبته الاوراد المستعملة لطلب الغذا فيجري منها
مجرى الغذا فيبطل عمله بل يجب ان يؤخر بعد تمام الهضم والمعدة خالية من الغذا والطبيعة .
في ذلك الوقت غير محتاجة الى استمراء غذا وليمتنع عند ابتداء عمله من النوم ان كان الدوا
ضعيفا حتى يستولي حركة الدوا وليمتنع ايضا من الفكرة والاشتغال بالكتابة والقراءة
ولعب الشطرنج ومحادثة من يجالسه ونحو هذه الاشيا ويجب ان يشرب على الدوا المسهل ان كان ي
حبا او معجونا ماء حارا فان ذلك يعين الدوا على فعله ويحلل الثفل ويحدره من المعدة سريعا
وان كان من الطبائخ والنقوعات فليشرب بعقبه ماء حارا لا سيما ان كان على هذه الصفة من الادوية
المسهلة فهي سريعة الانحدار من المعدة لا سيما ان شرب حارة فالحرارة اسرع حتى ربما
انحدرت قبل تمام عملها فان ظهر في الدوا قوة وتوقعت الزيادة في الاسهال فينبغي ان ترقد
رقادا يسيرا كي تنكسر حدته فاذا بدا بالعمل فليمتنع من النوم حتى يستولي فعل الدوا
وكذلك ليمتنع من كل شراب وطعام ما دام يجد للدوا طعما في الحشا او تاثيرا في المعدة
والمعا فان وجد المستعمل للدوا غثيانا وحركة في المعدة وتهوعا فليمصص الرمان المز
او التفاح المز او عساليج الكرم ويستعمل شم البصل ولياكل منه قليلا بالخل وتربط اسفل
رجليه بالملح والزيت في الماء الحار فان ذلك يجتذب قوة الدوا الى اسفل فان احس بمغص من قبل بامغاص

الرواسب فيشرب الماء الحار بالعسل او السمن والعسل ويكمد البطن بالماء الحار ويمرخ بالدهن اللطيف
ويديم الحركة والمشي غير العنيف فان متى كانت الامغاص في الامعاء العالية وان كانت امغاص
في الامعاء السفلية فليحقن بالحقن الرطبة السيالة لكي لا ترغ معها المولعة من اللغابيات ولماء دهن
ونحوها فان كان مع المغص قراقر ورياح فليجعل في الحقن شيء من الشراب وليس يجب ان تقصر
الى اسهال الطبيعة البتة مع المغص الا ان ضعفت القوة بل يجب ان يستعمل الاشياء المفرطة ويحفظ
ايضا متى امتنع الرواسب من العمل ان يزاد ذواتا لا ان ذلك غررا ويتوقع من ذلك اضطراب طبائع لم
يحتاج الى اخراجها بسبب مشاركة الرواان وقوة كل واحد منهما بصاحبه فحسن من اجل ذلك
امران رديه لا ان ابطا الرواسب لعلة تقع فليطلب التدبير ان كان ابطاؤه في المعدة وكم لبث ذلك
ان يوجد طعم الرواسب في الحشا بشرب الماء الحار بالعسل او الجلاب او ماء حار مع قليل ملح او يستعمل
اطلا سفرجله او من رمانه مزا او كمثرا فان كان الا ابطاء في الامعاء فيعرف ذلك من عدم طعم
الرواسب في الحشا وبحر حركة في الامعاء فيجب ان تقوى بشرب شراب النعنع المحلول فيه لب خيار شنبر
او نقيع الاجاص او نقيع العناب مع بعض الاشياء اللطاف. ويجب لمن شرب الرواسب المسهل ان يقلل
غذاه بعد شربه له مرة من ثلاثة ايام او اربعة ويحتمي من كل غذا ردي الغائلة ويقلل من شرب
الشراب ويجتنب من شرب الاشربة غير الموافقة ويجتنب ايضا الجماع وجميع الحركات المذكورة
انفا وليكن طعامه يوم قطع الرواسب ان كان محرورا واخرج المرة الصفرا حصرميه او سماقيه
ونحوهما من لحم كبش فتي او خروف او جدي او من لحم حيوان صغير جيد الطبيعة وليقلل منه
في ذلك اليوم بسبب ضعف الطبيعة فيه عن الهضم والبرير فيه قليلا قليلا مرة من ثلاثة ايام
كما ذكرنا حتى ينتهي الى عادته لكي تقل الفضول في بدنه وان كان الرواسب المستعمل لاخراج الاخلاط
الغليظة فليكن غذاؤه في ذلك اليوم الدجاج المعمولة بقليل من الابازير والكزبرة والبصل
القليل ايضا والزيرباجات المتخذة من اللحم السمين ونحوها وينبغي ايضا ان يستعمل من الشراب
بعد الرواسب المسهل ان كان محرورا وقصد بالرواسب اخراج المرة الصفرا وكان اسهاله متوسطا
بزر قطونا مغسولا بماء بارد قدر ثلاثة دراهم او اربعة مع اوقيتين جلاب لئلا تعلق بقايا الفضول
فينحدر بها فان كان الاسهال كثيرا فليشرب بعده بزر قطونا محمصا بالماء البارد وليشرب رب
السفرجل او رب الرمان او رب الريحان او نحوها فان كان المستعمل للرواسب بارد المزاج وقصد به

إخراج البلغم فإن توسط إسهاله فليشرب ماء العسل وبزر الكرفس بالماء الحار والزيت أو دهن الشيرج
فإن كان الإسهال كثيرا فليشرب ماء العسل المربى ببعض الأدوية اللطيفة وليشرب شرابا ممزوجا
فإن كان مزاج المستعمل للدواء باردا يابسا وقصد به إخراج المرار الأسود وكان إسهاله كثيرا
فليشرب بعده شرابا كثيرا ممزوجا أو يشرب ماء العسل فاترا وفيه مع درهمين من بزر الحبق
القرنفلي أو الأترجي وإن كان الإسهال الطبيعي فليشرب بعده ماء الجبن باردا أو ماء باردا على قدر ما
يريد من القوة والضعف وإذا قصر عمل الدواء ولم يبلغ المراد منه من إخراج ما قصد إخراجه
فليكرر شربه ثانيا بعد سبعة أيام أو خمسة أو أكثر قليلا وليكن ليعمل فعله ليخرج به
ما امتنع خروجه بالدواء الأول ويخرج أيضا ما بقي في البدن من الفضول وقد يكتفى بدخول
بدخول الحمام مرارا بعد شرب الدواء إذا لم يبلغ الغاية والنهاية عوضا وإثنائه ۝

القول في العلة التي دعت الأوائل إلى إبدال العقاقير وكيف حتى بلغوا إلى معرفة ذلك قال المؤلف

لم ترغب الأوائل إلى إبدال العقاقير إلا لضرورة عدم بعضها في بعض البلدان أو عدم الكثير منها
في زمان دون زمان أو فساد ما في نفسها لكنه بفساد ما في نفسها إما رطبا وجزئيا عفنا فقد ثبت
قوته وفسد مزاجه أما رطبه فقدم ممتنع وأما يابسه فقد استخرجت قوته في الماء بالطبخ مثل ما
يصنع كثيرا بالراوند الصيني وبكثير من الأدوية وذلك أن من الناس من يستخرج قواها في الماء
بالطبخ ويستعمل طبيخها في الأشربة والمعجونات ويبيعون أجرامها فتلك لا ما يبرى فيها
ويباع كثير منها امتحانها داخل الجزول في مواضع كثيرة وأما يابسه فقد غطس في البحر وغسله الماء
المالح فتذهب قوته الطبيعية وتكتسب قوة عرضية من الماء المالح فعند عدمه تدعو
الضرورة بسببها إلى الإبدال منها ولولا ذلك لتوقف العلاج وتعطلت النسخ وقد ذكر جالينوس
أنه طلب بالإسكندرية سراج القطرب لامرأة فراح يبغت ولم يصبه في ذلك الموضع فلولا أنه
استعمل الزجاج من ساعته بدلا منه لكانت المرأة قد هلكت فكان هذا من أعظم الأسباب إلى أن يذكر
إبدال كثير من الأدوية التي تكثر الحاجة إلى استعمالها في علاج الأمراض وتدعو الضرورة إلى
تصريفها في دفع الأعراض ۝ **قال المؤلف** إن الأوائل لما دعتهم الضرورة إلى إبدال العقاقير
للوجوه المذكورة إنما نظروا إلى الأدوية المفردة فوجدوها متعلقة من الأربع كيفيات

أعني الحرارة والبرودة والرطوبة واليبوسة وأن ليس لواحد منها بمجرده قوام دونها فقالوا
إن الدواء إذا عدم جعلنا عوضه دواء ثانيا في تلك الطبيعة بعينها من الحرارة أو البرودة أو
الرطوبة أو اليبوسة في تلك الدرجة بعينها أيضا فلما أنعموا النظر وأجمعوا الفكر رأوا
أن هذه القسمة غير صحيحة لأن كثيرا من الأدوية قد يكون في درجة ما من الحرارة أو البرودة أو
الرطوبة أو اليبوسة وكل واحد منها يخالف صاحبه في أعماله من قبل خواصها الكائنة فيها
ولولا ذلك لكان جميع الأشياء الحارة مثل حرارة التربد يسهل البلغم وليس الأمر كذلك لأنا قد نجد
السقمونيا في حرارة التربد وفي يبسها أيضا وهي تسهل المرة الصفراء فلما وجدوا فيهما هذا
الخلاف وطبيعتهما واحدة علموا أن فعلهما لخاصة في جواهرهما ولو كانت الأدوية إنما تفعل
بطبائعها دون خواصها التي تخفى عن العقل ولا توجد في الوهم لكان كل دواء حار في الدرجة الأولى
بدلا من دواء في تلك الدرجة بعينها من الحرارة وسائر الكيفيات على هذه الصفة فلما ثبتت في
الأدوية هذه الدلائل التي فعلها بخواص في جواهرها لا بطبيعتها فقط تلطف الأوائل في استخراج
الأبدال وذلك أنهم جعلوا الكثير من الأدوية عوضا من دواء واحد وزادوا في الأوزان ونقصوا
منها حتى يقوم مقامه وتوجد الخاصية التي في ذلك العقير الواحد كما فعل بديغورش في العا
الرند خاصته النفع من الفزع العارض للصبيان إذا علق عليهم فجعل بدلا منه ليؤدي عن خاصته
قشور الرمان وفرو السمور وعظام سوق الغربان فإن هذه الثلاثة إذا اجتمعت وفعل بها
ما يفعل بالفاوانيا أدت عن خاصته وكذلك البلاذر فإن من خاصيته إذهاب النسيان وتقوية
الذهن فإن جعل بدله إذا عدم وزنه خمس دراهم بندق ووزنه درهم بلسان وسدس وزنه نفط أبيض
قامت مقامه فعلى هذا المعنى قصد المتقدمون إلى أبدال الأدوية فإن وجدوا بدلا للدواء الذي
يرمون بدله من دواء واحد مثل وزنه بالسوا من دواء آخر كان ذلك بلوغ المطلوب ونهاية المعنى
على ما نجده في السقمونيا التي من خاصته إسهال المرة الصفراء ويجرد به المعدة ونجعل البدل
منها إذا عدمت وزنها لبن الشبرم لأنه يسهل الماء الأصفر والمرة الصفراء بقوة ومؤذي للمعدة أيضا
وكذلك قثاء الحمار يفعل قريبا من فعل السقمونيا ولكنه ليس يبلغ مبلغها إلا أن نجعل بدل
درهم سقمونيا وزن درهمين من عصارة قثاء الحمار أقل ذلك وسطه بدل الدرهم كان أمثاله
وما كان من الأدوية تفعل بطبائعها فقط جعل بدلها بالسوا ما كان في تلك الطبيعة نفسها

وفي تلك الدرجة بعينها من الحرارة والبرودة والرطوبة واليبوسة وأكثر ما يصيب ذلك
في ردع مادة او تصليب عضو او تغير مزاج الى آخر الكيفيات او جذب او تحليل او نحوهما
اعلم ان من الادوية ادوية جاذبة ٥ مثال السكطرامشير والدافسيا وشقائق النعمان
وبزر مرو والزبل والزفت والحلتيت والسكبينج واصل النرجس وعلك الانباط
وخثى البقر والفودنج وورق الكرنب وورق السوسن والاذن واغصان الخوخ و
الرمل والفراسيون والمرزنجوش وزهر الملح والسلق والقنة
والسمن والصابون والثوم كلها والعظام المحرقة ونحو هذه فاذا كان الطبيب لبيبا
مميزا عارفا بقوى الادوية المفردة نقل بعض هذه الادوية عن بعض اذا اعوزت في نسخة
ما مخصوصة بالجذب خاصة وان كانت تختلف الكيفيات منها في الدرجات وله النظر
في البدل منها بالزيادة والنقصان على حسب ذلك الدواء المبدل منه في القوة والضعف وعلى
حسب مزاج المستعمل له ٥ ومن الادوية ادوية قابضة مثال الزيتون البري
وحي العالم والاذخر والطرثوث والكرس والصبر وعجم الزبيب والخشخاش
والزعفران والحبة الخضراء والبنج والتمر وقشر البيض المشوي والزاج الجامد
والسعتري وعسالج الكرم والبلوط وانفحة الارنب والقمح المحرق والعوسج
ونحو هذه من الادوية المعروفة بالقبض ومفردة ايضا ادوية يجب للطبيب ان
ونقص في نسخة من النسخ ولا يعول فيها على درج الدواء متى فقد بذلك الدواء القابض
فاذا عدم في نسخة من النسخ المخصوصة بالقبض بعض هذه الادوية جعل العوض عنها ما وجد
ممكنا منها في ذلك الوقت وفي مثل هذه الادوية تظهر مباعدة الكيفيات لكنها كلها
من شأنها القبض والذي يجب للطبيب ايضا في مثل هذا ان ينظر الى بدن المستعمل لذلك الدواء
المركب من هذه الادوية هل حاد الى آخر الكيفيات ام لا فاذا ثبت عنده ذلك وعدم من
من تلك النسخة دواء ما بدله من جملة هذه واشباهها دواء يوافق ذلك المزاج الذي صار اليه
المستعمل للدواء فيكون المبدل منه في اكثر الامر اذا جرى على هذا القياس احسن من الدواء المذكور
في النسخة بعينها ٥ ومن الادوية ايضا ادوية مقيئة تدعو الضرورة
اليها في بعض الاوقات ليقصر بها التقيئ ٥ مثل الزرنيخ والشكاعى والزراريج

ولب الارز والخرنوب . ونحوها ه ومنها ادوية تنفع من زيادة اللحم مثل
اصل الحنظل واصل اللفاح الرطب ودهن قثا الحمار . وقشور النحاس والنشادر
والزنجار . ونحوها ه ومنها ايضا ادوية تدمل وتختم الجراحات مثل
النحاس المحرق المغسول والعفص . وقشور الرمان اليابسه . وحب الرمان والمرداسنج
والرصاص المحرق والاثمد المحرق . واسفيداج الرصاص . والنشادر والقلقطار المحرق
وقشور النحاس وقشور الجوز . والزنجار والقوره المحرقه . فهذه كلها تدمل
وتختم لا كنها تختلف في فعلها لان منها ما يفعل بلذع ومنها ما يفعل بلا لذع فيجب للطبيب
ايضا ان يتحرى في هذا الموضع متى اراد البدل لان الدوا الذي بلذع يحتاج الا يستعمل في بدن
حساس البنيه والدوا الذي لا لذع معه يقصر به البدن الحساس ه ومن الادوية ايضا
ادوية مفرحة لظاهر البدن . مثل اصل السلق والثوم وحب الما والخردل والزبل ه
وزبل الحمام وزهر النحاس وعاقرقرحا والحلتيت ولحا اصل الكبر والشونيز ه ه ه
ومن الادوية محللة للبدن مفتحة للاورام مثل البابونج والزيت العتيق
وشقائق النعمان والبصل والثوم ومرارة البقر ودهن السوسن والاقحوان ه
ومنها ادوية ايضا محلله للبدن مثل البابونج والزيت العتيق والخطمي
والفسط والطحرر . واصل الحنظل والبورق والشيح الارمني والملوخيه و
البرنطونا . ولحا الصنوبر وعرق الما ه ومن الادوية ايضا ادوية مقويه للاعضا
مثل السليخه . والعفص والمصطكي . والاسطوخودوس . والمر . والصبر ونحو هذه
ومن الادوية ايضا ادوية منضجة للمرة مثل الما الفاتر . او الزيت الممزوج
بالما الفاتر وحسو الحنطه والنشا وشحم الخنزير وشحم العجل والسمن والكثيرا
والزبيب الرطب والسمسم والكرنب ونحو هذه ه ومنها ايضا ادوية ملينه مثل
شحم الماعز وشحم الاوز وشحم الدجاج وشحم الثيران وشحم الجواميس وشحم الايل ه
والوشق والمايعه والعنبه والمقل ودهن قثا الحمار واصل الحنظل ودهن السوسن
وورق الخطمي والمصطكي . وعلك البطم وشقائق النعمان والجاوشير والسمن
والزبد والزوفا . ونحو هذه ه ومنها ايضا ادوية منفية لسطح البدن

ودهن النرجس والياسمين

ومفتحة وغسالة لوسخ الجراح ووسخ البدن كله مثل الكرسنة والشعير والباقلى
والترمس وبعر الماعز المحرق وماية اللبن واللوز المر واللوز الحلو وبزر اللوف
وشقائق النعمان • وورق لسان الحمل اليابس والزراوند وحب الراس واصل الاقاقيا
وبزر السرمق وعصارة الافسنتين والخربق الابيض والخربق الاسود والبسفايج
والحصرم والخردل البري وعلك الانباط والمصطكى والسكبينج
واصل الحنظل والسلق واليتوع والكمافيطوس وقرن الايل المحرق
ومرار ... المحرق ودقيق اصل النرجس والكثيرا وبياض البيض ، ومقدار الادوية كلها
وامثالها ... وتغسل وتفتح لا كيما تختلف في القوة والضعف فلذلك يجب متى قصرنا
البدل من واحد منها اذا عدم ان ننظر الذي في الدوا والمعروف مثل معروف من الادوية القوية
في ذلك المعنى لان فان البعيد من القوة جعلنا عوضه ما قارنه وبالضد وجعل الاصل
من المستعمل للدوا كما ذكرنا قبل ، ومنها ادوية تولد المني وتهيج شهوة الجماع
والباه مثل الحمص والباقلى والصنوبر والتين والجرجير والهليون وخصى الثعلب
والسقنقور والخولنجان والسنة العصافير والزنجبيل والشقاقل وبالجملة فان
الاغذية كل كثير الغذا والريح ومن الادوية كل مسخن مرطب ، ومنها ايضا ادوية
قاطعة للمني مثل القثا والخيار والبقلة اليمانية والبقلة الحمقا والسرمق والقرع
والبطيخ لا سيما الفلسطيني والتوت والكبر والجمار والسذاب والفلفل والفنجنكشت
وبالجملة كل ما يبس او يبرد او يرطب ، ومنها ادوية تسود الشعر مثل
اللاذن والمر وعصارة الاس والحمرة الجبلية ودهن الفستق والكرنب والزوفا الرطب
وسحالة النحاس وسحالة الحديد وشقائق النعمان وقشور الباقلى الاخضر المعفن في الزبل
والاقاقيا وقشور الجوز الاخضر المعفن في الزبل والعفص المحرق بالادوية والجلنوص
ونحوها ، ومنها ايضا ادوية منبتة لشعر الحاجبين ومسودة له مثل الصمغ
والاقاقيا والعفص والسماق وما طبخ الحنا وحب الاس والتوت وورق الكرم
وورق التين وحب شجر البلوط وقشور الجوز الاعلى وشقائق النعمان ونحوها
ومنها ايضا ادوية محمرة للشعر مثل الكلس والزرنيخ والارنب البحري

ولبن كلبة اول ما ينتج وقشور البلاقطي والقطران والزيت العتيق وصمغ الكرم
والبورق والقلقشورا ونحوها ❊ قال مسيح بن حكم بعمل الحيوان يسمى لاميران وهي دابة
تدخل في النار ولا تحترق فيطبخ بالزيت ويدهن بذلك الزيت الشعر فانه يحمره ❊ ❊
ومن الادوية ايضا ادوية لطيفة في مزاجها مثل الشيح الارمني المحرق
والقنجنكشت وبقلة اذخر والوج والحماما واصل السوسن والزراوند ولسان الحمل
واللوف والاسارون والزيت العتيق والعفص والفربيون والحمير والحنتيت وعلك
الانباط والفوذنج البري والفوذنج النهري وقصب الذريرة والفراسيون والشليخة
والجاورس والقطران والقسط والصمغ والمسك والمصطكي والشونيز والبلسان
والشراب والبسبايج والشطبيج والثوم والتين اليابس والبورق والزرنيخ الاصفر
المحرق والافسنتين والرماد والنورة وزهر الملح والحلزون المحرق والكرنب
والقلقطار والسنبل والزاج والزنجار وزهر النحاس والنشادر والزرنيخ الاحمر
وشحم الاسد وشحم النمر وشحم الضبع والحبرباذستر والمرزنجوش والقسط والنفط
القطران ونحو من ذلك ❊ قال المؤلف اما هذه الادوية فلم اجعلها هنا الا مقرونا بطبيعتها
في مزاجها فقط لا للوجود الذي عرض فيها القدم منها ومن اراد الابدال منها على حقيقة
ويقين فليطلبها في الجدول المعمول لها وهو الذي انا صانعه بعد فليدل على ذلك الله بعد
النظر الى مزاج المستعمل للدواء ❊ ومنها ايضا ادوية غليظة في مزاجها
مثل اصل لسان الحمل والجلنار وعجم الزبيب والرامك والقثا والخيار والبلوط واللعث
وما اشبهها ❊ ومنها ايضا ادوية ملطفة مرقية مثل البصل والثوم
والحرف والخردل والفلفل والعاقرقرحا والفوذنجان والجرجير والمقدونس والكرفس
الجبلي والكرفس البستاني والباذروج والبصل والكرنب والسلق والرازيانج والكر وبا
والسذاب وبزر السذاب والشبث والكمون والمصطكي والحبة الخضرا والزوفا
والانيسون والخردل البري والدارفلفل والفلفل الابيض والقاقلة والكبابة و
اشبهها ❊ وهذه الادوية ايضا لم اذكرها هنا الا على سبيل التقريب لما في الادوية
المرقية الملطفة ان شا الله تعالى ❊ ❊ ❊ ❊

تم جميع ما شرطناه ووعدنا به في صدر رسالة هذا الكتاب وبقي علينا الآن نبتدي بعمل
الجداول على ما ضمناه والله عز وجل اهل العون والناصر واليه ارغب في التوفيق
والتيسير بمنه

٣١

جبن فوة الامبرباريس شبيه بقوة الكمثرى ... فوة ...
تحرقها بالشوكة الجادة وهي شبيهة بشجر الكمثرى البري ٥ واما الاقاقيا فيعمل بعسل به
ذلك حتى تصفى الماء ثم تعمل منه اقراصا وقد تشوى على النار ويبقع عليه وقد يحرق في

[illegible]	[illegible]	تفسيرها باختلاف اللغات	الابدال	
امبرباريس	[illegible]	هو الشرشك وقيل هو الشرس بالشين المعجمة وهو البرباريس والانبرباريس وقيل انه اثوار ابو حنيفة هو الزرشك ويسمى بالفارسية الزرشك وهو اثرارة ٥ وبالبربرية ارغيس غير الام	[illegible]	hoc xiakantha
اقاقيا	[illegible]	هو رب القرظ بفتح القاف وبالظاء المعجمة والقرظ هو الشوكة المصرية لانها تنبت بمصر وهو سنط بالنوبيون	[illegible]	akacia ut akcia
اقحوان	[illegible]	يعرف بالعجمية غشولش وبعجمية سرقسطة بنلنيرة وهو صنفان احمر وابيض فالابيض يعرف اماربقول والاصفر امارنطون ابو حنيفة الواحدة اقحوانة وجمع الاقاحي بالتشديد والتخفيف ويقال الاقحوان والقحوان اذا القوا الالف واللام	[illegible]	يابونكار amaracino
[illegible]	[illegible]	قيل هو القرع الزنبق وقيل هو حب الزعرار ورايت حب القرعر هو حب الزعرار ويعرف بريانق وحبه احمر مدور خاصة النفع من المرة السوداء اصلاحه بالمصطكي اضراره بالقلب ... غير الام	[illegible]	arcteaucea thi dos. ldeit fabi na.
[illegible]	[illegible]	هو الحرشف والقرظ (?) وهو صنفان احدهما احسن واشد سوادا واغلظ ورق ويسمى هذا الصنف الوالية ناعرة ولقيرة العير الاسود والصنف الثاني يعرف بالعجمية ارتيفش اضراره بالكلى اصلاحه بالصمغ العربي ... غير الام	[illegible]	akalifi. lde ftorri ea
[illegible]	[illegible]	هو ثمرة الشجرة يسمى ورقها الانجران وصمغها الحلتيت واصلها المحروث ورايت الانجران ثمرة الحلتيت المنتن ويسمى مسفسطن ورايت في بعض الكتب الاسفيداج هو اصل الانجوان واصل الكاشم هو الاستغارة	[illegible]	ala ut laffa

احمرمنه ٥ والابيض صنفان منه ما ورقه شبيه بورق السرو وعليه الرائحة . الرتم يسهل لطافة
ولذلك يسهل الاجنة ٥ الانجرة في غاية من اللطافة وصحاح البيض والانجران له قوة لطيفة

العلل السيالة اذا اكل او شرب طبيخه غيره نعم لتستعمل في ادوية العين
بان يصب الماء وتصب الريح عليه وتابز العمل فررمز نواب في البول وفي الاجوان فقود
من قوى البابونج من تفتح وتحليل غيرانه

منافعها وخواصها ووجوه اشتعالها

لم يتفعا اذا شربت واذا اكل قطع الاسهال المزمن والرطوبات السائله من الرحم سيلانا مزمنا ويقطع العطش الكائن من الحر ونفود الكبد والمعده ومو جيد في الاضمده فاما اذا وضع على الاورام الحاره ٠ ويقال انه اذا الطخ به بطن الحبلى اسقط الجنين ٥

د فود الاقاقيا فانه مبرده ومي موافقه اذا وقعت في اخلاط ادويه العين وبواسير الحمره والنمله والراجس وقروح الفم وينفع من نتو العين ويقطع سيلان الرطوبات من الرحم وينفع من نتو المقعده والرحم ويعقل البطن ويسود الشعر

د اذا شرب بالسبانا مكنجبين وشي من ملح اسهل بلغما ومره سودا وينفع من كان به ربو واصحاب المره السودا واذا شرب بنانه دون زهره نفع من الحمى والربو ومن عليس النساء في طبيخه لصلابه الرحم وو الورم الحار العارض فيه فيبنبع من ذلك ومن تضمد به مع زهره للحمره والاورام ٭ الحاره

جـ جومره لطيف جرا وترهب تعفونه القروح الرديه الخبيثه لك فرتمكنت وطالت ومو ينفع القروح المسوده الوسخه اذا وضع عليها مع العسل ونرد الطمث اذا زاد كثيرا ويعسر الاجنه الاحيا ويخرج الاجنه الموتى واذا تضمد به نفى سواد الجلد ومن يتزحر به لاسقاط الاجنه ويحتمل الزلد ٭

ورق كل الصنعم اذا دق وتضمد به مع الملح ابرا القروح السرطانيه والقروح الوسخه والنوا العصب والخراجات والاورام العارضه في اصول الاذان ومن تضمد به مع الفيروطي الطحال الحاسي اذا دق الورق وصير في المتخرين قطع الرعاف ومن حتمل مع ادرار المرار ادرار الطمث واذا اخذ الورق ومو طري ووضع على الرحم الناتيه ردها وطبيخها مع المر يدر الطمث واذا اخذ مع السكنجبين نفع من الطحال ووجع الجنبين ٭

اذا اكل مع السكنجبين نفع من وجع قصبه الريه ونفع من الصوت المنقطع ومن يوكل بالخبز يدل الخزخير ومن يستخرج من الاعراق رطوبه بالرق والعصر ويخلط مع العسل ويتحنك له لورم اللهاه ويتغرغر به لورم اللوزتين فاذا تحسيت بيض نفع من السعال ومن تمضمض به لوجع الاسنان وباكل اللثات ومن تلقى الاستفراغ في الحل الحرث فيه جرافه ما يعالطف الاخلاط ويقطع السقطات ومو قاتل للشهوه مغم على ليعض الاعزبه

ومنه كره الرائحه وفي الانف فوه لقشرها حشكر لبته النار وان سرد ابال ويسبلها يدرع ما يلقاه من اعضاء البدن وحامضها مهيجان للجماع اذا اكلت بالبصل وتضر بالمعده والكرم

نوار السوسن هو المستعمل في الادهان وهو نافع من اوجاع العصب من البلغم ...
الابيرسا ... درهم الى اربعة دراهم بعد غسل وله رغبة الى البياض وذكر ابو جريج ان الاسفتين هو

[illegible]	الطبائع والدرج	تفسير معانيه باختلاف اللغات ؂	بدله والوزن
ايرسا	حار يابس في الاولى	هو السوسن الاسمانجوني ويقال له بالعجمية الليلية ولزهر هذا النبات الوان مختلفة فمنها ابيض وصفرة وفرفيرية فمن اجل اختلاف هذه الالوان سمي بهذا الاسم لان ايرسا هو القوس قزح ويعرف بالبربرية تافروت ويعرف بسوسن الالوان ؂	بدله سوسن ...
اورسيسا	حار يابس في الثانية	هو السوسن الابيض ومنه منه الربعي والبري هو اشريا	[illegible]
اذخر	حار يابس في ...	هو حب احمر مدور يشبه نور الجلبان وقال فيه ابن الجزار هو حب صغير منقط بسواد وبياض وقوم من الاطباء يصرفون الشونيز مكانه وهو الطاليقه بالعجمية وقوم يعرفونه بالبربرية وهو الابرين	نصف وزنه ... وزنه ...
اسفاقس	حار يابس في ...	هو بالعجمية شالبية له ورق شبيه بورق السفرجل الا انه اطول واقل عرضا عن ابن وافد وهو الناعمة ؂	نصف وزنه ...
افسنتين	حار يابس في ...	هو بالعجمية اسنانسه والشنانسه ويقال له ايضا بربه بطره وهو الشوب الرومي وهو الشيح الرومي وهو العنكس وهو الطباج ؂ اضراره بالمعدة اصلاحه بالانيسون من غير ... ؂	... وزنه ...
اراطل	...	هو بالفارسية الحرمار وهو نوع من الطرما ويسمى الغيرة ويعرف بالنصار بسبب الاوابد التي تخرجه ... شجرة الحرمل ... نصار	وزنه ...

irig gladiola

crinal dest lilio. ambrosia idest archimisia:-

Lilisfaco idest saluia:-

apsinthio idest aseño

carua

المخلوف من سطرس الكنفة الفاصة فيه ... واما ... قوة الحرارة فيها اقوى وورقه وزهره
اصغر من ورق ... انواع الافسنتين وزهرها ... وله رائحة عطرة ضعيفة شبيهة بالطرما
ابن عمران الا انه نوع من الطرما وقوتها ؂

المتولد من البلغم وينفع جميع اوجاع الرحم واذا احتقن به قرحة نفعت ودهن الران(؟) وابراء الاسعاس(؟)
ازاله حسوه(؟) لبسرة من خشونة الثياب لكن لم تعرف الكشوف(؟) الروبي وسوكان انواع عسره(؟)
انواع الافسنتين لا تخلوا كلها من كيفيتين وقوتين

منافعها وخواصها ووجوه استعمالها

اذا طبخ من اصله وزن مثقال وشرب بماء حار بالعسل سكن المغص العارض من البلغم واذا طبخ بدهن الورد ووضع على القروح جففها. واذا تضمد به الراس مع الخل ودهن ورد نفع من الصرع واذا اسلق وضمد به الراس مع الخل فعل مثل ذلك واذا اسلق وضمد به الخنازير والاورام الصلبه لينها ونفع القروح اذا ذر عليها او حمل بالعسل

اذا شرب بالخل نفع من نهش الهوام ونفع للسعال وينفع من اوجاع العصب العارض من البلغم ورطوبة الصدر وينفع من اوجاع الرحم بالخاصه واذا شرب بالشراب ادر الطمث واصله يفعل ذلك واذا احتمل به بطبيخه الشا(؟) نفع من اوجاع الرحم واذا احتمل احدر الجنين واصله يورث العمى. والحاجه ان يشرب بالماء والعسل المطبوخ ويسهل الماء الاصفر والصفرا والشربة منه من نصف الى ثلاثة مثاقيل ومن الاشياء الجوده(؟) كذلك ودهنه نافع من وجع العصب المتولد

هو مسهل للطبيعه يخرج الديدان وحب القرع وينفع فضول البلغم من الامعاء

اذا شرب طبيخ ورقه واغصانه ادر الطمث والبول ويخرج الجنين وينفع من الخراجات ويقطع الريح وينفع القروح الخبيثه واذا استنجي بطبيخه سكن الحكة العارضه للفروج من الزحير والانتشار(؟) ويسود الشعر

لتنقية الفضول المرية الكائنه في المعدة والبطن ويدر البول واذا شرب من مائه وعصارته نفع من اليرقان وينفع من الفهم(؟) واذا احتمل ادر الطمث واذا شرب بالخل وافق الاختناق العارض من الفطر ومن السم وان تضمد به الخاصره والمعدة والكبد للاوجاع المزمنه ويبرد من المرة السوداء لا سيما مع الافيثمون والشربه منه من خمسة دراهم الى سبعة اذا كان منقوعا

ينفع من ماكل الاسنان ويردع البله(؟) المتحلبه الى الاجسام وينزل اللحم الزائد ونعم حسه(؟) انه اذا طبخ اطراف الشجرة بشراب او بخل وشرب نفع من وجع الكبد منفعه عظيمه ويلين ورمها ومن لعقاد(؟) ذلك فلوب اطراف شجرتها وتنفع من وجع الاسنان

واحسنها للكبد والمعدة ما جرى به عنبر الزروق(؟) فضا لحا(؟) ومرارة يسيرة واللون ... الوحشيه
شجرة الاثل طوال في السماء ومنه تصنع القطاع والجفانز(؟) ورماد هذه الشجرة غسالة

وزعم قوم من الاطباء ان الصنف اللازوردي من انا غاليس اذا
للبس الوجعة سكن وجعها د . من اكليل الملك ما لونه الى لون الزعفران طيب الرائحة
ويحلل جـ طعم للاشنة قابض باعتدال وهو نافع الاول قوة لليبس بارده ... برودة قوته

ابدال الادوية	تفسير ما اختلف من اللغات	الدرجة	الاسم	
[illegible]	هي حشيشة الحيلق وبالعجمية الفردبالة والشنتبلة وهما صنفان ذكر وانثى فالذكر هو الشنتالة والانثى هو الفردبالة واللازوردي هو الانثى والاحمر هو الذكر	حار يابس في ٢	اناغاليس	Anagalus
[illegible]	قيل هو شجرة الحب وبالعجمية القرقلية وقيل هو القرط الزهراوي ليس القرقلية كان بينهما فرق لان اكليل الملك هو القرط واحاليله املس واكليل القرقلية خشن متلزقه ويقال له مليلوطس وهو نبات منتشر	حار يابس في ١	اكليل الملك	Mellilotu وهو حلبة برية
[illegible]	هي شيب العجوز وهي التي تصير على شجر البلوط والجوز والشربين واجود ما كان موجودا على الشربين الجبلي وكان طيب الرائحة ابيضا . ما اضعفها النفع من البلغم والسوداء اقراره بالمغا اضاحها بلاانيمون ... بغير الانام ٥	حار يابس في ١	اشنة	Urion:
[illegible]	هو الكبر وهو القبار ويسمى بالرومية القبوس ويعرفه العامة الكبار بالكاف والالف . ويعرف اصف بالام	حار يابس في ٢	اصف	Caparis:
[illegible]	هو الحرير ان ما سويه اذا نسج دود الحرير على نفسه ولم عشا ودود بان نفسه وخرج منه كان منه الابريسم والقز وان ترك في الشمس حتى يموت كان منه الحرير وهو الخام ٥	حار يابس في ١	ابريسم	Sirico; Metaxi:
[illegible]	هو الانسون وهو الحبة الحلوة وهو الرازيانج الرومي ۞ ومن عدم الانسون اقراره بالمغا اضاحه بالرازيانج بزره	حار يابس في ٢	انيسون	Aniso

مركب من طعوم ثلاثة مرارة وحرافة وعفوصة والمرارة والحرافة فيه اكثر والعفوصة ۞
اقل او ... ولمضغه نفع من وجع الاسنان ۞ بعض الاطباء الحرير حار ما كان منه حريث
كبير لخفة في الرائحة والنفع ما في الارات ... جـ ۞

زهره ويصبغ الريق بلون زهره احمر زاد فيها واذا استعط بعصارته في الشق ومنه شي شبيه بالحلبه
حقيق الحومعر الحاربيه اكثر من البارد وفي طبعه قبض وقوه بل في فرسه من العتود
وقوتها الثانيه قوه محلله مليّنه حب الاصف

منافعها وخواصها ووجود استعمالها .
فوتها الاول قوه تسخن قليلا وتجفف بغير لذع والثانيه قوه تجلوا كالبليغا وتجرب والثالثه قوه تخرج السل من نظر اللحم وعصارتها تنفع ما في الدماغ وتخرجه من المنخرين وتزكن الحاجات ولمسكان انتشار القروح الخبيثه في البدن واذا تغرغر بعصارته نقى الراس من البلغم ومن يستعط به للزكام واذا شرب بشراب نفع من نهشه الافاعي ومن وجع الكبد والكلى ٥
حشيش الكليل الملك قابض ملين الاورام الحاره ولاسيما الاورام العارضه في العين والرحم والمقعده والانثيين اذا طبخ بالمبختج وتضمد به وربما خلط معه صفره بيض او دقيق الحلبه او دقيق بزر الكتان واذا استعمل وحده شفى القروح الشهديه او استعمل بالعفص والشراب واذا شرب بالشراب سكن وجع المعده ٥
د يصلح لاوجاع الرحم اذا طبخ وجلس في مائها وهي نافعه اذا وقعت في اخلاط الدهن والادهان الى تحلل الاعيا ومن يقع في اخلاط دهن البان وسائر الادهان واذا انقعت في شراب ايام ذلك الشراب لونها عونها ونفعت المعده وطيبها واذا معبت ليخ البطن والقي ٥
هـ وتحلل قطاع منقي للرطوبات الزائده في المعده نعم لسدد الكبد ويحلله لحسا الطحال وعلته مدر للبول والطمث واقوى من الرواح اصله ويعده البشر ولحب ثم الورق والزهر واذا شرب لعسل وماء حار نفع من وجع النفس ولاورام ومن تضمد به الطحال برفق والشمع للورم العارض فيه ومن تحلل الخنازير ولاورام الصلبه
في الحرير تقويه للقلب وتصفيه لدمه وموجب للخفقان اذا استعمل في دوا المشي وبعض الاطبا يحرقه ليسهل سحقه وتزداد لطيبه وبعضهم لا يرى ذلك لئلا تضعف قوته ويعرضه قرصا رقيقا وسحق مع اللولو والكهربا والبسرحي يسحق وبعضهم يشرح قوه في الماء بالطبخ ولسقاية للماء الادويه ٥
ف وله بالجمله سخنه مييسه وهي تنفش الرياح عن البدن وتسكن الوجع وتحلله مدره للبول والعرق مزيله للفضول ونافع دوا السموم من الهوام وتقطع سيلان الرطوبات الى لونها البيض من الرحم وتدر البول واللبن وتهضم سهوه الجماع وقال الله حار بالمري في الدرجه الثالثه

افلو واجعها ومن الرصاص محلله للاورام الحاسيه الباطنه والظاهره واذا طبخ بالماء بالاعتدال لطيب حسن للقلب مقوي لجرمه في احود الاشيا من

الاسطوخودوس حريف الطعم مع مرارة يسيرة ح جوهره مركب من جوهر [illegible]
مرا العود ملس الاغاريقون صنفان احدهما يسمى الانثى والاخر يسمى الذكر واجودهما
الانثى شي واحر املس ج قوة الاغاريقون منقية مفتحة مقطعة لسدد الاحشا

اسطوخودوس	[illegible]	معناه موقف الارواح وهو الارشميشة بالبربرية وهي وشايع الشيح وقيل هو الاجاص من غير الاسم اضراره بالرئة اصلاحه بالكثيرا السربة خمسة دراهم	[illegible]
ازاذ	[illegible]	قيل الاصل هو حب المثنان ويقال له بالعجمية طرلشكه ويقال له ايضا ازرم ويسميه العرب الصنبق ❊	[illegible]
اغاريقون	[illegible]	هو اغارقه وهو عقير خفيف ابيض يوتى به من بلاد الروم وقيل انه عين شجرة وقيل انه ينبت كما ينبت الفطر . ومن غير الاسم اضراره بالمعا اصلاحه بالكثيرا خيرة الانى الخفيف	[illegible]
اسطوليون	[illegible]	هو العرس وهو البلسن عند جنيفة وذكر ذلك الزهراوي . ويسمى ابضا ❊	[illegible]
اجاص	[illegible]	هو العيون بقر ويعرف بالعجمية جرولش واذا قيل اجاص رطب يراد به العيون لعبر البالس المتمين الجلد ويعرف بالشاهلود . ومن غير الاسم اضراره بالراس اصلاحه بالعناب	[illegible]
اولحج وحوز	[illegible]	هو الزعرور ويقال انه ثمر شجر الدب ويقال له التشلس ورايت في بعض التفاسير انه ثمر الدب يشبه البرنجان وهو المشمش معطرا وجرته في كثير من الكتب والبعض هو عصير الدب . واما عصير الدب فهو فاتل ابيه ويسالذكره في حرب الغاف ❊	[illegible]

Pachádus
torbiscu
agaricón
[illegible]
pruna, damascena
nespula

اللوند اصلا الا انه مركب من قوتين متضادتين احدهما في قشره والاخر في جرمه قوة قابضة
مقوية للمعدة والمعا مانعة للاستهال المريي . ح الاجاص هو اشرها بردا وليينا وامساكا
للبطن و[illegible] شر اصول هذه الانواع اذ ❊

بسببه حار يابس وبسبب من ارده حار مسخنا للمعدة وبسبب لطافته جار .
ومعناه ان في جرمها طبقات مستقيمة والوكرمنه ليس من بده طبقات بل من [illegible]
مستقيم بزلك الحاب الزعفران . الحق الغالب على جرم الحرس البحرى وعلى جرم اللزوجه .. .

منافعها وخواصها ووجود استعمالها
الاسطوخودوس مركب من قوى مختلفة وهو منفع الشرود منضج ملطف منفع للاحشا كلها وبقوى الاعضا الداخلة وطبيخه صالح لاوجاع الصدر مثل الزكام وبقوى الاعضا الظاهرة وينفع من العفونة وملطف .
يسهل البلغم الغليظ وينفع من الحزن الزم المرتفعة الى الراس وينفع من المرة السوداء ويستعمل في دوا معده الله واذا طبخ اصله مع اشنان الزيت ولطخ به الجرب والقوبا والقرع في الراس نفع من ذلك . فزاد واشناو فال اذا اكثر منه لانه يسحج المعا ويطلب الخروج ولا شربه الا لاقوبا والغليظ الطباع .
يحلل مقطع لغلظ الكيموسات وخاصية اسهال البلغم ومضاده السموم واذا سقي منه مقدار مثقال نفع من وجع الصدر والربو وعسر البول ووجع الكلى والرحم ووجع الرحم الذي يعرض منه الاختناق ومن فساد لون البدن وينفع من ورم الطحال بالسكنجبين وينفع من وجع المعدة اذا مضغ وحده وينفع لعرق النسا ووجع المفاصل وبرد الطمث ويقويه
اذا خلط الحرس مع اكليل الملك وشعير حل ودهن ورد وحمل على العين حلل ورمها واذا حمل على اورام المقعدة فعل مثل ذلك واذا طبخ بالخل نفعت من النوى الوارم من لعسر اللبن واذا دق وعجن ببياض البيض وحمل على الورق نفع منه
ينفع كثيرا في البحانج المخصوصة بتنقية البدن وتصفية الدم ويصنع منها اشربة لتليين الطبيعة ونفع الصفرا د ردى للمعدة مضر للبطن د الاجام البري اذا نضج وجفف وطبخ بشراب ويغرغر بطبيخه فطع سيلان المواد الى اللهاة والعصبتين اللوزتين والله
يعقل الطبيعة ويربع المعدة ويقويها وينفع الغي والعطش ويجب لمن اراد ان يجرب فيها هذه المنافع ان يستعملها على ريق النفس .

جوهر جرمه لازم في قشره حرارة يسيره لها يعقل البطن للانطلاق وفي جوهر انواع منها الرمشع وهو اكثرها قبضا ومنها الارمني وهو اشرها كاره ومنها البري طبخه ويغرغر بها نفعت من ورم اللهاة واللوزتين .

ويدفن الكحل ... وينفع من الصرع والنافض ... [illegible]

ج ٤٠

الزنه يبعث من الاسارون انما هو اصله وقوه شبيهه بقوه الوج غيره
املس الكمر صا يبا الى الحمره وان يقطر منه في الاذن الوجعه يحلو اب الاذو به الموافقه
فان اراد شربا اخره فكما يستقى تحته وتلته بن رمل لوز حلو والمختار منه ما كان احمر رزينا

الاسم	الطبع	تفسيرها باختلاف اللغات	الابدال منها
اسارون	حار يابس في الثانية	هو الاسرو واطبا اسريقا معكرا وجربه للزهراوي ولسمه العجم اسره وبعض الاطبا تسميه ناردين بري	[illegible]
اذخر	حار يابس في الثانية	يسمى نواره تفاح اذخر وهو المعروف بتبن مكه ويعرف بتبن حرمي . المولف رايت الطبري قد سماه بجور حنثا ومن خواص اضراره يقلل الرحم ... الباذ زرد	[illegible]
افيون	بارد يابس في الرابعة	هو لابيون باليونانيه وهو المرفر وهو لبن الخشخاش البري ومن خواص اضراره بالريه اصلاحه بالفربيون	[illegible]
افيثيمون	حار يابس في الثالثة	هو الافيثيمون ويقال افيثيمون اقريطي لانه منسوب الى بلد ... اقرليس وهو الصعيتره وذكر الزهراوي انه الطيالة وليس كذلك انما سكون عليه وهو الشريش ... الافيثيمون هو الشريش وقال في الفيصوم هو الشرين	[illegible]
اترج	[illegible]	هو التفاح المائي وهو المنتن ولم ارد معنا بالاترج عن لحمه فقط وهو مع الطبع والرج معنا بالاترج وهل يا رد الماء هو عن لحمه ولهو الاترج	[illegible]
املج	بارد يابس في الثانية	هو من انواع الاهليلجات ... هو من كبار العنبر وقابل ... بعض الالسنة الماء اي المنشقق ويقال شير امج اي الاملج المربى باللبن لان شير اللبن بالفارسيه من خواص اضراره بالطحال اصلاحه بالعسل	[illegible]

Asare erbauachara

Scinathi

oppia

Epithimo

بط

citro

emelic

الى اربعه دراهم وبالسا من درهم الى درهمين . غيره فرايت به خلفا كثيرا مخلوطا فقشره
ولحمه وحماضه وحبه . المولف سياتي بالكلام على كل واحد منها في موضعه ان ذكره الباري
غيره تقطع العطش وتزيد القلب قوه وحيره وذكا

ترفع تنثر في اخلاط الطيب . سع الاذخر يشغل الراس اذا الحرارة اجوده الافيون ما كان لونه
سكن وجعها وسكن وجع النقرس ايضا . اسحق الا سمو حرث عطشا وجبا ما في العسر
محلوبا من افرنطيا او بيت المقرس عنبرة . يولد عما ومقال الشربة منه مطبوخا من درهم

منافعها وخواصها ووجوه استعمالها .

د سخن ويلدع اللسان جدا وهو مدر للبول ... صالحة لمن به حصى ولمن به عرق النسا
ويدر الطمث واذا شرب منه وزن سبعة دراهم او مثقال ما العسل اسهل مثل الخربق الابيض
ومن غير الاسم ينفع من وجع الوركين المتقادم ويقوي الاعضاء كلها

هو لطيف مقطع مدر للبول ملين للخشا مفتح للسدد مدر للطمث محلل للاورام وهو
نافع من نفث الدم ووجع المعدة والرئة والطحال والكليتين واصله مقوي للمعدة الواتيعت
شهوتها وينفع من الاستسقا وماطبخه ينفع من الاورام والاوجاع الكائنة
في الارحام ، ومن غير الاسم يفتت الحصا ،

اذا الخرمنه مقدار درهم اخرج الجاسه وارقو وسكن الالم وينفع من السعال والاسهال
المزمن واذا الخرمنه في كثير ايام يوما شربا جرا وان يحمل منه فتيله واحتمل من اسفل
جلبت يوما معتبرا وفعله في التنويم ، والخرد اكثر من الجون فيمن ضعفت حرارته
الغريزية وغلب على مزاجه البرد وان حل منه قليل في دهن ورد ومسح به الاطراف سكن

اذا شرب منه اربع درهمات بعسل وملح وشي يسير من الخل اسهل البطن بلغما ومرة سودا
ووافق خاصة المرة السودا . المؤلف الرحمه هو زنه مثقال واذا قبل الربع
درهمات فهو اربعة مثاقل ومن الاطبا من يقول انه درهم كيلا ودانق والمثقال اعم حيش ان الحسن
قوة الافيثمون شربه في قلع المرة السودا وهو صالح للمشايخ والمتحللين ، من غير الاسم
اذا شربه اصحاب المرة الصفرا قوي عليهم وقياهم والربهم ،

لحم الاترج يولد اخلاطا باردة لزجة لكنه يطفي حرارة المعدة وهو عسير الانهضام

يطفي حرة الدم وحرارة المرة الصفرا ويذهب العطش دابغ للمعدة مقو لها يشهي الطعام
ويعقل البطن وخاصته انه يسود الشعر ويمنعه من الانتثار وينفع من البواسير ويقطع النزف
واذا جمعت الملحان كلها غير الاصفر ملونه بزمن اللون الحلو محموده بالفعل بعض اذوا
السودا والبلغم وصفت اللون والجسم وامسك الشيب

الاسلس من المالحوليا جـ الاترج معتبر لغيره انه يختلف على اربعة اقسام عـلى
بحول الله ولان لم اذكره في الجدول المقابل لاترج اكثر من لحمه فقط . الزواهر الامـ لح

ابن ماسويه: خاصة الانزروت اسهال البلغم الغليظ الذي يجتمع في المفاصل والورك ـــــق الادوا غير الابدان وربما تنفع العين والامعا وجردها وبحجمها غرده فلذلك يجب الا منه مفردا مقدر عيني الى ثلاثة درهم وهو يصلح بالسكبينج والفليلج والتربد

اسماء الادوية	طبائعها ودرجاتها	تفسير معاني الاسماء واللغات	البدل منها	
انزروت	حار في الثانية يابس في الاولى	هو صمغ شجرة تنبت ببلاد فارس ويعرف بكحل فارس وهو العنزروت ويقال له ايضا اسر فيلش ومن خواصه اضراره بالمعدة اصلاحه بالصمغ العربي وقيل ان اصلاحه ان يتقع ما الشراب والحلتيت اصلاحه بدهن اللوز وذلك ان ينقع في المطبوخ حتى يتحلل ويخلط بالصمغ العربي	صمغ البطم	Sarcocolle
اسفنج البحر	حار يابس في الاولى	هو القيم وهو الغمام وهو رغوة الحجامين وتسمى بالعجمية اشفنجة	انزروت	Spogri
آس	حار في الاولى يابس في الثانية	هو الريحان وهو المرددان وهو المورد بانح وهو المرتة بالرومية وهو المارنة وقال ان هذه الاشياء كلها واقعة على حب الريحان دون الورق والاغصان. من غير الام اصلاحه بالكثيرا	حب الريحان او غيره	Iaris:
اشقيل	حار رطب في الثانية	قيل انها حشيشة تنفع في الغالية وهي ملتجة وهي مثل حب الريحان او الخردل والكبر لها عيدان صغار مثل الصعتر والاكبر ما اجودها وهو الريب بالرأي وهو رجل الجراد	مثقال بيلجه	
اسفاناخ	بارد رطب في الاولى	ويقال السبانخ بالبا واسفاناخ والعامة تعرفه اسبانخ	البقلة اليمانية	Spanachi
اظفار الطيب	حار يابس في الثانية	ابن وافد: هو عطر صنف من ذوات الاصداف وهو شبيه بضرب العرقيد ويقال له فارح عن الزهراوي وابن جناح	وزنه وثلث وزنه دار صيني ...	Vngulas my repsicas

حطرة جـ. افضل اسفنج البحر ما كان قريب العهد بالبحر وكانت فيه القوة ~~وهو ...~~ موه يجفف والثالثة قوة يرمل والثالثة قوة تلزق الجراحات الطرية. وقوة الاول

رائحة اظفار الطيب عطرية لان الحيوان الذي هو سنه يرعى الناردين فـ ــــــــرادا

والرطبيس وعرجه اخراجا لعود مع شي من المرة الصفرا ويستعمل للادويه اخراج
بشرب معردا ان بلت برمن اللون الحلو ويكون الوسن معرار وزنه عشرة مرات والشرد
والصبر والمقل والاشق وبزر الكرفس والنانخاه ونجود لها مان غايته كثيرة ونكاله

منافعها وخواصها ووجوه استعمالها

د له قوه ملزقه للجراحات ويقطع الرطوبه السايله من العين وينفع في اخلاط المراهم
الوجوح باكل اللحم العفن من الجراحات وله في الرمد قوه بالغه وخاصته اخراج الغذا
من العين لاسيما ان خلط بالنشا والسكر وكثيرا الوتي ويلحم القروح. ابن ماسويه
خاصيته اسهال البلغم اللزج واذا سحق بنيا في البيض او باللبن جبب لم يعود رويا نافع
من الرمد

ف وله قوه حاره يحلله والحراره له تو جر في الاسفنج للعرق فيها فوحيف
ويفتت الحصاه المتولده في المثانه والكلى رذلك عن الطبيب واذا وضع وهو
جاف في القروح الرطبه العفنه التي لها تحاليد في الاعضاء جففها واذا استعمل بالخل
قطع النزف وقد يحرق ويصلح للرمد والجلا وللعشى

هو ملزق للجراحات مدمل للقروح وفيه قوه تجفيف والورق اليابس اكثر من الرطب
وفيه النانخه قوه جالسه مانعه اذا وضع في خارج البدن وفيه بالجمله قابضه وما
طبخ نافع من سيلان الرطوبات من الرحم اذا اغتسل وعصارته تسيل اللثه وتحلو البهق
وتقطر في الاذن له تسيل منها القيح ويقطع الرعاف مع الخل ويقطع نفث الدم والاسهال
ويدر البول ويسكن اللذع الحادث في المثانه وينفع من نهش الرتيلا ولسع العقرب من غير ...

ق واما يخلعه في القبض والتحليل عن مسيح الزهرا وهو بزر يحبب الخردل وهو حاره
يابسه مقطعه للشرد العارضه في الراس مقويه للدماغ ومعهما شي من قبض وافضلها
اكثرها واشدها حراره وازانها ويدخل في اعمال الطيب ولا يدخل في اعمال النار

يلين الطبيعه وينفع من اوجاع الحلق والربو العارضه من الرم وينفع من الاوجاع
الحادثه من قبل المرة الصفرا ؟ ؟

مبحى منها شي من قبض مع لطافه وينفع من المعده والكبد والارحام بطبعها
وقال الرازي مسهل اكثر من حرها نلبه المراه التي بها اختناق الرحم واسهال القرع
وان شربت تحل حركات البطن ؟

اليه الكسبها منه محفوظه لانه اذا طالت به المرة ذهبت عنه ولم يجب ان يستعمل
برمها واذا ابل بالما والخل قطع انبعاث الدم العارض عن القطع والبط بعض الاطبا
يرحن بها كان في راحته شي يسير من راحه الجنر باشتر

قوة الابنوس جالية لظلمة البصر كافية جدا . قوة الحشيشة هو الاشنان ...
قوة تنفع ما كان فيه الحرقة لما تجمعها عن النظر . ابو زيد من الاعراب لم ار ...
غسله وربما استعمل ... وحطب جد اكثر الناس يستعملون الارز لقطع الاسهال

الاسم	الطبع	تفسيرها باختلاف اللغات	المنافع
الابنوس	حار يابس في الاولى	هو صنفان حبشي وهندي والحبشي اسود ليس فيه طبقات يشبه في ملاستها قرنا محكوكا واذا كسر كان كسره كثيفا يلذع اللسان ويقبضه ⊕	[illegible]
الاشنان	حار يابس في الثانية	هو حشيشة القلي ومنها يصنع شب العصفور ابن جلجل رايت في بعض التراجم انه البرباطه المولف هو اخضر والاشنان هو الحمض ابو جريج هو الحمض وهو اشنان القصارين ومن غير التراجم اضراره بالمثانة اصلاحه بالعسل ⊕	يقطع [illegible]
الارز	حار يابس في الاولى	الارز بالعجمية يعرف بريج وبالبربرية فانبه	[illegible]
الاشقيل	حار يابس في الثالثة	هو العنصل والعنصلان ويسمى بصل الفار لانه يقتل الفار وهو بصل الخنزير وهو بالعجمية الاشكله وقيل ان الاشقيل ما شوي منه خاصة وهو قاطع جالس عن الزهراوي	[illegible]
اسقولوقندريون	حار يابس في الثانية	سميت بهذا الاسم لشبهها بالدود لانه يقال لها سقولوقندريون ومعناه اربعة واربعون رجلا ويعرف بالحشيشة الرودية ويقال لها عقربان ويسمى باليونانية اشقلمش . ابن الجزار يقال هو الثوم	[illegible]
الراسن	حار يابس في الثالثة	هو والزنجبيل يقال لها بالعجمية البربطوره	[illegible]

Ellenos

Orizi

Scila

Ascolopendrion

Rasdio ut elenio est enula

الاحمر الرديء منه ⊕ والاشقيل على ضربين ابيض واحمر والابيض اخص بالنفع من الاسقيل
مدر للبول منفعة لما في الصدر والرئة من الرطوبات الغليظة جدا الاسقولوقندريون جيد
العفن في غير ما كتاب في باب السين ⊕ جد اكثر ما يستعمل من البربطوره اصلها خاصة وقد يستعمل

كما يفعل بعض الاحجار بالحط وجوهر له لطيف وقوتها الاول قوة مسخنة والثانية قوة تجلو والثالثة
بيا ضا من جوهر يثبت بالبهامة وهو بواد لها يفارقه حر الحصاه وهو قوة مقبول الاطباء وشهرته

منافعها وخواصها ووجوه استعمالها

جلا ملطف يجلو غشاوة البصر وينفع من البله المتقادمة والظلمة العارضة في المعدة واذا احرق ينفع من الرمد وتشاربه نافعة من وجع العينين ويخلط مع ادوية العين التي تنفع من قروح العين العتيقة والبثور التي تحدث في العين من جلس النعافان

يعمل الاطباء يفعل من حداثة المقام وان شربت امراة من الاشنان العارسي وزن خمسة دراهم اسقطت ولدها حيا او ميتا وان شرب منه من نصف درهم الى درهم انزل البول والحيض وان سقي المستسقي منه ثلاثة دراهم اسهله ماء ويذهب الباهم ويقتل منه عشرة دراهم

يجلو جلا حسنا اعني ولسنوا على جلائه بلا نعتبه لظاهر البدن اذا اطلي عليه من خارج وهو موافق للجراحات الرطبة فاذا طبخ بالدبس زاد في لطفه زيادة بينة واذا اغتسل به نقى البدن من الاوساخ

هو نافع من البهق والربو والقشرة والسعال العارض من الرطوبة الغليظة ويجب ان لا يمنع عنه من كان في صدره وريته ومعاه شيء من قروح لانه يلذع عند تحركه ويؤذيها واذا اكثر منه قتل ومن يستعمل للغسل المركوب بان يدق وينقع ويخلط ماؤه لغسل ويصنع منه للعرق وتكون الغسل مثل ورق العصارة مرتين ومن يشوى فيخلط في المعجونات مثل اللوغاذيا ويشربا بالخل ويصنع منه شراب

حب ورق بقرة الحشيشة اذا طبخ بخل وشرب اربعين يوما حلل ورم الطحال وينفع ايضا ان يضمد به الطحال ومن نافع من تقطير البول واليرقان ويفتت الحصاة التي تكون في المثانة ومن يظن انه ينفع الحبل فينبغي ان يقلعه في يوم لم يكن في ليلته القمر فيه

ينفع من العلل الحادثة في الصدر والربو من قبل الاخلاط الغليظة اللزجة اذا شرب واذا يتجرد به واستنشق دخانه واذا وضع في المواضع المالكولة من الاسنان سحق وجعها مرارا كثيرة من ساعته ولبن بقر النبات احمر وتراللد ويسقى من الطحال الصلب ومن نافع جرا للقروح الخبيثة الردية اذا جب وسحق ونثر عليها في دهنه بقر النبات اذا انطلى به الرأس بالخل ودهن الورد وافق من به البرغش والسدر والصرع والفالج

لان فيه حرارة محرقة مقطعة لقطيعا بليغا من غير اسخان قوي ولولا ذلك صار مطلقا مليناً للبطن لطيف وقوتها الاول حارة والثانية والثالثة قوة تقتل الحصاة وتحلل صلابة الطحال المؤلف ايضا وعصارته وذلك انه يشرط الاطباء بسحقه ويستخرج الرطوبة التي فيه وتجفف الظل

رابعها بقرا
ويستعمل

pitie

كل انفحة وبينها اجزاء غريبة وحرارة عرضية ومكتسبة من العفونة المتولدة من غذاء الحيوان التي هي منه لان
اليه من عفونات البدن . اسحق انما اكتسبت مقررة الحرارة والحرافة التي فيها من العفونة المتولدة من ...

الابدال منها	تفسير معانيها واختلاف اللغات	الطبائع والدرج	اسم
انفحة [illegible]	الانفحة هو اللبن من كل حيوان وهو بالحا المعجمة ويقال الانفحة بكسر الالف وتشديد الحا والانفحة بكسر الالف ايضا وتخفيف الحا	حارة يابسة في الثانية	انفحة الارنب
انفحة الخرانق?	يقال انفحة كما ذكرنا ومنفحة بالميم وتخفيف الحا عن يعقوب بن اسحق السكيت	حارة يابسة في الثالثة	انفحة الخشف?
انفحة الارنب	والانفحة ايضا بالعجمية فواليه وهو الذي يعقد به اللبن	حارة يابسة في الثانية	انفحة ابن ايل?
انفحة الكبش?	الشيء المعروف بالانفحة هو ثفل في الرضع والحمل هو الكبش والظبي والغزال	حارة يابسة في الثالثة	انفحة الجمل?
انفحة [illegible]	الانفحة بالفارسية هو الفرشق ويقال بالفارسية فرشو حسب ... ان الفراس لان حسب عندهم الفرس لتشرب الباء	حارة يابسة في الثانية	انفحة الخيل
انفحة السبع?	يقال بالفارسية فرشو صهو ومعناه انفحة الكلب لان صهو هو الكلب وفرشو الانفحة كما ذكرنا فيما قبل	حارة يابسة في الثالثة	انفحة الكلب

بانها في الدرجة الثالثة وحكمها اذابة كل جامد وتجميد كل ذائب ومعناه انفحة الكلب
جلله ذكر الا يبعانه في الاجواب وكل انفحة محللة ملطفة ومع ما فيه من جميع ما ذكرنا اضطرارا ومن
نزف النساء وتحلل الورم وليس انفحة الارنب فقط بل انها في كل حيوان ومن خاصة انفحة الارنب

يتغذى به الحيوان الرضيع اكثره من اللبن فيتولد الانفحة من عفونة ذلك اللبن بما ينصاب
الحيوان الذي هي منه كاكتساب النضج حرارة من المعا فيتولد فيه منه العفونة والرود ولحل الغمه

منافعها وخواصها ووجوه استعمالها

ان المراة اذا شربتها بعد طهرها ثلاثة ايام متواليه منعت الحبل واذا احتملتها بعد
بعد طهرها اعانت على الحبل وقيل ان شربها ينفع المصروع وتنفع من قروح المعا والاسهال
المزمن والنسا اللواتي يسلن من ارحامهن الرطوبات وخاصتها قطع الطمث وينفع
من نفث الدم وتحلل اللبن المتجبن في المعدة وتذيب الدم الجامد في البطن واذا شربت منه

اذا شربت نفعت من السموم القاتلة واذا شربت انفحة العجول والجواميس
نفعت من الدم الجامد في المعدة وتنفع من لدغ الحيات ه

اذا احتملتها المراة بعد الطمث ثلاثة ايام متواليه منعت من الحبل ذكر ذلك
اسحق بن سليمن • وانفحة الارنب تفعل ذلك عن كثير من الاطبا

اذا شرب بشي من خل نفعت من اللبن المتجبن في الجوف والدم المنعقد فيها ايضا
وانفحة الارنب تفعل ذلك ايضا •

تابعة من قروح المعا والاسهال المزمن واذا شرب بخل نفعت من جمود اللبن
في البطن والدم المنعقد فيه ايضا ه

ذكر مسيح بن حكم ان يوخذ جرو كلب رضيع فيشق بطنه ويوخذ ويخرج انفحته
وتجفف في الظل ويسقى المعضوض من الكلب الكلب منها مثل الحمصة بما وما العسل
ويبرى من شرب ذلك سبعة ايام او اربعة عشر يوما نفعت منفعة عظيمه ه

ذلك فيما عاينا اذا عقدنا بها اللبن فيتجبن واذا احللنا منها شيا وطرحناه على الدم المنعقد
وذكر بعض الاطبا انه سقى من انفحة الارنب مرارا بخل ثقيف لمعضوض به الصرع فنفعه وزعم
النفع من نهش الهوام ولا سيما المسن من عامة الاكثر نافع في الجزول ه

اللبن

ابو ماسويه من حرق الارنب كما هو صحيح ويستعمل للحصاة المتولدة في الكلى وصفة حرقه ان يجعل في قدر ويسد
بارد في الدرجة الثانية وفيه غلظ وبعض رطوبة والرصاص من جملة الفضة ولكنه دخل عليه في
الرصاص المصري وبالملح وبالمرقشيثا والزرنيخ على ما يبيع ادهن عند مقدمة الاسرار ... فمن

			تفسير مفردات اختلاف اللغات	
Leporis lago	ارنب	[illegible]	يقال له بالعجمية لبير وبالرومية لبرم ويعرف بالفارسية مرفشط بالرا الغير معجمة	الف منها
Sirico mineo 1 plumb[o]	اسرب	بارد رطب [illegible]	هو الرصاص وقيل الاسود خاصة والابيض هو الانك المعروف بالقصدير وبالعربية الصرفان وهو الابار وهو الاسرب بالفارسية هو اشر اجناس الرصاص	[illegible]
Plarca psimuthi	اسفيداج	[illegible]	هو البياض يعرف بلسان جلوند وهو من كلام العامة يدينع من الرصاص على صفة يصنع الزنجار من النحاس ويعرف باسفيداج الرصاص والمحروق منه صرقون والاسفيداج هو البارود وهو البرافع	[illegible]
Siricon mini	اسرنج	[illegible]	هو الشرقون وهو الزرقون وهو الحجر يصنع من الاسرب بالنار	[illegible]
Tymeo 1 anti[...]neo	اثمد	[illegible]	هو الحجر الاسود وهو الكحل الاسود والعامة تعرفه بكحل الحجر وهو الاصبهاني والمغربي والزغولة وهو كثير بالاندلس ومنه كحل الحبلا تشلوندي نوع اخر	[illegible]
	[illegible]	[illegible]	هو حجر رمليه العاج عن مسح	[illegible]

وهو سفنجوس وتحرك حركة دائمة فاذا يلون بلون الرمد يرد واستعمل وقد يحرق
يعود حتى يلون بلون الزرنيخ الاحمر ويرفع ويستعمل او يحجر الاسرنج حارث من الاسرب اذا
اذا عدت وكان ذا اصباغ لغسيله الاهي اي وافر وقد يشوى الاثمد بان يحشى الشحم وللصبغة حتى يحترق

حي ويطبخ او يطين او يعجن وبدخل الفرن ولنقا حتى يحترق ويستعمل ا ر طبع الرصاص معه لثلاثة اجزاء منه وزرنيخ ومرتك. ار في كتاب الاحجار مزدبر الرصاص لعصير لشوى الاسفيداج على مقدار الصفيحة يوخذ جزء جزء فيحصر على جمر وينثر عليه الاسفيداج.

منافعها وخواصها ووجوه استعمالها

عـ ومما ينتفع بجملته من الحيوان اذا اشوي واكل دماغه من الارتعاش العارض لعقب مرض واذا ام لدت به لثة الطفل واطعم لهم نفع من الوجع العارض لهم من نبات الاسنان واذا احرق راسه وخلط بشحم دب او خل ابرا داء الثعلب عن اسحق بن سليمن لحمه اذا طبخ او عجن في فرن نفع مـــن قروح المعا

ار اذا احرق وذر او دبلستا ونجعب البله من العين ويحمل في المراهم فيبرد الجراح والقــروح التي تكون في اعيون الناس والحيوان كلها فـــولش يصلح للسرطان والاورام الرديه والاورام التي تكون في المقعده والاورام الحارة التي تكون في المذاكر والخصا والثدي: وان ضرب منه صفح والزيت الصلبه ابرا ها ازالها واذا سحق بدهن ورد نفع من القروح

يبـــرد الاورام الحاره ويردع مادتها ويحلل ويتبس ويملي القروح لحما انقيا ويقلع اللحم الزايد في القـــروح فلعلها رفيعا ويدملها اذا وقع في الغبروطي والمراهم وقوته الاولى قـــوة مبرده والثانيه مغريه ومن تعمل كما يغسل الاقليميا ويستعمل ويقوم من الادويه الغســـاله ۞

ينفع القـــروح ويلزق الخراجات وينزعب باللحم المتعفن ويبرد ويلطف الكثير يعرض لمن شرب اسرنج ما يعرض لمن شرب المرتك من ثقل المعده واشراد البطن وضيق النفس والخناق وما اشبه ذلك .

حـ لمن انحجر منه يغسل مع قوة العامسيه لنا يجعب في قوة الاثمد مغريه وانضه مبرده يرصف باللحم الزايد في القـــروح ويدملها وينفع ا وسالحــــها واوساخ القروح العارضه في العين ويقطع الرعاب العارض من الجب الرية فوق الرماع واذا خلط ببعض الشحوم الطريه ولطخ على حرق النار لم يعرض فيه جشحو لشه وادمـــل

مـــ وله قوة تبليس وتنقي الاوساخ وتنزعب بالكلف ودرن البرون وتجلو الاســـنان

على مقدار الصفيه يوخذ فيحصر في طنجير عميق ومن مخروق ويوخذ الطنجير على جمر ويجعل او حل في النار واحميت عليه فليسحق ويصير الى الحمرة ه واجود الاثمد واجواده اشده تر يعما فيه الاز لم يذهب لم يوخذ ويطفى بلبن امراة ولدت ذكرا او ببول الصبيان او بخمر عتيق وفي تعمل

ذكر جـ انه جزء حجر الحية وقال جعلته في قلادة وعلقته في عنق المارن ه وجع
النبيذ قال ابن الجزار في البسر عن جالينوس مثل هذه الخاصة وذلك انه قال ان الحجر

الاسم	الطبائع والدرج	تفسير ما فيه من اختلاف اللغات	الابدال منه
الراتينج	حار يابس في الدرجة الثانية	هو شجر الارز في وهو على النور اعن صمغ ابن حجم	[illegible]
غاغاطيس	حار يابس في الدرجة الثانية	الزمراوي هو حجر يستعمله الاساكفة ومنافعه غير فائضة ولا اخر لعه حجرا	[illegible]
ارومعاطوس (Corali)	حار يابس في الدرجة الثانية	هو حجر الحية	[illegible]
اسفنزن (Asforlithos)	حار يابس في الدرجة الثانية	حجر اسيوز حجر لما تقب الى الرخاوة تثقب سريعا ويكون على ظهرها شبه غبار الرحا يقال له زهرة حجر الاسيا ومنافعها ما حية ويقال لها حجر اللبوس وهو حجر الاسيا	[illegible]
ابراقليطوس	حار يابس في الدرجة الثانية	صمغ بن حجم هو وحجر مقلب	[illegible]
تم	حرف	الالف والحمد لله كثيرا	[illegible]

عليها وقال جـ قد امتحنت ذلك مرارا كثيرة وكثيرا ما الخرز منها
منفعة عظيمة المولف مثل ما ذكر في حجر الحية صمغ يقال ان حجر الحية
مفتاح اسنا وليس حجر زهرة حجر المجلوب من اسيوس

المعدة ثم استطبخها مزيدا من بطنه فينتفع من ذلك نفعا بينا من غير ان الفش فيه صورة
الزيد يسمى البسر مما ينتفع به في جميع اوجاع المعدة وخاصة جوهره اذا علق

منافعها وخواصها ووجود اشتعالها

يجلو البصر وينفع من ورم الشريين والانثيين اذا طليت به مرفوقا
مرومها

فسوده تختلفه فباضه تحلله ينفع من اورام اللهاة ويستعمل
في ادويتها والزيت اللحم المنتن نعل وتحلله من غير لذع

اذا احرق كان فيه قوة مفتتة للحصاة اذا شرب بشراب ابيض وخاصتها النفع من
وجع المعدة بالتعليق ومن الناس من يركب مغزا الحجر في خاتم وينقش عليه تنينا
له شعاع ذكر ذلك مسيح عن سليمان الملك انه ذكره في مقالته الرابعة عشر وذكر عن
جالينوس انه جرب نفع مغزا الحجر من غير ان ينقش فيه تنينا

هو حجر لطيف من بلد النجوم العمية بالزنج والافوه الزمهر والخضرة منتفار به
بها ان الزمهر افوى فعلا عن مسيح فود مغزا الحجر وزمرده مفتتة لغقينا
يسيرا محلله للجراحات واذا خلط كل واحد منهما نصح البطم بالزيت
وينفع النفس من اذا ضمد به فم البلغم وينفع من وجع الطحال اذا خلط بالكلس والخل

اذا شرب نفع من لذع العقارب وينفع من النواسير

الباء على بركة الله وعونه بسم الله

شربها بالعادة وعلقتها في العنق وجعلت لماس الحجر في المعدة ما يسمع بذلك
اذا علق على الانسان نفع من لذع الافاعي . بعض الاطباء يسمى زمرده حضرت اسبا

اصول عمران البشنين قشور جوز لك بوزن الغليظ واجودها الحمر واذا ناقها السود

مركب من جواهر مختلفة احتره جوهر ارضي فانه جوهر حار . واما بزر البادا ورد فجوهره لطيف

وجع المعدة ويدر البول ويصلح الاورام البلغمية ويقال انه اذا علق طرد الهوام من البيت

الاسم	الطبائع والدرج	تفسيرها واختلاف اللغات	البدل
البسباسة	حار يابس في الثانية	هي بالفارسية الرازيانج وزانب الرازيانج ... وبالرومية العربية وهي ايضا ارسعن وقيل انها قشور جوز الطيب وقيل هي الجاروس ومن غير الام اضراره بالمعدة ويصلح بالرامك وصلاحه بالعسل ومن الكرفس	[illegible]
اطراقطيلس	حار يابس في الاولى	تاويله بالفارسية ريح الورد وهو العصفور البري وقال ... هو الشكاعى وخطاه الزعفراني ونسمى اقنثا الوقى ومعناه هو الاشم باليونانية الشوكة البيضاء ويعرف بالشوكة العربية	وزنه ... وزنه [illegible]
بزر قطونا	بارد رطب في الثانية	هو اشفيلس وزائده بالسين الغير معجمة وغير ... وبالسين المعجمة وهو اسم فارسي . قيل بارد رطب	بزر البقلة الحمقاء / بزر [illegible]
[illegible]	حار في الاولى يابس في الثانية	هو الأحزر وخبـــــوز	باذروج
بابونج	حار يابس في الاولى	هو البابونج وبالرومية لماملو وتفسيره تفاح الارض ويقال حماملون وهو حمالس ويقال له فراس ومن الجاوب ... لشجو هو جامالاون خاصة النفع من وجع الطحال ...	الاقحوان
باذرنجبويه	حار يابس في الثانية	حـ تسمى مفرح المحزون وهو الحبق الترنجاني وقيل بزره هو ترنجويه والنبات باذرنجبويه ويقال له المرماخور ومن غير الام اضراره بالارنبة اصلاحه بخل خمر .	[illegible]

ما الشرب منها درهمين منقوع في الماء حتى يخرج لزوجته ويشرب مع السكر والجلاب والـ

لون الزعفران ومنه ما لونه اصفر حـ جوهره لطيف وقوته اولى قوة تلين وتجفف وقوته الثالثة

في الاعراب عندهم كره علي الزيت . واذا خلط تمام الازار البابونج وبالكرا فعل كرا ... ابرل

Machyr

Tractilis

Psilon

Chamemulon

Basilico cytrato:

PLATES

The Arcadian Library manuscript, pp. 1–52